Clinics in Developmental Medicine No. 166
CENTRAL NERVOUS SYSTEM TUMOURS
OF CHILDHOOD

© 2005 Mac Keith Press
30 Furnival Street, London EC4A 1JQ

Editor: Hilary M Hart
Managing Editor: Michael Pountney
Sub Editor: Pat Chappelle

First published in this edition 2005

British Library Cataloguing-in-Publication data:
A catalogue record for this book is available from the British Library

ISSN: 0069 4835
ISBN: 1 898683 38 7

Printed by The Lavenham Press Ltd, Water Street, Lavenham, Suffolk
Mac Keith Press is supported by Scope

Clinics in Developmental Medicine No. 166

Central Nervous System Tumours of Childhood

Edited by

EDDY ESTLIN

Royal Manchester Children's Hospital
Manchester
England

and

STEPHEN LOWIS
Royal Hospital for Sick Children
Bristol
England

2005
Mac Keith Press

Distributed by 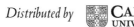 **CAMBRIDGE**
UNIVERSITY PRESS

CONTENTS

AUTHORS' APPOINTMENTS

Ute Bartels

Paediatric Brain Tumour Program, Division of Haematology–Oncology, Hospital for Sick Children, Toronto, Canada

Jaclyn A Biegel

Professor of Pediatrics, Dept of Neuropathology, The Children's Hospital of Philadelphia, and University of Pennsylvania School of Medicine, Philadelphia, PA, USA

Eric Bouffet

Professor, Paediatric Brain Tumour Program, Division of Haematology–Oncology, Hospital for Sick Children, Toronto, Canada

GA Amos Burke

Consultant Paediatric Oncologist, Cambridge University Hospitals NHS Trust, Addenbrooke's Hospital, Cambridge, England

Gary Butler

Professor of Paediatrics, University of Reading, England

Andrew Curran

Consultant Paediatric Neurologist, Alder Hey Children's Hospital, Liverpool, England

Peter B Dirks

Assistant Professor, Paediatric Brain Tumour Program, Division of Neurosurgery, Hospital for Sick Children, Toronto, Canada

Eddy Estlin

Macmillan Consultant in Paediatric Oncology, Royal Manchester Children's Hospital, Pendlebury, Manchester, England

Jean-Pierre Farmer

Professor of Neurosurgery, McGill University, Montreal, Quebec, Canada

Carolyn R Freeman

Professor of Oncology and Pediatrics, McGill University, Montreal, Quebec, Canada

Richard J Gilbertson

Assistant Member and Director, Molecular Clinical Trials Core, St Jude Children's Research Hospital, Memphis, TN, USA

Adam Glaser

Consultant Paediatric and Adolescent Oncologist, Leeds Teaching Hospitals NHS Trust, England

Annie Huang

Assistant Professor, Paediatric Brain Tumour Program, Division of Haematology-Oncology, Hospital for Sick Children, Toronto, Canada

Douglas J Hyder

Assistant Professor, Paediatric Brain Tumour Program, Division of Haematology-Oncology, Hospital for Sick Children, Toronto, Canada

Stephen Lowis

Macmillan Consultant in Paediatric Oncology, The Hospital for Sick Children, Bristol, England

Erica Mackie

Formerly Consultant Paediatric Oncologist, Southampton General Hospital, Southampton, England

Shelley Renowden

Consultant Neuroradiologist, Frenchay Hospital, Bristol, England

Susanne J Rogers

Senior Research Fellow, Institute of Cancer Research, Sutton, Surrey, England

Lucy B Rorke-Adams

Clinical Professor of Pathology, Neurology and Pediatrics, University of Pennsylvania, and Senior Neuropathologist, Division of Neuropathology, The Children's Hospital of Philadelphia, Philadelphia, PA, USA

Jerard Ross

Specialist Registrar, Dept of Paediatric Neuro-surgery, Royal Hospital for Sick Children, Edinburgh, Scotland

Frank H Saran

Consultant Clinical Oncologist, Royal Marsden NHS Foundation Trust, Sutton, Surrey, England

John Thorne

Consultant Neurosurgeon, Dept of Paediatric Neurosurgery, Royal Manchester Children's Hospital, Manchester, England

SECTION ONE

INTRODUCTION, AND OVERVIEW OF DIAGNOSIS, BIOLOGY AND THERAPY

1
INTRODUCTION

Eddy Estlin and Stephen Lowis

Cancer occurring in childhood is rare. The total, age-standardized annual incidence in the United Kingdom has been estimated to be 118 per million children under 15 years of age, with a risk of developing malignancy in childhood of 1 in 581 (Stiller et al. 1995). Primary CNS tumours as a whole form the second largest group of malignancies in childhood, accounting for approximately one quarter of the total number of cases.

In contrast to adult practice, the majority of paediatric patients can expect to be cured, with a high anticipated quality of life. The overall figure for cure of paediatric patients – in excess of 70% – is driven largely by the high success seen in management of leukaemias, but progressive improvements in survival are being produced by the large national and international collaborations involved in treatment of solid tumours such as soft tissue sarcoma, Ewing's tumour and neuroblastoma. For some paediatric tumours, such as Hodgkin's and non-Hodgkin's lymphoma or germ cell tumour, the prognosis is so good that the major thrust of current studies is to reduce morbidity while maintaining the high overall survival of patients. Despite this, within developed economies, cancer remains one of the main causes of death in infancy and childhood.

Children with CNS tumours provide healthcare professionals with unique challenges in terms of diagnosis, treatment and follow-up, and the management of these children is increasingly recognized as requiring national and international collaboration. The possibility of cure is less than for most other tumours and even then, overall survival figures are boosted by the inclusion of patients with cerebellar and optic pathway pilocytic astrocytomas, for which the likelihood of long-term survival approaches 100%. For many primary brain tumours, the possibility of cure remains low, and when it is achieved, carries a burden of late effects far greater than for other types of malignancy. Injury to a developing brain may be associated with profound and under-recognized disability in later life, and this may go undetected until beyond childhood. The importance of a systematic approach to the management of these patients is therefore higher perhaps than for any other group of patients.

Sadly, the development of such systems has been slow. Within the UK, neurosurgical specialization in paediatrics is still limited. Compared with models of care in mainland Europe and North America, treatment has historically been less frequently centred on the small number of regional cancer treatment centres, with the result that children's ongoing care has not been supervised by a paediatric oncologist. Registration of primary CNS tumours with the UK Childhood Cancer Study Group has remained below that for other tumours, and recruitment into clinical trials has been similarly poor (Anonymous 1997). The improvement

3

TABLE 1.1
**Professionals working within the multidisciplinary team for
management of children with brain tumours***

Tertiary healthcare team
Paediatric oncologist
Paediatric neurosurgeon
Paediatric neuro-anaesthetist
Paediatric radiotherapist, with appropriate team of radiographers
Neuropathologist
Neuroradiologist, paediatric radiographers
Paediatric endocrinologist
Paediatric ophthalmologist
Paediatric neurologist
Paediatric surgeon
Paediatric surgical specialties (ENT, maxillo-facial, plastic surgery)
Paediatric neurosurgical and oncological nursing teams
Clinical nurse specialists
Specialist chemotherapy pharmacy support
Play therapist
Specialist social worker
Specialist rehabilitation team (physiotherapy, occupational therapy)
Speech and language therapist
Neuropsychologist
Child psychiatrist
Clinical psychologist

Primary and secondary healthcare team
General practitioner
Community paediatrician
Community children's nursing service
Specialist paediatric nursing teams in hospital and community
Audiometrist
Dietician
Educational psychologist
Liaison teacher
School nurse, health visitor, district nurse

*Royal College of Paediatrics and Child Health (1997) guidelines.

in survival seen for almost every other tumour type has not been seen for neuro-oncology, and the late morbidity of treatment has, until recently, remained high. Nor is this situation confined to the United Kingdom. A recent North American study suggested that the Combined Oncology Group was identifying only 71% of children under the age of 15 years and 24% of adolescents aged 15–19 years with cancer (Liu et al. 2003).

As with all areas of care for children diagnosed with cancer, the management of children with brain tumours needs to be multidisciplinary. Specific guidelines relevant to the UK were published in 1997, and this document continues to provide a useful description of the structure of an effective multidisciplinary team for the management of children with brain tumours (Anonymous 1997). The presence within the team of so many different specialist workers (Table 1.1) means that effective communication is essential, and usually this role falls to the paediatric oncologist.

The last decade has seen considerable progress in the management of neuro-oncology patients. Neurosurgical specialization has become more common. Neuroimaging has improved dramatically, with effectively universal access to high-Tesla MRI, MR spectroscopy, functional MRI, and more recently, positron emission tomography. Neurosurgical techniques have developed in line with improved technology. As a direct consequence of this, surgeons achieve macroscopically complete resections, with less intraoperative damage, far more often than in previous years. The philosophy of second look surgery for many tumours, particularly ependymoma, is now widely accepted, further improving the chances of achieving surgical remission.

Radiotherapeutic techniques have also progressed, and will very likely lead to reduced late morbidity. Stereotactic targeting of the radiation field, limiting the exposure to normal tissues, is generally available. Intensity modulated radiotherapy, which is further able to limit unwanted tissue exposure is slowly becoming available, and will doubtless be the standard for all patients within the next few years. Hyperfractionated radiotherapy schedules are being explored with the intention of increasing survival, or reducing long-term sequelae. The concurrent use of chemotherapy has led to a reduction in the dose of radiotherapy needed for cure of medulloblastoma in particular; and the possibility is being glimpsed that some tumours, for which radiotherapy was once considered essential, may soon be curable with other therapies such as high dose chemotherapy and autologous marrow reconstitution.

The role of chemotherapy in most paediatric tumours has been accepted for many years, and progressive improvements in survival from many such tumours stems largely from improvements in chemotherapy. The place of chemotherapy in the management of brain tumours is less well defined, but is becoming clearer as better coordinated clinical trials open. The rarity of individual subtypes of paediatric CNS tumours means that meaningful information about advances in diagnosis, treatment and follow up can be made only with national, and often international cooperation. In the UK, clinical trials involving children with CNS tumours are coordinated through the United Kingdom Children's Cancer Study Group (UKCCSG) Data Centre in Leicester. In the USA, the Children's Oncology Group (COG), formed in the year 2000 from the four pre-existing national paediatric cancer research organizations, is supporting a wide variety of clinical and scientific studies in the area of paediatric oncology (Estlin and Ablett 2001). In addition, the International Society of Paediatric Oncology (SIOP) links many European and non-European groups in multinational studies.

Clearly defined staging and response criteria allow comparison between different therapeutic strategies. Central pathological review and consensus between investigators regarding diagnostic criteria mean that like can be compared with like. Finally, the recognition within a given diagnostic group of biological subgroups carrying favourable or unfavourable prognoses extends normal diagnostic criteria, and will allow more rapid recognition of beneficial change.

In the UK and France, early clinical studies of new chemotherapy agents in paediatric CNS tumours are conducted by the National Paediatric Brain Tumour Committees of the UKCCSG, the French Society of Paediatric Oncology (SFOP) and the UKCCSG/SFOP New Agents Groups. In North America, early clinical trials are conducted by the Children's

Oncology Group, but the Paediatric Brain Tumour Consortium – comprising centres in North America that are able to provide a high level of support in areas of science and imaging – also conduct early clinical studies.

Within Europe, the organization of international phase III studies for paediatric CNS tumours has been a relatively recent event, and has been generally confined to clinical study protocols involving low-grade glioma and medulloblastoma. In North America, phase III studies have also mainly focused on medulloblastoma, but it is hoped that these 'lead' studies will allow the development of international collaborative group studies for other childhood CNS tumours such as ependymoma, high-grade glioma and diffuse intrinsic pontine glioma.

The histopathological diagnosis of certain CNS tumours is sometimes controversial. The importance of accuracy in diagnosis, and increasingly, in grading of tumours is central to the development of improved treatment strategies. Large histology databases have been established by organizations such as the Children's Brain Tumour Consortium, and these are helping to define limitations for the current classification of certain childhood CNS tumours (Gilles et al. 2000). National and international organizations have been formed to coordinate the increasingly complex studies. Biological, psychological and supportive care and epidemiological studies are now integrated into treatment strategies (Estlin and Ablett 2001). Further efforts are needed, however, to ensure that all children with CNS tumours have access to collaborative group studies.

The aim of this book is to introduce issues concerning the contemporary diagnosis, treatment and follow-up of children with CNS tumours. This will be achieved by means of discussion of the cause and diagnosis of CNS tumours, the management of specific CNS tumours of childhood, the contemporary management of neurorehabilitation, the care of late effects, and the general principles involved in palliative care of children with CNS tumours.

In the first section of the text, the epidemiology of CNS tumours will be described, including those syndromes and diseases that are known to predispose to the development of a CNS tumour in childhood. Also included in this section are chapters providing an overview of the principles of neuroradiology, focusing on the appearances of specific diseases, and an overview of the contemporary diagnostic pathology and molecular oncology of CNS tumours. Some emphasis is placed upon radiological diagnosis, given the importance of radiological – principally MRI – assessment of brain tumours in defining treatment and prognosis. Following this, a discussion of the principles that are important in the study of cellular biology of CNS tumours, and how these may lead to novel targeted therapies and improved risk stratification, will be given. The section will be completed by overviews of the general principles of surgery, chemotherapy and radiotherapy in relation to childhood CNS tumours, and a discussion of some of the most important areas relating to acute management of patients with newly diagnosed brain tumours.

In the second section, tumour-specific chapters will be presented that will focus on the epidemiology, clinical presentation, investigation, treatment and prognosis for individual tumour types. It is intended to provide a review of the large majority of paediatric brain tumours, acknowledging that some rarer subtypes are perhaps only peripherally covered.

The management of very rare paediatric tumours, such as atypical teratoid rhabdoid tumours, is not clearly defined.

The morbidity of patients suffering a brain tumour is recognized to be different, and for many children greater than for other malignancies. Neuropsychological late effects may be profound, poorly recognized and progressive, and have a major effect on the abilities and quality of life of the developing child. Physical disability – paresis, secondary musculo-skeletal change, sensory impairment – although often not progressive, affect normal development, education and socialization. Neuroendocrine effects secondary to pituitary damage affect growth and sexual development in particular. Many of these late effects occur together, disrupting the life of survivors to a greater extent than would be seen if they occurred individually. The third section of this book therefore focuses on the effects of brain tumours on the developing brain, the late effects experienced by survivors and ways in which rehabilitation may limit these. Finally, issues relating to the care of patients at the end of life are discussed.

The centralization of neurosurgical and oncological resources, which has improved overall outcome for children with cancer in general, leads to less familiarity in non-specialist centres. Most paediatricians will see children with brain tumours only infrequently, but these patients are amongst the most vulnerable and potentially unstable to be encountered. We hope that this book will make the principals of managing brain tumours in childhood clearer and more accessible than perhaps has been the case, and hopefully increase awareness and understanding of the needs of children with brain tumours.

REFERENCES

Estlin EJ, Ablett S (2001) Practicalities and ethics of running clinical trials in paediatric oncology – the UK experience. *Eur J Cancer* **37**: 1394–1398; discussion 1399–1401.
Gilles FH, Brown WD, Leviton A, Tavare CJ, Adelman L, Rorke LB, Davis RL, Hedley-Whyte TE (2000) Limitations of the World Health Organization classification of childhood supratentorial astrocytic tumors. Children Brain Tumor Consortium. *Cancer* **88**: 1477–1483.
Liu L, Krailo M, Reaman GH, Bernstein L (2003) Childhood cancer patients' access to cooperative group cancer programs: a population-based study. *Cancer* **97**: 1339–1345.
Royal College of Paediatrics and Child Health (1997) *Guidance for Services for Children and Young People with Brain and Spinal Tumours. Report of a working party of the United Kingdom Children's Cancer Study Group and the Society of British Neurological Surgeons.* London: Author.
Stiller CA, Allen MB, Eatock EM (1995) Childhood cancer in Britain: the National Registry of Childhood Tumours and incidence rates 1978–1987. *Eur J Cancer* **31A**: 2028–2034.

2
THE EPIDEMIOLOGY OF PAEDIATRIC CNS TUMOURS

GA Amos Burke

Incidence of primary CNS tumours

Tumours of the CNS are the second most common malignancy in childhood, accounting for around 20% of the total. The international incidence of childhood CNS tumours shows marked variation between differing populations, with the highest incidence being seen in Europe (3.14 per 100,000 in Nordic countries, Denmark, Finland, Norway and Sweden) and lower rates in South America, Africa and Asia. The lowest rates are those for ethnic Chinese populations (Shanghai, Taipei, Hong Kong and Singapore), with 1.31 per 100,000, and blacks in Africa (1.12 per 100,000) (Stiller and Nectoux 1994). Whilst the reported incidences for Western industrialized countries such as the United Kingdom (2.7 per 100,000, Stiller et al. 1995) and Canada (2.76 per 100,000, Keene et al. 1999) are similar, differing rates for different ethnic groups within these populations are seen. In the USA the age-adjusted rate for black Americans (2.17 per 100,000, SE 1.15) was found to be significantly lower than for white Americans (2.64 per 100,000, SE 0.56; p<0.001), but still significantly higher than for blacks in Africa (Stiller and Nectoux 1994). In the UK, similar lower frequencies of CNS tumours have been observed among children of south Asian and West Indian ethnic origin, although these do not reach statistical significance (Stiller et al. 1991). The data on international incidence of brain and spinal cord tumours suggests that genetic factors primarily and then environmental factors play aetiological roles.

The incidence of all CNS tumours is apparently rising in Western industrialized countries (McKinney et al. 1998, Keene et al. 1999). The reasons for this remain unclear. Enhanced diagnostic yields must contribute only marginally in these countries, and it is likely that environmental exposures to ill-defined causal agents are responsible.

Age and site distribution of primary brain and spinal tumours

Approximately 10% of tumours occur in children under 2 years of age, 20% between 2 and 5 years, 25% between 5 and 10 years, and 45% over 10 years (Keene et al. 1999). Most tumours (52%) are supratentorial and histologically astrocytic (33%).

Figure 2.1 shows the relative incidence of brain tumour types in childhood by age group from an analysis of 2899 childhood brain tumours in England, Scotland and Wales 1978–1987 by Stiller et al. (1995). What can be seen is that the percentage of tumours with astrocytic histology rises throughout childhood, whereas the percentage of tumours that are either primitive neuroectodermal tumours (PNETs), medulloblastomas or ependymomas falls. The sex ratio shows a male bias for all tumours except astrocytomas (Stiller et al. 1995).

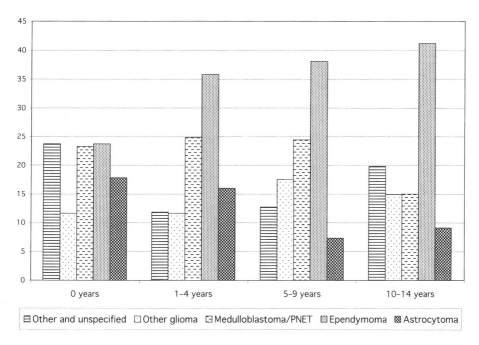

45
40
35
30
25
20
15
10
5
0

| 0 years | 1–4 years | 5–9 years | 10–14 years |

⊟ Other and unspecified   ☐ Other glioma   ⊟ Medulloblastoma/PNET   ⊞ Ependymoma   ▩ Astrocytoma

Fig. 2.1. Percentage incidence of paediatric brain tumours by age group in the UK (from data reported by Stiller et al. 1995).

Incidence of secondary and metastatic tumours

The precise incidence of secondary brain tumours after primary therapy for childhood malignancy is difficult to ascertain from the literature. Furthermore, the incidence is likely to rise with increasingly intensive therapy. Since many secondary CNS tumours will not present until adulthood, the risk of developing a tumour is always assessed on the basis of historical treatment.

It appears that having a first CNS tumour in childhood increases the risk of a second (benign or malignant). Among children who have therapy for a malignancy other than acute lymphoblastic leukaemia (ALL), exposure to ionizing radiation and a diagnosis of a genetic disorder (principally neurofibromatosis type 1 (NF1) also elevates the risk of a second CNS tumour (Little et al. 1998).

The largest group of children who have received therapeutic irradiation to the craniospinal axis is those treated for ALL. The cumulative incidence of secondary brain tumours after treatment for ALL is reported to vary between 0.4% at 10 years and 1.39% at 20 years in various studies (Walter et al. 1998, Loning et al. 2000, Bhatia et al. 2002). This incidence is up to 20 times that seen in non-cancer control populations. In each of these studies, a clear dose relationship is seen between craniospinal radiation and the development of secondary CNS tumours. The histological subtypes of tumour occurring are diverse and include glioblastoma multiforme, anaplastic astrocytoma, PNET, meningioma and medullo-

9

blastoma. The median latency between initial treatment and the development of CNS tumour varies from 7 to 12 years, with longer latency for meningioma and shorter for high-grade gliomas. Young age at irradiation may (Loning et al. 2000) or may not (Walter et al. 1998) be associated with a higher incidence of secondary brain tumours. A further contributory factor to the development of secondary CNS tumours after ALL therapy is defective thiopurine methyltransferase phenotype in children receiving antimetabolite based therapy. A study of 52 children from St Jude Children's Research Hospital, Memphis, demonstrated that children who received prophylactic cranial irradiation for acute lymphoblastic leukaemia and had a genetic defect in thiopurine metabolism experienced a significantly higher 8 year cumulative incidence of brain tumours than those who did not (42.9% vs 8.3%, p=0.0077) (Relling et al. 1999).

Epidemiological evidence for aetiological factors in primary childhood brain tumours

INFECTIOUS AGENTS

Several studies have investigated the possible role of (viral) infectious agents in the aetiology of childhood brain tumours. Following the widespread contamination of polio vaccine with simian virus (SV40) during the late 1950s and early 1960s, and the finding of SV40 DNA in pathological specimens of ependymoma and choroid plexus tumours, several epidemiological studies have concluded that there is no link between the incidence in SV40 contamination and childhood brain tumours (Strickler et al. 1999). Recently, a small study found evidence of the related JC polyoma virus late gene VP1 DNA in one of 11 cases of medulloblastoma compared to none in 5 samples of normal cerebellum (Khalili et al. 1999). JC virus is named after the initials of the patient from whom it was first isolated. The possible role for JC virus requires further epidemiological investigation.

Evidence from analysis of space–time clustering of childhood brain tumours gives the most robust direct evidence to support a possible infectious agent in the aetiology of at least some CNS tumours. In a recent study conducted in the north-west of England covering the period 1954–1998, McNally et al. (2002) examined data for 1467 childhood brain tumours (ages 0–14 years). Significant space–time and cross-clustering of astrocytomas and ependymomas was demonstrated as well as seasonal peaks in month of birth occurring in November, December and January. The authors suggest that taken together, their data provide consistent evidence for an environmental agent (or agents) in the aetiology of astrocytoma and ependymoma. The patterns of incidence they found were not consistent with a sustained environmental exposure either geographically or over time, but more consistent with an agent exhibiting temporary occurrence at many points in time and space. They conclude that an infectious agent is the most plausible explanation of the findings. Population mixing studies, such as that of Parslow et al. (2002) have not yet shown firm epidemiological evidence of an infectious aetiology for CNS tumours in the same way as they have for ALL. This may be because of the many histological subtypes of CNS tumours and small numbers included in these studies. Further research considering specific candidate infections and the factors determining sensitivity is required to advance the understanding of a potential infectious aetiology for childhood brain tumours.

TABLE 2.1
The National Institutes of Health (NIH) criteria for NF1*

Diagnosis of NF1 requires two or more of the following:

- Six or more café au lait spots greater than 5 mm diameter in prepubertal, and greater than 15 mm in diameter in postpubertal individuals
- Two or more neurofibromas of any type or one plexiform neurofibroma
- Axillary or inguinal freckling
- Optic nerve glioma
- A distinctive osseous dysplasia such as dysplasia of the sphenoid wing, thinning of long bone cortex, with or without pseudoarthrosis
- A first-degree relative with NF1 according to the above criteria

*Anonymous (1988).

OTHER AGENTS

A wide variety of possible aetiological agents have been proposed for the childhood CNS tumours based on epidemiological studies. These include: exposure to ionizing radiation as discussed above, but not proximity to nuclear installations (in Scotland) (Sharp et al. 1999); prenatal and early postnatal exposure to N-nitroso compounds (Preston-Martin et al. 1982); prenatal or childhood farm residence leading to an increased risk of PNET, also associated with maternal exposure to pigs or poultry (reviewed by Yeni-Komshian and Holly 2000); and the use of inhaled anaesthetic gas during delivery (McCredie et al. 1999).

Tumour syndromes

Genetic factors are thought to account for only 2–4% of childhood CNS tumours (Narod et al. 1991). However, the incidences of particular types of CNS tumour are greatly increased in some tumour syndromes. All of these syndromes share autosomal dominant inheritance and are described below.

NEUROFIBROMATOSIS TYPE 1 (NF1)

NF1 has an incidence of 1:4000, with the responsible NF1 gene being located on chromosome 17q12 (Seizinger et al. 1987). Fifty per cent of cases are due to new mutations. Diagnostic criteria are given in Table 2.1.

Whilst these criteria are robust for adults, a study of 1402 patients with NF1 younger than 21 years (DeBella et al. 2000) found that although nearly 95% of all patients have two cardinal features by the age 8 years and 100% have these features by the age of 20 years, 30% of children aged under 1 year have only one cardinal feature and so cannot be confidently diagnosed. In a further analysis of 39 patients with an average age of 1.6 years who did not meet the criteria for NF1 at first examination but did so subsequently, it was found that at least two cardinal clinical features were found at an average age of 4.6 years. The inclusion of other predictive criteria to allow the diagnosis of NF1 to be made in younger children is the subject of ongoing study. Additional criteria might include short stature, macrocephaly or the finding of unidentified bright objects on magnetic resonance imaging (DeBella et al. 2000).

TABLE 2.2
Diagnostic criteria for NF2 as used in the Manchester NF2 database*

Bilateral vestibular schwannomas *or* a family history of NF2 *and*
Unilateral vestibular schwannoma *or* any two of:
meningioma, glioma, neurofibroma, schwannoma, posterior subcapsular lenticular opacities
Additional criteria
Unilateral vestibular schwannoma *and* any two of:
meningioma, glioma, neurofibroma, schwannoma, posterior subcapsular lenticular opacities *or*
multiple meningioma (two or more) *and*
unilateral vestibular schwannomas *or* any two of:
glioma, neurofibroma, schwannoma, cataract

*Evans et al. (1999).

Fifty per cent of individuals with NF1 will develop a neurological complication during their lives (Creange et al. 1999). In the childhood years, 15–20% of individuals with NF1 have CT or MRI evidence of optic pathway gliomas. Of these, 30–50% will become symptomatic with the majority becoming evident before the age of 6 years (reviewed by Listernick et al. 1999). Histologically, the vast majority of these tumours are pilocytic astrocytomas, although diffuse astrocytomas and glioblastomas are also described.

NEUROFIBROMATOSIS TYPE 2 (NF2)
Described by JH Wisheart in 1820, this disorder (now known to be autosomal dominant) is more commonly associated with adult CNS tumours in the form of vestibular schwannomas (formerly known as acoustic neuromas) than with paediatric CNS malignancies. The responsible gene is located at chromosome 22q12.2, encoding a product known as merlin or schwannomin that functions as a tumour suppressor gene. Several types of mutation occur in the gene that lead to the formation of a truncated product. The population prevalence in the UK is believed to be approximately 1:200,000, making it much less common than NF1. What is believed to be the world's largest database recording clinical information on affected individuals with NF2, the UKNF2 was set up in Manchester in 1989 and has over 300 patients recorded. Diagnostic criteria used by the UKNF2 are given in Table 2.2.

A recent study from this database (Evans et al. 1999) has revealed that 18% of patients with NF2 (61/334) presented in the paediatric (0–15 years) age group. Twenty-six of the 61 presented with features of vestibular schwannoma, 19 with symptoms of meningioma and 7 with a spinal tumour. It has been suggested by others that a search for other features of NF2 should be made in any child presenting with meningioma (Perry et al. 2001).

TUBEROUS SCLEROSIS (TS)
This disorder complex is characterized by the presence of hamartomas and 'benign' neoplastic lesions that invariably affect the CNS and well as other organs. Clinical manifestations are usually present before the age of 10 years (Ahlsen et al. 1994). Neurological symptoms predominate at the time of presentation. In infancy, infantile spasms are the characteristic

TABLE 2.3
Diagnostic criteria for von Hippel–Lindau Disease*

CNS and retinal haemangioblastomas, *or*

CNS or retinal haemangioblastomas *plus* one of the following:

    multiple renal, hepatic or pancreatic cysts

    phaeochromocytoma

    renal carcinoma

or

A definite family history *plus*

    CNS or retinal haemangioblastomas, *or* one of the following:

    multiple renal, hepatic or pancreatic cysts

    phaeochromocytoma

    renal carcinoma

*Robertson (2002).

seizure disorder, while in older children, seizure disorders are often accompanied by developmental delay and learning disorders. The incidence is between 1:5000 and 1:10000, and a positive family history is found in almost 50% of cases. Genetic studies have identified two TSC loci, one at chromosome 16p13.3 (Anonymous 1993) and the other at 9q34 (van Slegtenhorst et al. 1997). The commonest CNS neoplasm in TS is the subependymal giant cell astrocytoma arising from the wall of the lateral ventricles (Nabbout et al. 1999). It occurs in 6–16% of individuals with confirmed TS. Presentation is usually in the first two decades of life although presentation in infants has been reported. These tumours are associated with massive intracranial haemorrhage.

Von Hippel–Lindau Disease (VHL)

In this disease, capillary haemangioblastomas of the CNS and retina occur. There are protean clinical manifestations of this disorder, with more than 25 distinct lesions being identified. The diagnostic criteria for vHL are given in Table 2.3.

    Other pathological lesions are renal cell carcinoma, phaeochromocytoma and visceral cysts. The incidence of VHL is 1:40,000 to 1:50,000. Approximately one quarter of all cerebellar haemangioblastomas occur in patients with VHL disease. VHL associated haemangioblastomas tend to peak in occurrence in the third decade, although childhood presentation in the second decade is recorded (Hemminki and Collins 2001).

Turcot Syndrome

This describes a heterogeneous group of disorders for which both autosomal dominant and autosomal recessive inheritance has been proposed. They are characterized by the coexistence of colorectal neoplasms with either (predominantly) medulloblastoma or glioblastoma. Some cases are variants of the familial adenomatous polyposis (FAP) syndrome, while others are variants of the hereditary non-polyposis colorectal carcinoma (HNCC) syndrome (Cavenee 1997). The population incidence of Turcot syndrome is not known and only 100–200 cases have been reported. At least two defined clinical groupings can be seen within the syndrome.

13

TABLE 2.4
Diagnostic criteria for Gorlin (NBCC) syndrome*

Diagnosis of NBCC syndrome is made in the presence of two major or one major and two minor criteria

Major criteria

- More than 2 basal cell carcinomas or one under the age of 20 years
- Odontogenic keratocysts of the jaw proven by histology
- Three or more palmar or plantar pits
- Bilamellar calcification of the falx cerebri
- Bifid, fused or markedly splayed ribs
- First degree relative with NBCC syndrome

Minor criteria

- Macrocephaly determined after adjustment for height
- Congenital malformations: cleft lip or palate, frontal bossing, 'coarse face', moderate or severe hypertelorism
- Other skeletal abnormalities: Sprengel deformity, marked pectus deformity, marked syndactyly of the digits
- Radiological abnormalities: bridging of the sella turcica, vertebral anomalies such as hemivertibrae, fusion or elongation of the vertebral bodies, modelling defects of the hands and feet, or flame shaped lucencies of the hands and feet
- Ovarian fibroma
- Medulloblastoma

*Kimonis et al. (1997).

In the first, medulloblastoma is associated with FAP. Where FAP does occur, the finding of congenital hypertrophy of the retinal pigment epithelium (CHRPE) is a predictor of the presence of polyps. In Turcot syndrome, CHRPE has been reported to be bilateral (Robertson 2002). In these cases, there is mutation in the APC gene (found in all but one family) found on chromosome 5q21. The gene encodes a 300kDa protein that is ubiquitously expressed and modifies the interaction between the beta catenin protein and the E-cadherin cell adhesion molecule. In the second clinical group, glioblastoma is seen in patients without FAP, some of whom have HNCC and mutations in DNA mismatch repair genes.

GORLIN SYNDROME (NAEVOID BASAL CELL CARCINOMA SYNDROME, NBCC)
Gorlin syndrome is characterized by naevoid basal cell carcinomas and jaw keratocysts (developing during the first decades of life), palmar and plantar pits, skeletal abnormalities, ectopic calcifications and ovarian fibromas. Diagnostic criteria are given in Table 2.4.

The characteristic CNS tumour is medulloblastoma, which occurs in approximately 5% of mutation carriers. These occur in the first half of the first decade and tend to be of desmoplastic variant histology (Schofield et al. 1995, Cowan et al. 1997).

While the inheritance of Gorlin syndrome is autosomal dominant with high penetrance, there is variable expression. The incidence is 1:57,000, and approximately 40% of new cases represent new mutations (Evans et al. 1991). The affected gene is PTCH, which lies on chromosome 9q31.

14

COWDEN SYNDROME

This rare syndrome is associated with hamartomatous and neoplastic lesions such as dys-
plastic gangliocytoma of the cerebellum (Lhermitte–Duclos disease), verrucous skin lesions,
papules and fibromas of the oral mucosa, multiple trichilemmomas (benign skin appendage
tumours), hamartomatous polyps of the colon, thyroid neoplasms and breast cancer. The
affected gene is PTEN/MMAC1, located on chromosome 10q23. The gene product may
be involved in cell growth and differentiation (Wiestler et al. 1997).

LI–FRAUMENI SYNDROME

Classical Li–Fraumeni syndrome (LFS) is characterized by the "presence of bone or soft
tissue sarcoma presenting at less than 45 years of age in an individual henceforth described
as the proband; presence of other cancers in the first degree relatives of the proband presenting at less than 45 years of age and one first or second degree relative of the proband
in the same familial line presenting with cancer before 45 years or sarcoma at any age"
(Marsh and Zori 2002).

There are two genetic determinants of LFS. The first of these is germline mutation of
the TP53 gene located at 17q13. This gene has 11 exons and encodes a 53 kDa nuclear
phosphorprotein that has a key role as a transcription factor for genes involved in cell cycle
control and apoptosis.

The second gene, hCHK2 (checkpoint kinase 2), located at 22q, has been identified
recently as another susceptibility gene for LFS. It has been shown that the gene product
directly phosphorylates p53, indicating its involvement in p53 regulation of DNA damage
(Marsh and Zori 2002).

Among 108 families with TP53 germline mutations, 551 tumours were reported of
which 67 (12.2%) involved the CNS (the third most common tumour type after breast
cancer and sarcomas). The paediatric brain tumours associated with LFS carrying TP53
germline mutations are medulloblastoma/PNET, choroid plexus tumour and ependymoma,
with mean age of presentation of these tumours being 5.2, 1.0 and 8.0 years respectively
(Ohgaki et al. 1997).

Summary

The incidence of primary brain tumours in childhood shows international variation and is
increasing in Western industrialized countries. Reasons for this increase are unclear, but
environmental exposures to unknown noxious agents characteristic of modern living are
implicated. With increasing success in the treatment of other childhood cancers it is likely
that more secondary CNS tumours will be seen, especially as a consequence of therapeutic
craniospinal radiotherapy. Genetic syndromes account for only a small percentage of
childhood brain tumours but are important because individuals with these syndromes have
increased frequencies and sometimes increased aggressiveness of childhood brain tumours.

REFERENCES

Ahlsen G, Gillberg IC, Lindblom R, Gillberg C (1994) Tuberous sclerosis in Western Sweden. A population
study of cases with early childhood onset. *Arch Neurol* **51**: 76–81.

Anonymous (1988) Neurofibromatosis. Conference statement. National Institutes of Health Consensus Development Conference. *Arch Neurol* **45**: 575–578.

Anonymous (1993) Identification and characterization of the tuberous sclerosis gene on chromosome 16. The European Chromosome 16 Tuberous Sclerosis Consortium. *Cell* **75**: 1305–1315.

Bhatia S, Sather HN, Pabustan OB, Trigg ME, Gaynon PS, Robison LL (2002) Low incidence of second neoplasms among children diagnosed with acute lymphoblastic leukemia after 1983. *Blood* **99**: 4257–4264.

Cavenee WK (1997) Turcot syndrome. In: Kleihues P, Cavenee WK, eds. *Pathology and Genetics of Tumours of the Nervous System*. Lyon: International Agency for Research on Cancer, pp. 191–192.

Cowan R, Hoban P, Kelsey A, Birch JM, Gattamaneni R, Evans DG (1997) The gene for the naevoid basal cell carcinoma syndrome acts as a tumour-suppressor gene in medulloblastoma. *Br J Cancer* **76**: 141–145.

Creange A, Zeller J, Rostaing-Rigattieri S, Brugieres P, Degos JD, Revuz J, Wolkenstein P (1999) Neurological complications of neurofibromatosis type 1 in adulthood. *Brain* **122**: 473–481.

DeBella K, Szudek J, Friedman JM (2000) Use of the National Institutes of Health criteria for diagnosis of neurofibromatosis 1 in children. *Pediatrics* **105**: 608–614.

Evans DG, Birch JM, Ramsden RT (1999) Paediatric presentation of type 2 neurofibromatosis. *Arch Dis Child* **81**: 496–499.

Evans DG, Farndon PA, Burnell LD, Gattamaneni HR, Birch JM (1991) The incidence of Gorlin syndrome in 173 consecutive cases of medulloblastoma. *Br J Cancer* **64**: 959–961.

Hemminki K, Li X, Collins VP (2001) A population-based study of familial central nervous system hemangioblastomas. *Neuroepidemiology* **20**: 257–261.

Keene DL, Hsu E, Ventureyra E (1999) Brain tumors in childhood and adolescence. *Pediatr Neurol* **20**: 198–203.

Khalili K, Krynska B, Del Valle L, Katsetos CD, Croul S (1999) Medulloblastomas and the human neurotropic polyomavirus JC virus. *Lancet* **353**: 1152–1153.

Kimonis VE, Goldstein AM, Pastakia B, Yang ML, Kase R, DiGiovanna JJ, Bale AE, Bale SJ (1997) Clinical manifestations in 105 persons with nevoid basal cell carcinoma syndrome. *Am J Med Genet* **69**: 299–308.

Listernick R, Charrow J, Gutmann DH (1999) Intracranial gliomas in neurofibromatosis type 1. *Am J Med Genet* **89**: 38–44.

Little MP, de Vathaire F, Shamsaldin A, Oberlin O, Campbell S, Grimaud E, Chavaudra J, Haylock RGE, Muirhead CR (1998) Risks of brain tumour following treatment for cancer in childhood: modification by genetic factors, radiotherapy and chemotherapy. *Int J Cancer* **78**: 269–275.

Loning L, Zimmermann M, Reiter A, Kaatsch P, Henze G, Riehm H, Schrappe M (2000) Secondary neoplasms subsequent to Berlin–Frankfurt–Munster therapy of acute lymphoblastic leukemia in childhood: significantly lower risk without cranial radiotherapy. *Blood* **95**: 2770–2775.

Marsh DJ, Zori RT (2002) Genetic insights into familial cancers – update and recent discoveries. *Cancer Lett* **181**: 125–164.

McCredie M, Little J, Cotton S, Mueller B, Peris-Bonet R, Choi NW, Cordier S, Filippini G, Holly EA, Modan B, Arslan A, Preston-Martin S (1999) SEARCH international case–control study of childhood brain tumours: role of index pregnancy and birth, and mother's reproductive history. *Paediatr Perinat Epidemiol* **13**: 325–341.

McKinney PA, Parslow RC, Lane SA, Bailey CC, Lewis I, Picton S, Cartwright RA (1998) Epidemiology of childhood brain tumours in Yorkshire, UK, 1974–95: geographical distribution and changing patterns of occurrence. *Br J Cancer* **78**: 974–979.

McNally RJ, Cairns DP, Eden OB, Alexander FE, Taylor GM, Kelsey AM, Birch JM (2002) An infectious aetiology for childhood brain tumours? Evidence from space–time clustering and seasonality analyses. *Br J Cancer* **86**: 1070–1077.

Nabbout R, Santos M, Rolland Y, Delalande O, Dulac O, Chiron C (1999) Early diagnosis of subependymal giant cell astrocytoma in children with tuberous sclerosis. *J Neurol Neurosurg Psychiatry* **66**: 370–375.

Narod SA, Stiller C, Lenoir GM (1991) An estimate of the heritable fraction of childhood cancer. *Br J Cancer* **63**: 993–999.

Ohgaki H, Hainaut P, Hernandez T, Kleihues P (1997) TP53 germline mutations and the Li–Fraumeni syndrome. In: Kleihues P, Cavenee WK, eds. *Pathology and Genetics of Tumours of the Nervous System*. Lyon: International Agency for Research on Cancer, pp. 185–187.

Parslow RC, Law GR, Feltbower R, Kinsey SE, McKinney PA (2002) Population mixing, childhood leukaemia, CNS tumours and other childhood cancers in Yorkshire. *Eur J Cancer* **38**: 2033–2040.

Perry A, Giannini C, Raghavan R, Scheithauer BW, Banerjee R, Margraf L, Bowers DC, Lytle RA, Newsham IF, Gutmann DH (2001) Aggressive phenotypic and genotypic features in pediatric and NF2-associated meningiomas: a clinicopathologic study of 53 cases. *J Neuropathol Exp Neurol* **60**: 994–1003.

Preston-Martin S, Yu MC, Benton B, Henderson BE (1982) N-Nitroso compounds and childhood brain tumors: a case–control study. *Cancer Res.* **42**: 5240–5245.

Relling MV, Rubnitz JE, Rivera GK, Boyett JM, Hancock ML, Felix CA, Kun LE, Walter AW, Evans WE, Pui CH (1999) High incidence of secondary brain tumours after radiotherapy and antimetabolites. *Lancet* **354**: 34–39.

Robertson DM (2002) Non-cancerous ophthalmic clues to non-ocular cancer. *Surv Ophthalmol* **47**: 397–430.

Schofield D, West DC, Anthony DC, Marshal R, Sklar J (1995) Correlation of loss of heterozygosity at chromosome 9q with histological subtype in medulloblastomas. *Am J Pathol* **146**: 472–480.

Seizinger BR, Rouleau GA, Ozelius LJ, Lane AH, Faryniarz AG, Chao MV, Huson S, Korf BR, Parry DM, Pericak-Vance MA (1987) Genetic linkage of von Recklinghausen neurofibromatosis to the nerve growth factor receptor gene. *Cell* **49**: 589–594.

Sharp L, McKinney PA, Black RJ (1999) Incidence of childhood brain and other non-haematopoietic neoplasms near nuclear sites in Scotland, 1975–94. *Occup Environ Med* **56**: 308–314.

Stiller CA, Allen MB, Eatock EM (1995) Childhood cancer in Britain: the National Registry of Childhood Tumours and incidence rates 1978–1987. *Eur J Cancer* **31A**: 2028–2034.

Stiller CA, McKinney PA, Bunch KJ, Bailey CC, Lewis IJ (1991) Childhood cancer and ethnic group in Britain: a United Kingdom Children's Cancer Study Group (UKCCSG) study. *Br J Cancer* **64**: 543–548.

Stiller CA, Nectoux J (1994) International incidence of childhood brain and spinal tumours. *Int J Epidemiol* **23**: 458–464.

Strickler HD, Rosenberg PS, Devesa SS, Fraumeni JF Goedert JJ (1999) Contamination of poliovirus vaccine with SV40 and the incidence of medulloblastoma. *Med Pediatr Oncol* **32**: 77–78.

van Slegtenhorst M, de Hoogt R, Hermans C, Nellist M, Janssen B, Verhoef S, Lindhout D, van den OA, Halley D, Young J, Burley M, Jeremiah S, Woodward K, Nahmias J, Fox M, Ekong R, Osborne J, Wolfe J, Povey S, Snell RG, Cheadle JP, Jones AC, Tachataki M, Ravine D, Kwiatkowski DJ, et al. (1997) Identification of the tuberous sclerosis gene TSC1 on chromosome 9q34. *Science* **277**: 805–808.

Walter AW, Hancock ML, Pui CH, Hudson MM, Ochs JS, Rivera GK, Pratt CB, Boyett JM, Kun LE (1998) Secondary brain tumors in children treated for acute lymphoblastic leukemia at St Jude Children's Research Hospital. *J Clin Oncol* **16**: 3761–3767.

Wiestler OD, Kleihues P, Vital A, Padberg GW (1997), Cowden disease and dyspalstic gangliocytoma of the cerebellum/Lhermitte–Duclos disease. In: Kleihues P, Cavenee WK, eds. *Pathology and Genetics of Tumours of the Nervous System*. Lyon: International Agency for Research on Cancer, pp. 188–190.

Yeni-Komshian H, Holly EA (2000) Childhood brain tumours and exposure to animals and farm life: a review. *Paediatr Perinat Epidemiol* **14**: 248–256.

3
PAEDIATRIC CNS TUMOURS: NEUROIMAGING

Shelley Renowden

The neuroimaging appearances of individual brain tumours are rarely specific, and the differential diagnosis of abnormalities identified by imaging must take into account patient age and tumour location. All tumours present as mass lesions and most are seen as areas of low density on cranial computed tomography (CT), low signal on T_1-weighted (T1W) magnetic resonance imaging (MRI) and high signal on T_2-weighted (T2W) MRI, with distortion of normal structures. They may show abnormal enhancement following intravenous contrast. The presence or absence of haemorrhagic changes, necrosis and calcification, and the extent of contrast enhancement, will vary among tumours of different but also *similar* histologic type, as will be appreciated from the images reproduced in this chapter. In general, however, malignant tumours are *more likely* to be heterogeneous with foci of necrosis, areas of haemorrhage, heterogeneous contrast enhancement and oedema (Fig. 3.1). Benign tumours are *more likely* to be homogeneous and without haemorrhage or oedema (Fig. 3.2).

The role of imaging is therefore not to provide a precise histologic diagnosis (that is the role of the neuropathologist) but rather to make the correct diagnosis of a 'brain tumour' and differentiate it from other mass lesions – acute or subacute infarcts (Fig. 3.3), focal cortical dysplasias (Fig. 3.4), abscess and inflammatory lesions. This is not always straightforward. Imaging is also important for precise tumour localization and determining the relationship to eloquent cortex (Fig. 3.5) and therefore is necessary for surgical planning and also in follow-up.

Neuroimaging techniques

COMPUTED TOMOGRAPHY
Cranial CT is usually the first imaging test to be done because it is more available. Scans should be obtained both pre- and post-intravenous iodinated contrast. Spiral CT ensures fast scanning and enables multiplanar reconstruction.

MAGNETIC RESONANCE IMAGING
MRI is usually also necessary for defining the full extent of the tumour, planning treatment, aiding prognosis and follow-up – hence the preponderance of MR scans illustrating this chapter. Prognosis is dependent upon not only histologic type and grade but also tumour size, extent of disease, location, type of treatment and treatment response. MRI sequences will vary from centre to centre but at our institution T1W sagittal spin echo (SE), T2W fast spin echo (FSE) axial and gadolinium enhanced T1W scans in the planes appropriate to

tumour location are routinely employed followed by gadolinium enhanced T1W sagittal spinal images in selected tumours. Additionally, planning MRI scans (heavily T1W gadolinium enhanced, 3D thin slice gradient echo volume acquisition sequences) for image-guided resections or biopsies are obtained. Alternative protocols are available in the literature (Griffiths 1999).

Intravenous gadolinium-containing compounds are paramagnetic agents that increase tissue contrast in conventional MR studies. They shorten T_1 relaxation times and the effect, that of contrast enhancement (Fig. 3.12b), is seen in blood vessels and normal structures that lack a blood–brain barrier (pituitary gland, infundibulum, pineal gland, dura, choroid plexus) and also with any pathology that disrupts the blood–brain barrier.

MRI has superior soft tissue contrast and spatial resolution to CT. Additionally, it is free from artefact commonly seen in the posterior fossa on CT. It is the preferred modality for assessment of spinal leptomeningeal spread of disease (see later). CT may give useful additional information about tumour density: whereas astrocytomas are always hypodense with respect to brain (except the highly malignant ones), iso- or hyperdense tumours are more commonly small round cell tumours such as medulloblastomas (Fig. 3.6), germinomas, primitive neuroectodermal tumours (PNETs) and ependymomas. These are very cellular tumours with high nuclear to cytoplasmic ratio and less free water. The presence of fat density may also be a useful clue, seen in lipomas, dermoids (Fig. 3.7) and teratomas. Calcification, readily demonstrated on CT, is poorly seen on MRI (Fig. 3.45) but is useful to positively identify craniopharyngiomas (Fig. 3.8), teratomas, dermoids (Fig. 3.7) and oligodendrogliomas.

MR PROTON SPECTROSCOPY (MRS)
A detailed account of MRS is beyond the scope of this text. Basically, MRS provides a relative measurement of the amount of certain metabolites within a small volume of brain tissue. Different disease processes alter the spectrum obtained in certain recognizable ways.

MRS will not accurately determine tumour type as tumour spectra overlap considerably (Warren et al. 2000). Initial surgical resection or biopsy will determine both the tumour type and grade. Neither is MRS completely specific for 'tumour'. In a small percentage of cases there is overlap with spectra of multiple sclerosis and infarction. MRS therefore serves as an adjunct to routine MRI but is potentially useful for tumour grade, assessing response to treatment and differentiation from radionecrosis. It will also usefully distinguish cystic tumour from abscess (Dev et al. 1998, Burtscher and Holtas 1999).

N-acetyl-L-aspartate (NAA), choline (Cho), creatine (Cre), lactate and lipid peaks are usually determined. NAA is found in neurons and axons, and levels indicate neuronal function. Low NAA levels are found in tumours reflecting parenchymal replacement or destruction by neoplastic cells. Choline is found in cell membranes, and increased choline levels in tumours reflect membrane turnover associated with glial proliferation and neuronal and axonal destruction. Creatine and phosocreatine are important in energy metabolism, and in tumours, creatine peaks are variable. Loss of phosphocreatine possibly suggests ischaemia or alteration in the activity of creatine kinase. Lactate, reflecting increased glycolysis or ischaemia, is more likely to be found in high-grade tumours but its presence cannot be used as a reliable indicator of malignancy as it is also seen in low-grade tumours such as pilocytic astrocytoma. Neoplasms involving or destroying white matter will demonstrate elevated lipid levels due to myelin breakdown.

Tumours therefore tend to have a lower NAA/Cho ratio than normal brain and sometimes elevated lactate and lipid peaks (Tzika et al. 1997). The more malignant the brain tumour, the higher the Cho and the lower the NAA, which becomes markedly decreased or absent. High NAA/Cho and high Cr/Cho ratios are therefore associated with a good prognosis (Byrd et al. 1996, Girard et al. 1998, Warren et al. 2000), and low NAA/Cho levels are associated with a poor prognosis and shorter survival. A notable exception to this pattern is the juvenile pilocytic astrocytoma, which also has a low NAA/Cho ratio and may also demonstrate a lactate peak (Hwang et al. 1998). Lactate and lipid are more characteristically elevated in malignant tumours irrespective of cell type (Byrd et al. 1996). During follow-up, sequential increases in tumour Cho may be indicative of malignant degeneration, whereas decrease in Cho, lactate and lipids and increase in NAA and Cr are associated with a good response to treatment. A change in Cho may be seen as early as 2 weeks after beginning treatment whereas assessing response on imaging grounds alone relies on changes in tumour size which may take months.

MRS may usefully differentiate radiation necrosis from recurrent tumour. Radiation necrosis shows absent or marked decrease in all metabolites except lactate, which may be elevated. MRS can also differentiate post-surgical changes and scar formation from residual tumour. Post-surgical tumour bed without tumour demonstrates a decrease in all metabolites including Cho.

It is important to note that the magnitude of the Cho peak is reduced by about 15% after gadolinium in enhancing tumours (Sijens et al. 1997) and so spectra should be obtained consistently either all before or all after contrast.

Those centres using MRS need to be aware of potential problems in acquiring spectra contaminated by recent tumour-related haemorrhage producing magnetic susceptibility effects and air, fat or bone within the voxel.

Tumour types
POSTERIOR FOSSA TUMOURS
In the paediatric population, posterior fossa tumours account for just under half of children's CNS tumours. Medulloblastomas, cerebellar astrocytomas, ependymomas and brainstem gliomas comprise 95% of these.

Medulloblastomas (PNET-MB)
These account for 30–40% of posterior fossa neoplasms. These tumours probably arise from germ cells from the roof of the fourth ventricle and hence 70% are midline vermian lesions (Fig. 3.9), but some, classically the desmoplastic variant, may occur laterally in the cerebellar hemisphere (Figs. 3.10, 3.14) usually in older children and young adults (Levy et al. 1997). They may also present as an exophytic mass in the cerebellopontine angle (CPA), extending through the foramina of Luschka or Magendie.

CT typically demonstrates a midline, vermian, well-defined solid mass, iso- or hyper-dense and with homogeneous contrast enhancement (Fig. 3.11). The density before contrast and clinical short history should facilitate the correct diagnosis. Cysts are present in about 60–80% and calcification in approximately 20%.

With MRI (Fig. 3.9), the signal on T1W scans is variable and may be hypointense or isointense with respect to grey matter. The T2W signal is heterogeneous with iso- to moderately hyperintensity with respect to grey matter. The hyperdense appearance on CT and isointense appearance on T2W MRI is attributed to its marked cellularity and high nuclear to cytoplasmic ratio. A heterogeneous appearance is common on T2W, reflecting the presence of cysts, necrosis and calcification (Figs. 3.12, 3.13, 3.14). Ninety per cent will demonstrate contrast enhancement that may be homogeneous or patchy. Some do not enhance at all (Fig. 3.12). There is mild to moderate oedema, generally more than usually seen with cerebellar astrocytomas.

The presence of cysts and calcification make it difficult to differentiate medulloblastoma from ependymoma, choroid plexus carcinoma, PNET or atypical teratoid rhabdoid tumours. Haemorrhagic changes are uncommon in medulloblastoma (Fig. 3.14) and is more commonly present in these other malignant posterior fossa tumours.

CSF dissemination of PNET-MB is common, and hence it is important to image the spine at presentation using gadolinium-enhanced MRI (Fig. 3.9). Spinal drop metastases occur in about 15–20%. Occasionally, the primary tumour does not enhance but the lepto-meningeal disseminating tumour does.

Cerebellar astrocytoma
These account for about one third of childhood posterior fossa tumours. The majority are benign, pilocytic tumours – juvenile pilocytic astrocytoma (JPA) or diffuse fibrillary astrocytoma (Fig. 3.15), but anaplastic and malignant astrocytomas may occur. They are typically slow growing and are large at presentation. Although benign, they may break through the adjacent pia and extend into the subarachnoid space. The JPA may be cystic or solid, and is typically a well-defined cystic midline mass (Fig. 3.16) with a solid enhancing mural nodule. The cyst wall does not enhance as it is not part of the primary tumour and need not be resected. Importantly, this must be distinguished from the solid tumour with necrosis in which the 'wall' of the necrotic area does enhance (Fig. 3.17). Ten percent are completely solid tumours (Fig. 3.18). The tumour may extend from the vermis into the hemisphere in 30%. Approximately 15% involve the hemisphere only.

CT and MRI demonstrate a well-defined smoothly marginated cyst with a solid iso- or hypodense but avidly enhancing nodule and with little oedema. The endothelial cells have open tight junctions and fenestrations enabling this marked enhancement. Fleck-like calcification may be seen in 20% on CT. There is usually obstructive hydrocephalus.

On MRI, the cyst usually appears proteinaceous, and slightly hyperintense on both T1W and T2W. The solid components tend to be hyperintense with respect to grey matter on T2W and enhance avidly. Haemorrhage is rare.

The diffuse fibrillary type astrocytoma (10–15%) is more invasive and occurs more commonly in adolescents. Diffuse infiltrating astrocytoma may be solid or partially cystic and may or may not enhance. Occasionally they may mimic a JPA. The infiltrative types tend not to enhance.

Ependymomas

Around 60–70% of ependymomas are infratentorial, the remainder supratentorial. The posterior fossa lesions (which comprise 10–15% of posterior fossa tumours in children) have a peak incidence at 1–5 years and a second peak later in the adult at 30–40 years. These tumours, generally slow growing, arise from well-differentiated ependymal cells most often from the floor of the fourth ventricle (but also from the roof of the fourth, third and lateral ventricles) or from ependymal rests elsewhere in the neuroaxis. These rests may be found at sites where the ventricles are sharply angulated (posterior to the occipital horns), the ventral spur of the aqueduct, adjacent to the foramen of Luschka and the cerebellopontine angle (Fig. 3.19), along the tela choroidea, central canal spinal cord and filum terminale. The tumours may infiltrate though the ependymal layer into the adjacent brain, making excision difficult.

Fourth ventricular tumours may sometimes be soft and pliable and extend through the foramina of Luschka and Magendie into the CPA in 20% (plastic ependymoma). The tumour insinuates into the subarachnoid space around blood vessels and cranial nerves. It may adhere to the brainstem and can be difficult to remove.

On CT, they are usually iso- or hyperdense or heterogeneous, ill defined, expansile fourth ventricular masses with cysts. Calcification is present in 50% (Comi et al. 1998, Lefton et al. 1998). Contrast enhancement is extremely variable (heterogeneous in 40%, homogeneous in 40% and absent in 10–20%). Intratumoural haemorrhage is seen in 10%.

On MRI, ependymomas are usually heterogeneous lesions due to the presence of cysts (Fig. 3.20), calcification and haemorrhage. The solid components are iso-or hypointense with respect to grey matter on T1W and heterogeneously hyperintense on T2W. Heterogeneous enhancement is present in most.

Choroid plexus tumours

These rare tumours arise from the epithelium of the choroid plexus, presenting in young children and infants. Ten to 20 per cent are malignant. Location follows that of normal choroid plexus, and about 80% of these tumours occur in the lateral ventricle. The second most common site is the fourth ventricle (Figs. 3.21, 3.22) (McEvoy et al. 2000), and the author has seen only CPCs at this site. They may also originate in the CPA and third ventricle. Both CPPs and CPCs may show CSF dissemination (Fig. 3.23).

CPCs are invasive, generating oedema in the adjacent brain, and the tumour margins tend to be irregular and poorly defined. The tumour is more heterogeneous than the CPP, the result of necrosis, calcification and haemorrhage (Figs. 3.21, 3.22).

In my experience, the solid components of the tumour are iso- or hypointense with respect to grey matter on T2W MRI and the diagnosis is further suggested by an aggressive, haemorrhagic, cystic tumour in a very young child.

CPPs are well circumscribed, smooth, lobular intraventricular and non-invasive cauliflower-like masses (Fig. 3.46). They appear dense on CT, usually with homogeneous enhancement, but occasionally with cystic areas due to tumour degeneration. Calcification occurs frequently and bone formation is also described (Sarkar et al. 1999).

CPPs are large vascular tumours supplied by choroidal, superior cerebellar or posterior inferior cerebellar arteries, and MRI occasionally demonstrates the serpiginous vascular

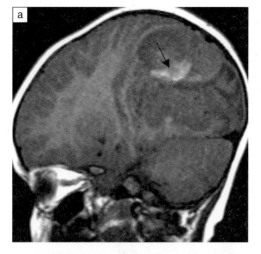

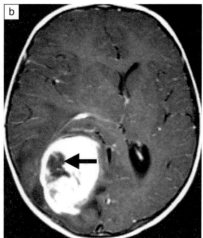

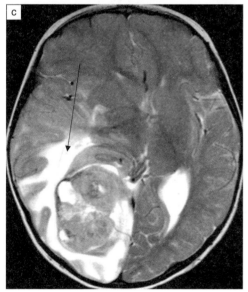

Fig. 3.1. T1W parasagittal (a), T1W axial post-gadolinium (b) and T2W axial (c) MR scans of a typical malignant tumour, in this case a PNET. There is a heterogeneous mass in the right occipital lobe, with extensive oedema (long arrow – c). There is enhancement, foci of necrosis (arrow – b) and evidence of haemorrhagic change (arrow – a). The latter is hyperintense on T1W and hypointense on T2W, and therefore represents intracellular methaemoglobin.

This was a rapidly growing tumour – scans 3 months previously demonstrated a small amount of rather nonspecific signal change involving the cortex and white matter without contrast enhancement. The patient had experienced a few seizures only and the scans shown are as a result of routine follow-up.

flow voids on T2W. With MRI, the tumour is of intermediate signal intensity on T1W and intermediate or increased on T2W (Sarkar et al. 1999). There is usually intense but often heterogeneous gadolinium enhancement. The pathophysiology of associated hydrocephalus is still debated. In a few it will be obstructive. Large amounts of CSF are produced by tumour causing a communicating hydrocephalus in many, but the hydrocephalus can persist after complete resection of the tumour (McEvoy et al. 2000). This may be explained by protein secretion by the tumour into the CSF, or tumour related haemorrhage producing a functional obstruction at the arachnoid granulations or adhesions around the exit foramina of the fourth ventricle.

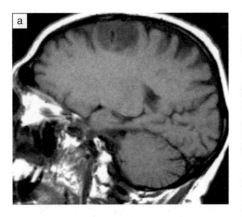
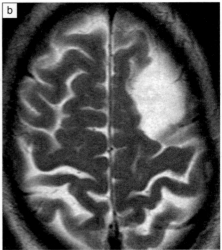

Fig. 3.2. T1W (a) and T2W (b) axial MR scans of a typical low-grade glioma. There is a mass in the left middle frontal gyrus, low signal on T1W and high signal on T2W. The lesion distorts the superior frontal gyrus, returns homogeneous signal, did not enhance with gadolinium and is not associated with oedema.

Brainstem glioma

These represent 15% of all paediatric infratentorial brain tumours and 75–85% present before the age of 10 years. Most are diffuse fibrillary astrocytomas located in the pons, and these carry a very poor prognosis. They have a characteristic imaging appearance and biopsy is therefore often be avoided. JPAs may also occur as may anaplastic and high-grade gliomas. Focal tumours, particularly tectal gliomas, dorsal exophytic tumours and cervico-medullary tumours, are associated with a significantly more favourable prognosis. A non-pontine epicentre and uniform gadolinium enhancement (suggesting a pilocytic tumour) are also favourable prognostic factors (Farmer et al. 2001). Partial resection of dorsal exophytic tumours is recommended, and these patients may achieve long-term remission. Cervicomedullary lesions are amenable to radical resection, and here tumour growth is limited by fibres of the pontomedullary barrier and cervicomedullary junction.

MRI is important to demonstrate optimally tumour definition (focal or diffuse), nature (solid or cystic), site, extent and direction of growth.

Diffuse gliomas (hypodense on CT) return low signal on T1W and high signal on T2W (Figs. 3.24, 3.25). They are poorly marginated on imaging with faint irregular contrast enhancement (Selvapandian et al. 1999). Prominent enhancement may occur in response to radiotherapy (Fig. 3.25). Calcification is very rare.

Focal lesions are well defined and may enhance (Fig. 3.26). They are either solid or partially cystic, often abutting an aspect of the fourth ventricle. Although complete surgical excision may not be possible, the residuum may not progress.

(continues on p. 90)

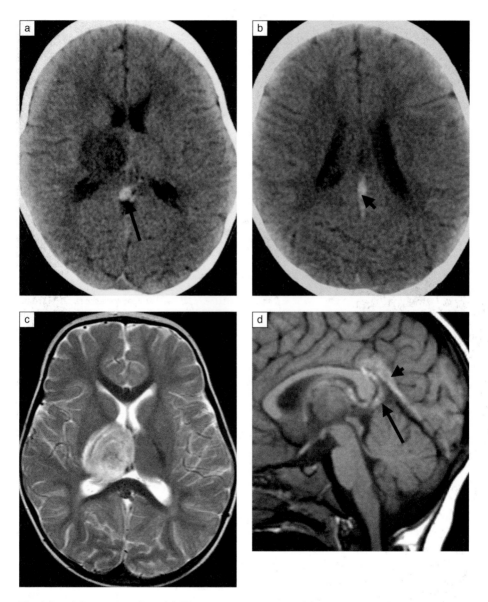

Fig. 3.3. Axial uncontrasted cranial CT scans (a, b) and T2W axial (c) and T1W sagittal (d) MR scans in an 18-month-old girl with a 2 week history of headaches and vomiting and a 2 day history of left-sided weakness, demonstrate a mass lesion involving the right thalamus and posterior limb of the internal capsule. It shows low density on CT and returns heterogeneous high signal on T2W MRI. There was no enhancement on CT. A tumour at first might be suspected but the presence of dense thrombus in the right internal cerebral vein, vein of Galen (arrow) and straight sinus (arrow head) indicates that the correct diagnosis is one of deep venous sinus thrombosis with a venous infarct. The hyperintense signal of intracellular methaemoglobin in the thrombosed venous structures on T1W MRI and its hypointense signal on T2W MRI confirm the diagnosis.

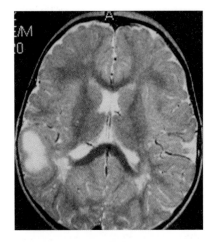

Fig. 3.4. T2W axial MRI in a 10-year-old with intractable seizures demonstrates homogeneous hyperintense signal in the white matter of an expanded gyrus in the right parietal lobe. Note that the signal is tapering towards the ventricle. This is cortical dysplasia of the balloon cell type. Cortical dysplasias may enhance and calcify, and the radiological differentiation from tumour is sometimes very difficult, necessitating follow-up imaging or biopsy.

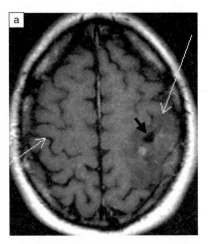

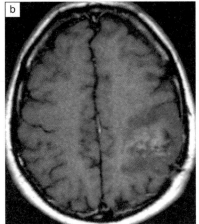

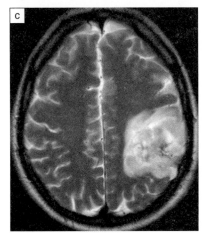

Fig. 3.5. Axial T1W (a, b) and T2W (c) MR scans in a patient with an oligodendroglioma. MRI is often useful to precisely localize the tumour to aid neurosurgical planning. The central sulcus near the vertex has a characteristic sigmoid shape (long white arrows), localizing this tumour to the left parietal lobe and involving the postcentral gyrus. (A full account of gyral localization using MRI is beyond the scope of this text).

There are no imaging features specific for oligodendrogliomas. Here the tumour involves cortex and white matter. It is heterogeneous with a small cyst (short black arrow). There is also patchy high signal on T1W and low signal on T2W indicating either haemorrhagic change (with intracellular methaemoglobin) or calcification. There is no oedema.

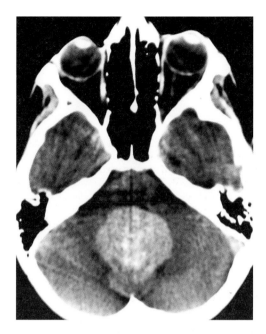

Fig. 3.6. Axial uncontrasted cranial CT demonstrates a dense homogeneous midline posterior fossa mass in a 5-year-old boy. There was homogeneous contrast enhancement (not shown). The hyperdense nature of this tumour makes the diagnosis of medulloblastoma highly probable.

27

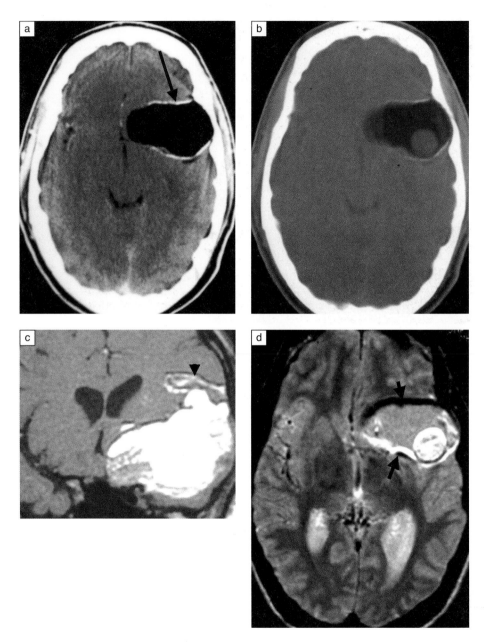

Fig. 3.7. Axial uncontrasted cranial CT scans (a, b) using different window (density) settings demonstrate calcification (long arrow) in the wall of a fatty extra-axial left perisylvian mass. Extra-axial masses arise outside the brain parenchyma from meninges, nerves or blood vessels and tend to displace the brain. On CT, fat is of much lower density (darker) than CSF but not as low as air. Note the soft tissue hair ball within the lesion. This mass is typical of a dermoid.

→

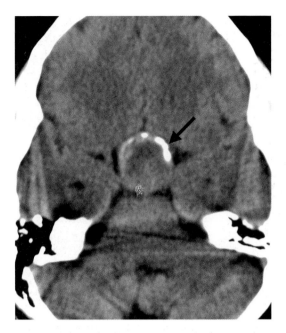

Fig. 3.8. Uncontrasted cranial CT in a 12-year-old girl with visual loss demonstrates a partly cystic/solid suprasellar mass compressing the chiasm. The presence of peripheral calcification in the wall (arrow) makes the diagnosis of craniopharyngioma almost certain.

←

Coronal T1W MRI (c) demonstrates that fat is of very high signal (white) on T1W MRI. Here, it has ruptured into the subarachnoid space (arrowhead). The T2W axial image (d) demonstrates chemical shift artefact (short arrows) – an MR misregistration artefact that arises at a fat–fluid interface, in the frequency encoding direction.

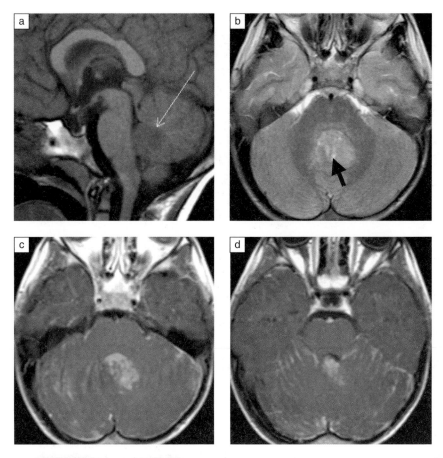

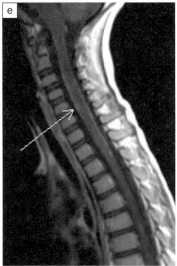

Fig. 3.9. These MR scans – T1W sagittal (a), T2W axial (b), T1W post-gadolinium (c,d) in the posterior fossa and gadolinium enhanced T1W sagittal through the cervical spine (e) – demonstrate typical features of a medulloblastoma: a small midline inferior vermian mass arising from the roof of the 4th ventricle, hypointense (arrow) on T1W (a). The mass is mildly hyperintense on T2W (b) and contains small cysts (arrow). There is moderate and fairly homogeneous enhancement with gadolinium (c). Note also leptomeningeal enhancement within the posterior fossa (d) and over the cervical spinal cord (e) (arrow), indicating leptomeningeal tumour dissemination. The leptomeningeal enhancement is thick, irregular and discontinuous, and this appearance helps to differentiate it from the normally enhancing venous plexus.

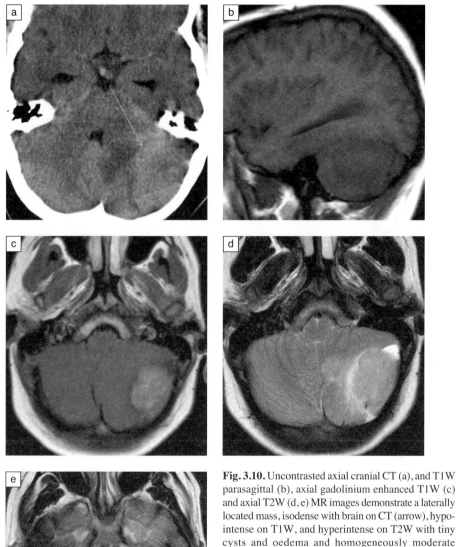

Fig. 3.10. Uncontrasted axial cranial CT (a), and T1W parasagittal (b), axial gadolinium enhanced T1W (c) and axial T2W (d, e) MR images demonstrate a laterally located mass, isodense with brain on CT (arrow), hypointense on T1W, and hyperintense on T2W with tiny cysts and oedema and homogeneously moderate enhancement. There is distortion of the 4th ventricle. This is a typical desmoplastic medulloblastoma in a 17-year-old boy.

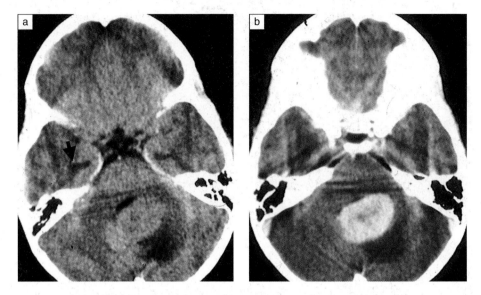

Fig. 3.11. Axial cranial CT pre- (a) and post- (b) contrast demonstrate a midline posterior fossa mass in a 5-year-old girl. The mass is isodense before contrast with almost complete homogeneous contrast enhancement. There is oedema and the mass effect with compression of the 4th ventricle causing mild hydrocephalus (note enlargement of the temporal horns).

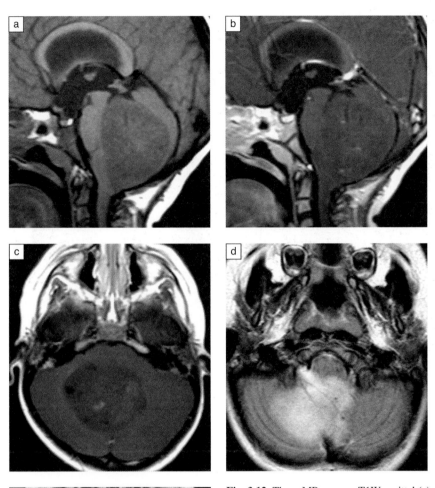

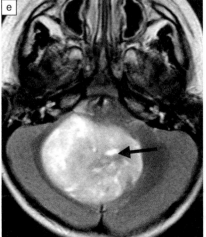

Fig. 3.12. These MR scans – T1W sagittal (a), T1W sagittal (b) and axial (c) post-gadolinium and T2W axial (d,e) – of a large inferior vermian medulloblastoma demonstrate minimal enhancement of this posterior fossa mass which extends through the foramina of Luschka and Magendie. Ten per cent of medulloblastomas enhance minimally or not at all. Note again the small cysts best seen on T2W (arrow – e). There is moderate hydrocephalus due to compression of the 4th ventricle and aqueduct with dilatation of the 3rd and lateral ventricles. Note the depression of the floor of the 3rd ventricle (the hypothalamus) and enlarged 3rd ventricular recesses.

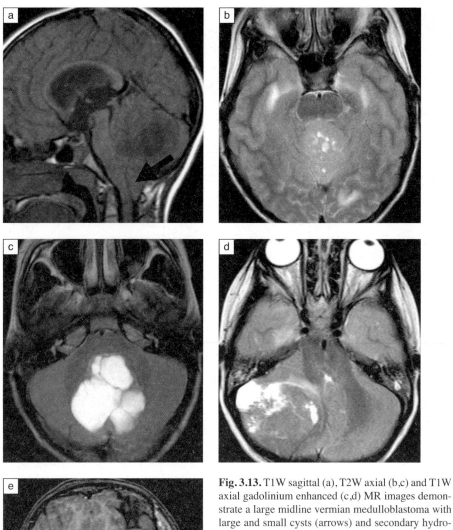

Fig. 3.13. T1W sagittal (a), T2W axial (b,c) and T1W axial gadolinium enhanced (c,d) MR images demonstrate a large midline vermian medulloblastoma with large and small cysts (arrows) and secondary hydrocephalus. Note also herniation of the cerebellar tonsils (arrow) through the foramen magnum due to the mass effect – an acquired Chiari 1 malformation.

This might be confused with an astrocytoma, but the tumour was dense on CT (not shown) facilitating the correct diagnosis.

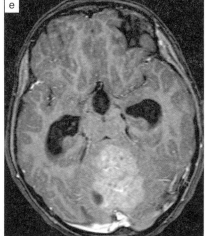

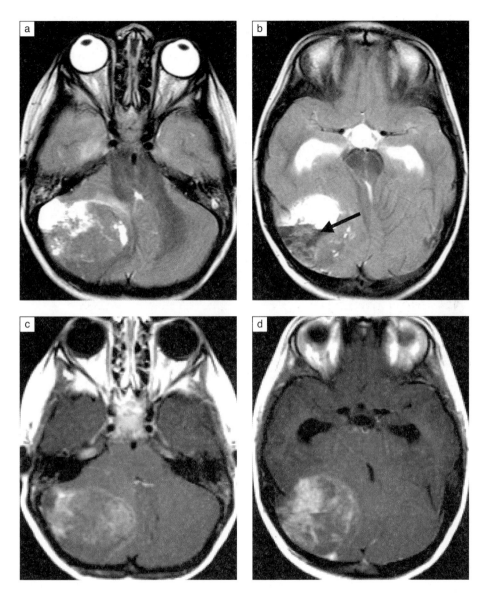

Fig. 3.14. T2W axial (a,b) and T1W axial gadolinium enhanced (c,d) MR images demonstrate a laterally located cystic desmoplastic medulloblastoma with hydrocephalus in a 16-year-old girl with haemorrhagic fluid levels (arrow – b), hypointense on T2W, the characteristic signal of intracellular methaemoglobin or deoxyhaemoglobin. Haemorrhage in medulloblastomas is unusual. There is irregular enhancement of the solid component.

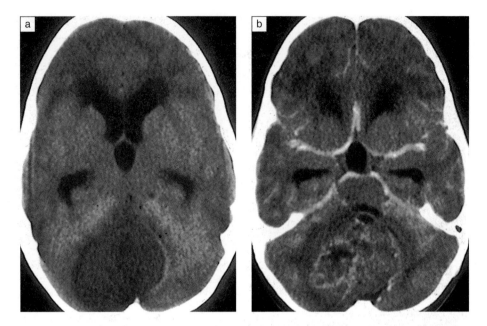

Fig. 3.15. Axial cranial CT pre- (a) and post-contrast (b) demonstrate a large midline hypodense irregularly enhancing posterior fossa mass in a 10-year-old child with oedema, compression of the 4th ventricle and obstructive hydrocephalus. This is an infiltrating fibrillary astrocytoma.

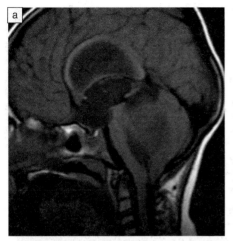

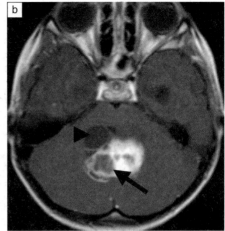

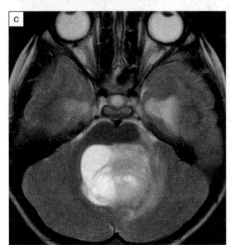

Fig. 3.16. T1W sagittal (a), T1W axial gadolinium enhanced (b) and T2W axial (c) MR images demonstrate a juvenile pilocytic astrocytoma in a 9-year-old child. There is marked enhancement of the solid component, which also contains necrotic areas (arrows – b). The tumour-related cyst walls (arrowhead – b) do not enhance. There is oedema, compression of the 4th ventricle and aqueduct and obstructive hydrocephalus with tonsillar herniation, enlarged 3rd and lateral ventricles, and bowing and thinning of the corpus callosum. Note again the dilated recesses and depression of the floor of the 3rd ventricle.

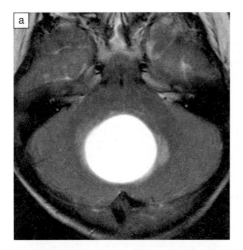

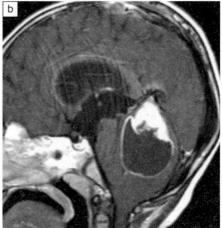

Fig. 3.17. T2W axial (a), T1W sagittal (b) and axial (c) gadolinium enhanced MR images of a solid but largely necrotic juvenile pilocytic astrocytoma showing avid enhancement of the solid nodule superiorly and enhancement of the solid walls encasing the necrotic area. There is obstructive hydrocephalus.

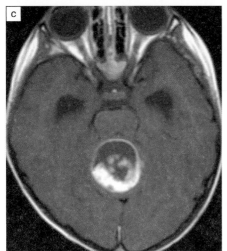

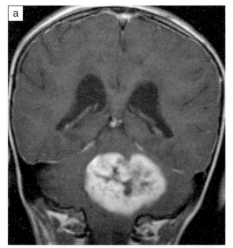

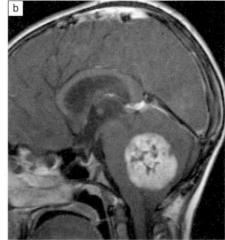

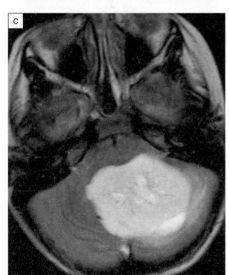

Fig. 3.18. T1W coronal (a) and sagittal (b) gadolinium enhanced and T2W axial (c) MR images demonstrate a solid juvenile pilocytic astrocytoma in a 4-year-old boy, with some small areas of necrosis.

Differentiation from a medulloblastoma may be more difficult here, but one might expect the latter to enhance less intensely.

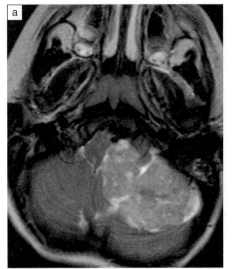

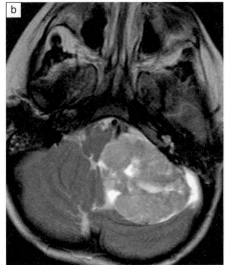

Fig. 3.19. T2W axial (a,b) and T1W axial gadolinium enhanced (c) MR images demonstrate an
ependymoma arising in the left foramen of Luschka
and extending into the cerebellopontine angle. The
tumour is hyperintense on T2W and contains cysts.
There is bright enhancement of the solid component.

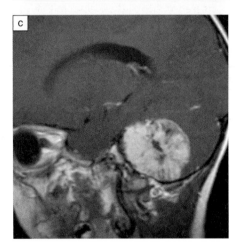

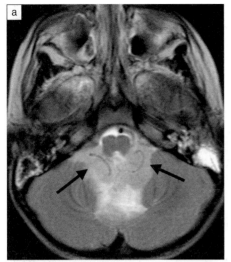

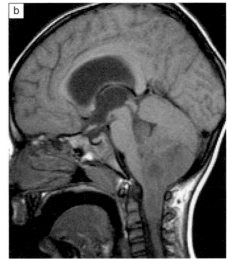

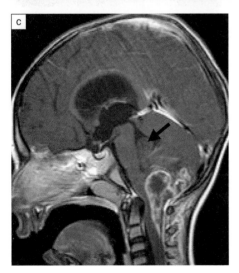

Fig. 3.20. T2W axial (a) and T1W sagittal MR images, the latter pre- (b) and post-gadolinium (c) demonstrate the typical appearance of a 4th ventricular ependymoma in a 3-year-old boy. The tumour is heterogeneous, hypodense on T1W before contrast, and inhomogeneously enhances with non-enhancing areas (arrow) and cysts. The tumour extends out through the foramina of Luschka (arrows) and insinuates around the cranial nerves and blood vessels, and also passes through the foramen magnum into the cervical spine. These features are typical of but not exclusive to an ependymoma.

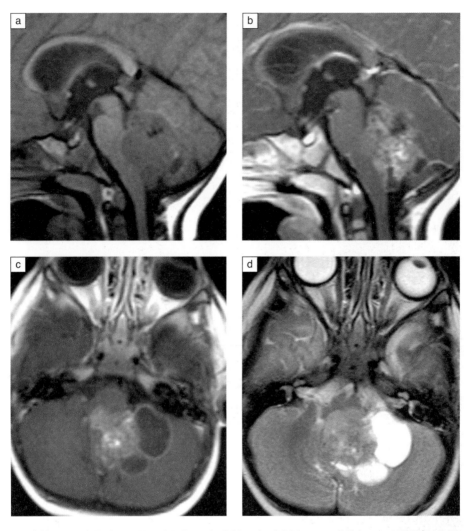

Fig. 3.21. T1W sagittal pre- (a) and T1W sagittal (b) and axial (c) post-gadolinium and T2W axial (d) MR scans in a 7-month-old, demonstrate a 4th ventricular irregularly enhancing mass with cysts extending into the left foramen of Luschka. This appears similar to an ependymoma but the age at presentation would favour a choroid plexus carcinoma.

Fig. 3.22 *(opposite).* T1W sagittal (a) and parasagittal (b) MR images pre- and T1W sagittal (c) and axial (d) images post-gadolinium and T2W axial images (e,f) in a 13-month-old girl demonstrate an in-homogeneous, irregularly enhancing mass with cysts arising in the 4th ventricle and extending into the right foramen of Luschka. Foci of hyperintensity on T1W before contrast (arrow – b) represent areas of

$\rightarrow$

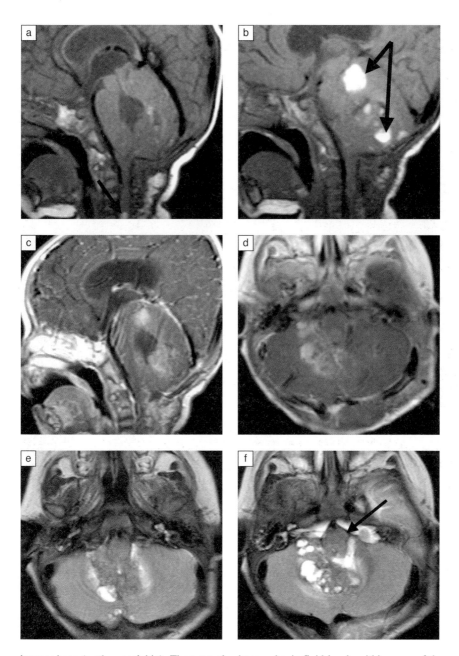

haemorrhage (methaemoglobin). There are also haemorrhagic fluid levels within some of the small cysts. Note an area of haemorrhage in the cervical cord (arrow – a). On T2W, the solid tumour is hypo-intense with respect to cortex and there is evidence of siderosis with haemosiderin (black) staining of the brainstem (arrow – f) indicative of chronic haemorrhage from the tumour. There is mild oedema. This is a choroid plexus carcinoma.

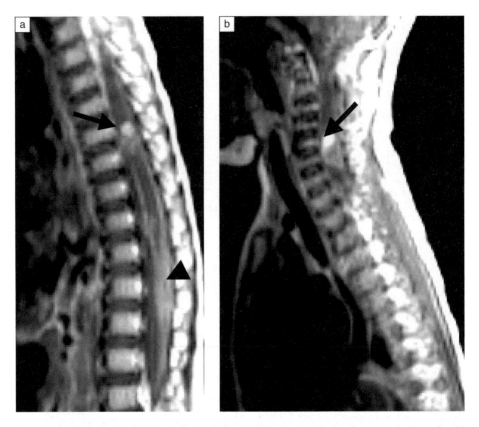

Fig. 3.23. T1W sagittal gadolinium enhanced spinal MR images (lumbosacral – a; cervicothoracic – b) in the same patient as in Figure 3.22 demonstrate leptomeningeal enhancement over the cord surface and enhancement of the lumbosacral nerve roots (arrowhead – a), indicating leptomeningeal spread of disease. There are also intramedullary metastases (arrows) with secondary syringomyelia. CSF dissemination here has occurred via the central canal of the cord.

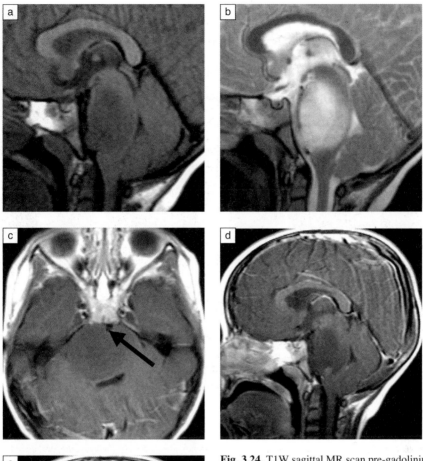

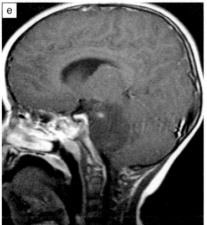

Fig. 3.24. T1W sagittal MR scan pre-gadolinium (a), T1W axial and sagittal scans post-gadolinium (c,d) and T2W sagittal scans (b,e) in a 7-year-old presenting with a progressive history of VIth nerve palsy and long tract signs, demonstrate the typical features of a diffuse pontine glioma – a mass with low signal on T1W and high signal on T2W, expanding the pons and causing posterior displacement and distortion of the 4th ventricle. There are two small areas of enhancement. These lesions have a characteristic appearance and are not usually biopsied. The tumour is seen to wrap itself around the basilar artery (arrow – c).

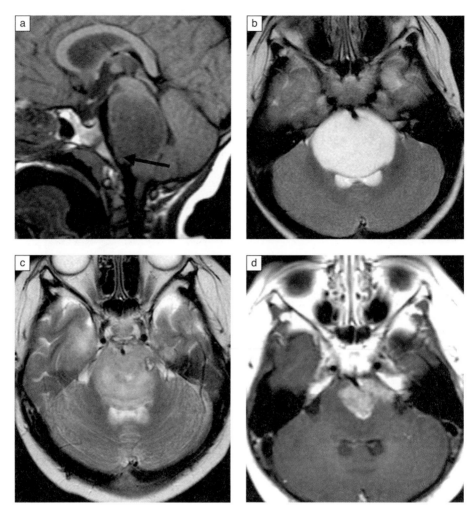

Fig. 3.25. T1W sagittal (a) and T2W axial (b) images in another patient with a diffuse pontine glioma, this time with an exophytic element (arrow). The glioma once again is seen to expand the pons with posterior displacement of the 4th ventricle and wrapping around the basilar artery.

T2W axial (c) and T1W axial (d) gadolinium enhanced MR scans obtained after radiotherapy show a reduction in T_2 signal change and now, enhancement. The latter is common after radiotherapy.

→

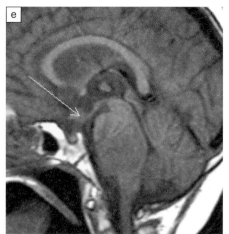

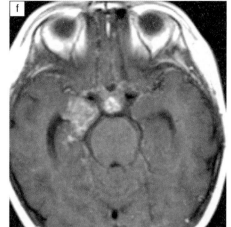

Fig. 3.25 *(continued)*. Unfortunately, T1W sagittal
(e) and gadolinium enhanced axial scans (f,g) in this
patient some months later, following clinical deterioration, show leptomeningeal spread of tumour.
Note the nodular leptomeningeal enhancement and
a hypothalamic mass (e,f).

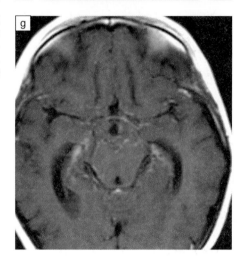

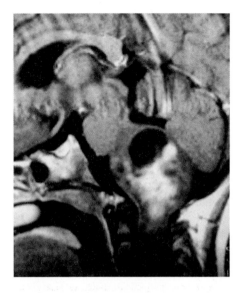

Fig. 3.26. T1W gadolinium enhanced sagittal image demonstrates a cervicomedullary glioma. It is a cystic tumour with a well defined, brightly enhancing solid component suggesting that it is a pilocytic astrocytoma. It abuts the 4th ventricle, is amenable to surgery and is associated with a more favourable prognosis.

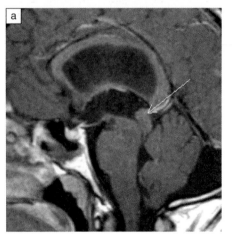
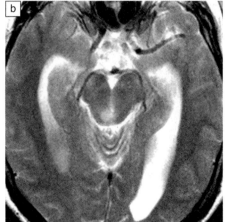

Fig. 3.27. T1W gadolinium enhanced sagittal (a) and T2W axial (b) MR scans demonstrate a typical tectal plate glioma with a non-enhancing mass on T1W (arrow) that returns hyperintense signal on T2W. The aqueduct is compressed, resulting in obstructive hydrocephalus. It is easy to see how such a small tumour would be missed on CT.

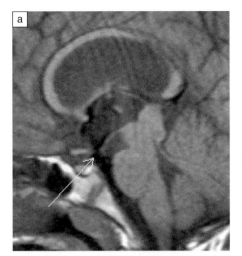

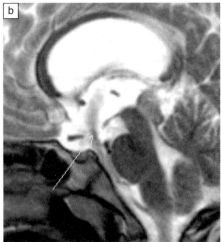

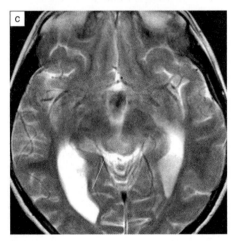

Fig. 3.28. T1W (a), T2W (b) sagittal and T2W axial (c) MR scans in a patient with a tectal plate glioma and treated hydrocephalus. The latter has been treated using neuroendoscopic 3rd ventriculostomy. Note the hypointense 'flow void' (arrows) indicating the moving passage of CSF through the defect in the floor of the third ventricle. This feature may be used to confirm patency of the 3rd ventriculostomy.

49

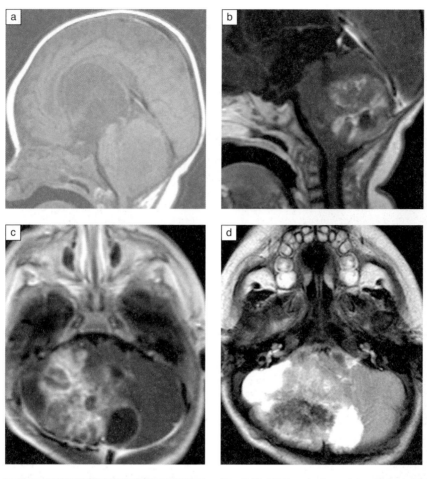

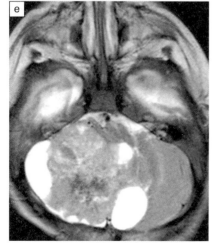

Fig. 3.29. T1W sagittal pre- (a) and post-gadolinium (b), T1W axial (c) post-gadolinium and T2W axial (d,e) MR scans, in a 3-month-old infant with irritability, a rapidly increasing head circumference and signs of hydrocephalus, demonstrate a large right cerebellar hemisphere mass. It is heterogeneous, irregularly enhancing with containing cysts and is producing severe obstructive hydrocephalus. Hypointense signal on T2W (d,e) is likely to represent deoxyhaemoglobin (hypointense on T1W also), suggesting haemorrhage.

This is a malignant atypical teratoid rhabdoid tumour (ATTR). There was no evidence of leptomeningeal spread intracranially or in the spine.

There are no specific features to suggest ATTR, and a similar appearance at this age might be seen in a choroid plexus carcinoma or PNET.

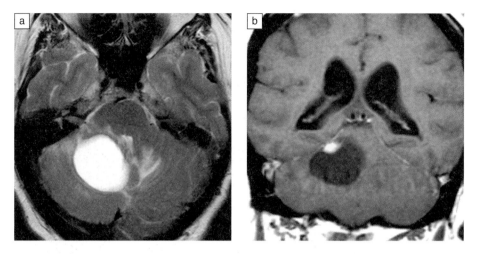

Fig. 3.30. T2W axial (a) and T1W gadolinium enhanced coronal (b) MR images demonstrate a common appearance of an haemangioblastoma, a peripherally located tumour with a large cyst and an enhancing nodule. There is also associated oedema.

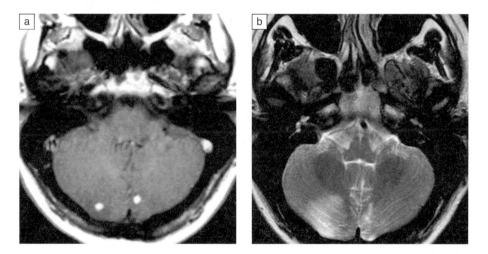

Fig. 3.31. T1W gadolinium enhanced (a) and T2W axial (b) MR images in a patient with von Hippel–Lindau syndrome demonstrate two small enhancing solid haemangioblastomas, one associated with oedema.

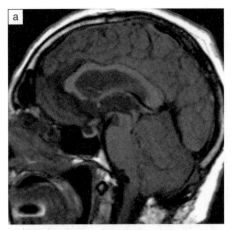

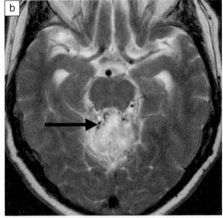

Fig. 3.32. T1W sagittal (a), T2W (b) and T1W gadolinium enhanced axial (c) MR images demonstrate a large solid haemangioblastoma with enlarged feeding arteries seen as large vascular flow voids (arrows – b). Angiography and embolization may be useful preoperatively in such a patient.

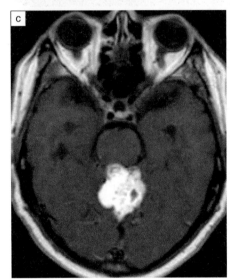

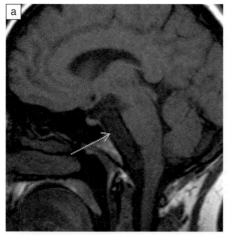

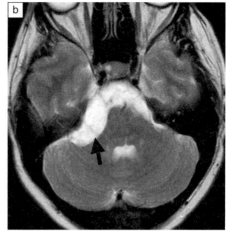

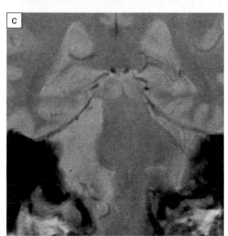

Fig. 3.33. T1W sagittal (a), T2W axial (b) and coronal proton density (c) MR images demonstrate the typical appearance of an extensive epidermoid. These are extra-axial lesions composed of keratin and cholesterol. They appear as non-enhancing lobulated masses, returning similar signal to CSF, insinuating in the subarachnoid space around blood vessels and nerves making complete excision often impossible. They return similar signal to CSF on T1W (arrow – a) and T2W (arrow – b) images but often return a little higher signal than CSF on proton density (c) and FLAIR sequences (a T2W sequence with water suppression). Here the tumour, originating in the right CPA but extending into the pontine cistern up to the hypothalamus, is noticed mainly by its mass effect. The brainstem is displaced posteriorly and is distorted on the right.

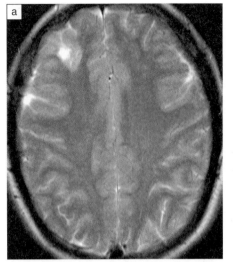

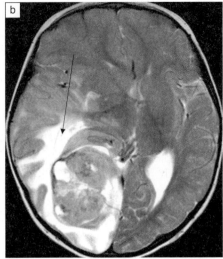

Fig. 3.34. T2W axial (a) and coronal (b) and T1W coronal (c) MR images in a patient with seizures demonstrate a mass lesion, with high signal on T2W and low signal on T1W, without oedema and without contrast enhancement. There is scalloping of the overlying skull vault (arrow), and this is seen in patients with peripheral long-standing lesions – any benign tumour. This tumour was a low-grade astrocytoma.

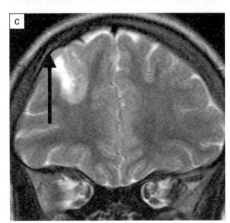

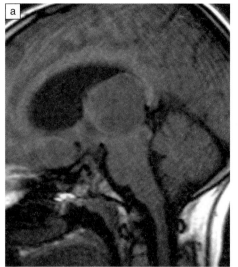

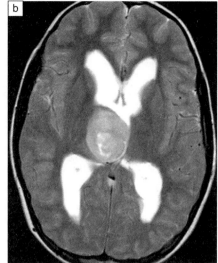

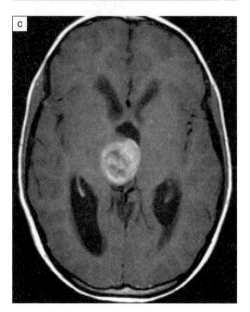

Fig. 3.35. T1W parasagittal (a), T2W axial (b) and gadolinium enhanced T1W axial (c) MR images demonstrate a heterogeneous mass in the right thalamus compressing the 3rd ventricle and causing obstructive hydrocephalus. There is marked contrast enhancement, some evidence of necrosis but no oedema. This proved to be an anaplastic astrocytoma.

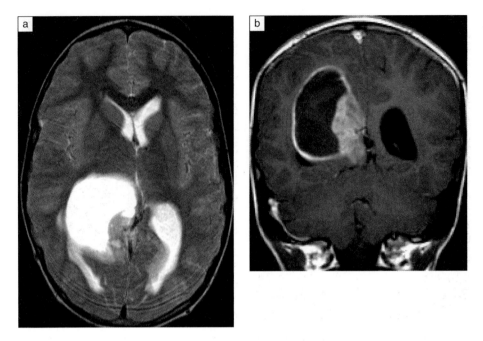

Fig. 3.36. T2W axial (a) and T1W coronal gadolinium enhanced (b) MR images in a patient with a supratentorial ependymoma. Such a diagnosis should be considered in a child with a paraventricular mass. These are usually cystic with an enhancing solid component and calcification, which may be seen on CT.

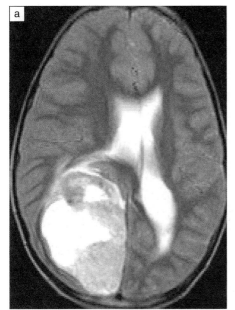

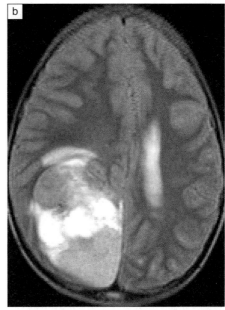

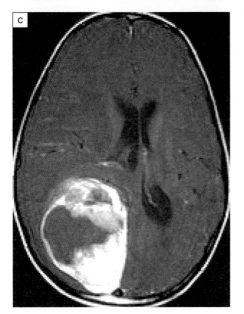

Fig. 3.37. T2W (a,b) and T1W gadolinium enhanced (c) axial MR images in a child with an ependymoma. The typical site, cystic and solid enhancing component are emphasized. There is mild oedema.

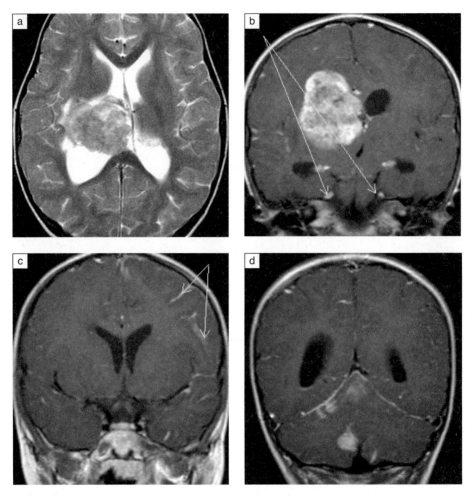

Fig. 3.38. T2W axial (a) and T1W coronal (b,c,d) MR images demonstrate features of a highly malignant brain tumour centred on the right thalamus. It is enhancing heterogeneously with areas of necrosis. There is oedema. Note also extensive leptomeningeal enhancement indicating tumour dissemination (arrows). Note the large leptomeningeal posterior fossa deposit (d).

This was a malignant atypical teratoid rhabdoid tumour. A PNET or malignant germ cell tumour would look similar. I have not seen extensive leptomeningeal disease in glioblastoma multiforme.

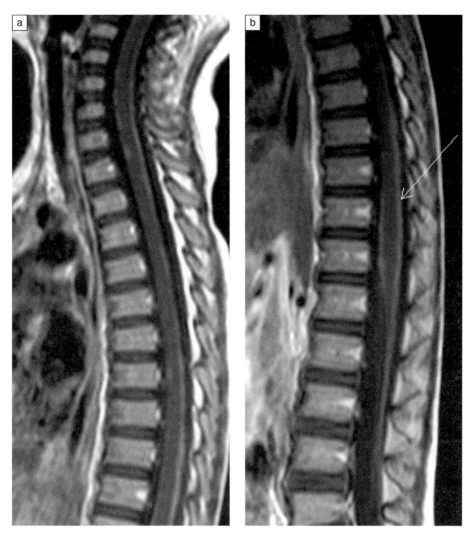

Fig. 3.39. Gadolinium enhanced T1W sagittal images of the cervicothoracic (a) and thoracolumbar (b) spine, in the same patient as Figure 3.38, demonstrate leptomeningeal spread of tumour with irregular thickened enhancing meninges over the cord (arrow).

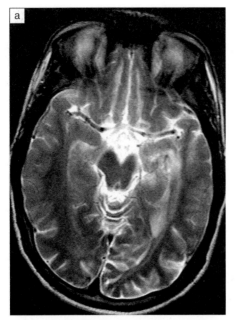

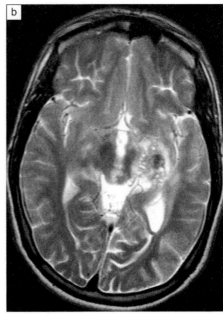

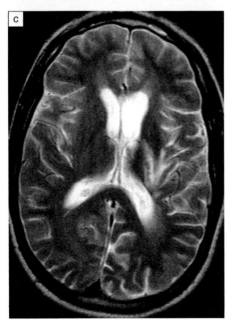

Fig. 3.40. T2W axial MR images in a 17-year-old boy with a progressive right hemiparesis and cognitive decline demonstrate an inhomogeneous mass in the medial aspect of the left temporal lobe extending into the basal ganglia, with hypointense foci and small cysts. Note atrophic changes in the left cerebral hemisphere with pallor in the white matter, enlargement of the sulci and left lateral ventricle and Wallerian degeneration in the left brainstem. There was moderate enhancement of the mass on CT and MRI (not shown). Biopsy of the mass diagnosed germinoma. The atrophic changes commonly seen almost certainly reflect involvement of the white matter tracts by tumour.

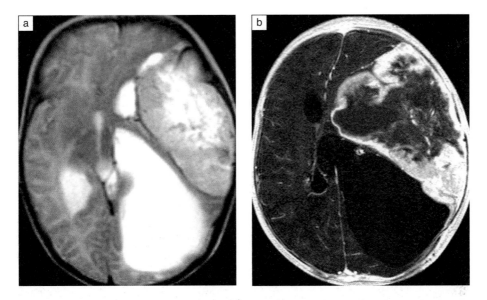

Fig. 3.41. T2W axial (a) and T1W axial gadolinium enhanced (b) MR images in a 16-month-old with seizures and an increasing head size demonstrate a large enhancing but necrotic left cerebral hemisphere mass with small cysts anteriorly and medially. There is compression of the left lateral ventricle and obstruction of the left occipital horn which is markedly dilated. The solid component has an extensive peripheral attachment. This tumour appears aggressive but was a desmoplastic infantile ganglioglioma and was successfully resected.

61

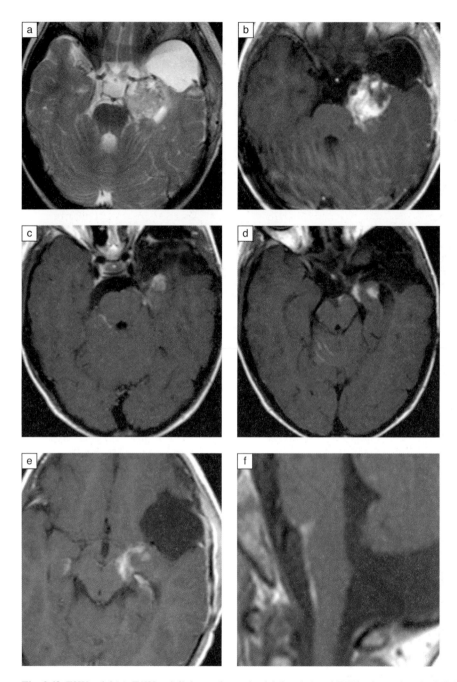

Fig. 3.42. T2W axial (a), T1W gadolinium enhanced axial (b,c,d,e) and T1W enhanced sagittal (f) MR images from a 3-year-old boy with a previously operated and partially excised desmoplastic infantile ganglioglioma. They demonstrate residual solid enhancing tumour in the medial aspect of the left temporal lobe, again with a leptomeningeal attachment and leptomeningeal dissemination of this benign tumour.

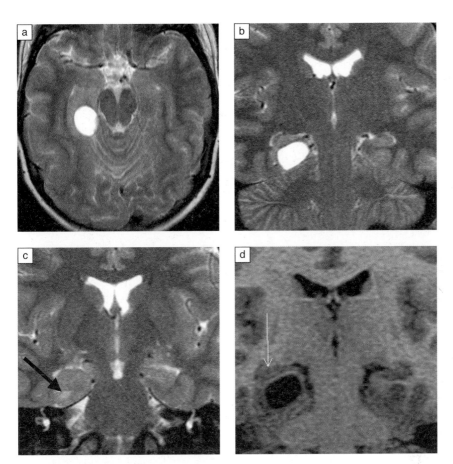

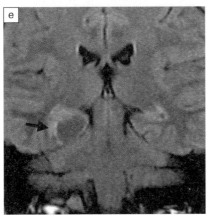

Fig. 3.43. This young patient has seizures. T2W axial (a) and coronal (b,c), T1W (d) and FLAIR (e) coronal images demonstrate a very high T_2 signal lesion in the right parahippocampal gyrus, separate from the hippo-campal formation (arrowhead – d). It returns higher signal than CSF on T1W and FLAIR. There is a little surrounding T_2 signal change in the white matter (arrow – e). This proved to be a cystic ganglioglioma but cannot be differentiated on imaging from a cystic astro-cytoma or DNET.

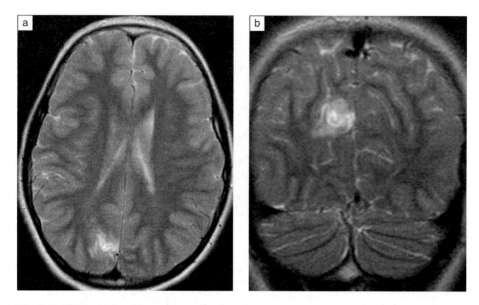

Fig. 3.44. T2W axial (a) and coronal (b) MR scans from a patient with refractory seizures demonstrate a small cortically based lesion in the medial right occipital lobe superiorly. There is no oedema and there was no enhancement. This was found to be a DNET.

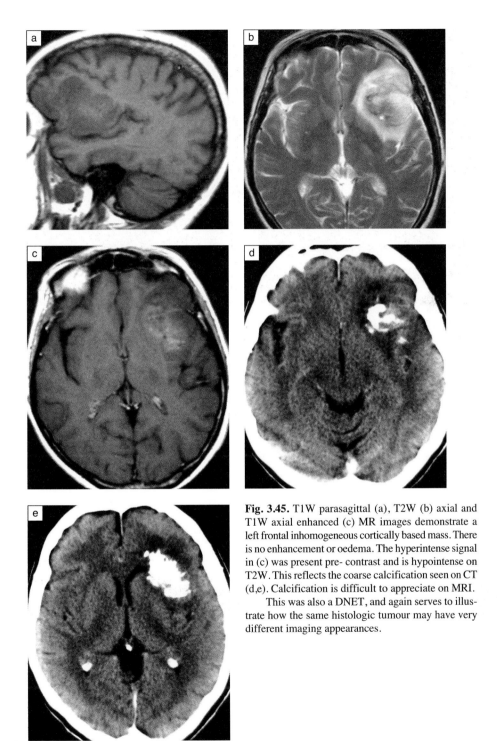

Fig. 3.45. T1W parasagittal (a), T2W (b) axial and T1W axial enhanced (c) MR images demonstrate a left frontal inhomogeneous cortically based mass. There is no enhancement or oedema. The hyperintense signal in (c) was present pre- contrast and is hypointense on T2W. This reflects the coarse calcification seen on CT (d,e). Calcification is difficult to appreciate on MRI.

This was also a DNET, and again serves to illustrate how the same histologic tumour may have very different imaging appearances.

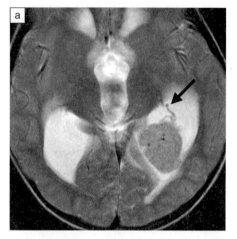

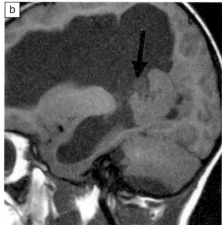

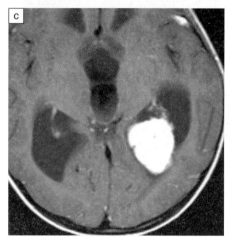

Fig. 3.46. MRI in a 14-month-old boy imaged because of developmental delay demonstrates marked non-obstructive hydrocephalus. The cause is a choroid plexus papilloma arising from the choroid plexus of the trigone of the left lateral ventricle. T2W axial (a), T1W parasagittal (b) and T1W gadolinium enhanced (c) MR images demonstrate the typically avidly enhancing trigonal mass. The mass has a small proteinaceous cyst returning higher signal than CSF on T1W (arrow – b). Note the enlarged feeding arterial pedicle (arrow – a) optimally seen on the T2W axial image.

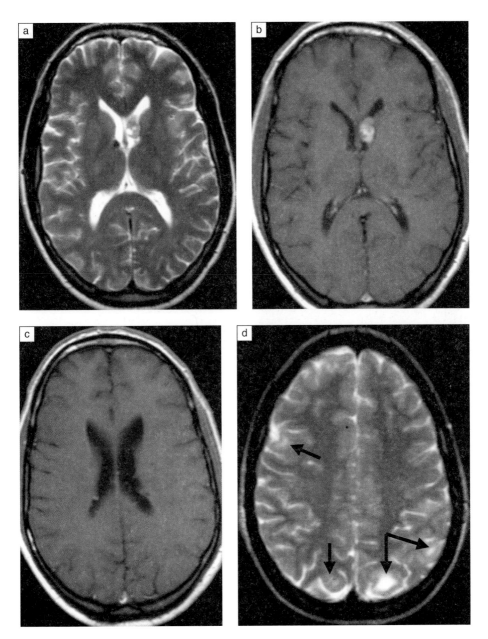

Fig. 3.47. T2W axial (a, d) and enhanced T1W axial (b,c) MR images in a 10-year-old with seizures demonstrate a mass in the region of the left foramen of Munro. It is enhancing on T1W (b) and isointense with cortex on T2W (a) with small cysts.

Note other subependymal non-enhancing nodules protruding into the lateral ventricles (c). There are also multiple subcortical hamartomas (arrows) seen as high signal in the subcortical white matter (d) within an expanded gyrus. These appearances are diagnostic of tuberous sclerosis with a giant cell astrocytoma near the left foramen of Munro.

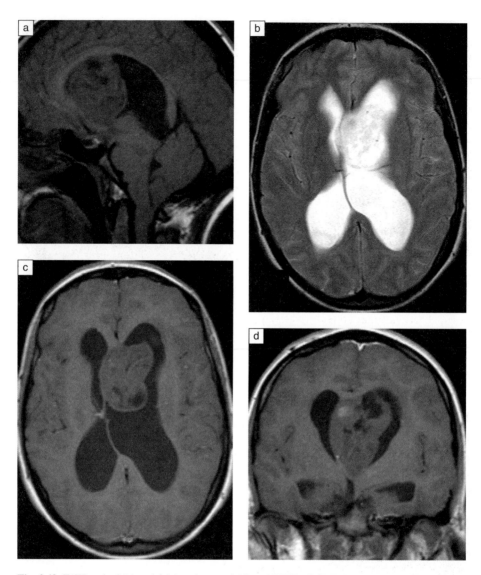

Fig. 3.48. T1W sagittal (a), axial (c) and coronal (d) and T2W axial MR images demonstrate a mass within the left lateral ventricle, attached to the septum pellucidum. It has many small cysts and was calcified on CT (not shown). This tumour did not enhance, although enhancement is well known to occur in such tumours. This was a neurocytoma. Here it is causing obstruction at both foramina of Munro. The 3rd ventricle and hypothalamus are markedly compressed with downward herniation of both the hypothalamus and cerebellar tonsils, the result of obstructive hydrocephalus involving the lateral ventricles. The corpus callosum is bowed and thinned by the obstructed ventricles.

The differential diagnosis would include oligodendroglioma, subependymoma, and astrocytoma.

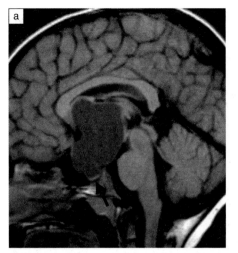 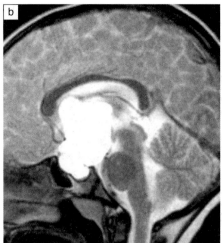

Fig. 3.49. T1W (a) and T2W (b) sagittal MR images in a child demonstrate the typical appearance of a craniopharyngioma. This is seen as a large, cystic suprasellar mass extending upwards, compressing the hypothalamus, optic chiasm and third ventricle. The signal is that of proteinaceous fluid on T1W, being slightly higher signal than CSF. Gadolinium was not given. However, you would expect a solid component to enhance.

Note that the pituitary fossa (arrow), containing anterior pituitary tissue only, is of normal size consistent with the suprasellar (not intrasellar) tumour origin. The normal high signal of the posterior pituitary is absent, reflecting the hypothalamic disturbance and central diabetes insipidus.

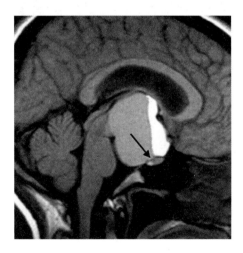

Fig. 3.50. T1W sagittal MRI also of a suprasellar craniopharyngioma but this time the cyst fluid is of much higher signal reflecting very elevated protein levels. Note there is a fat–fluid level and the very hyperintense component is probably fat. Fat returns very high signal on T1W.

Both the anterior and posterior pituitary glands are seen within a normal size pituitary fossa (arrow).

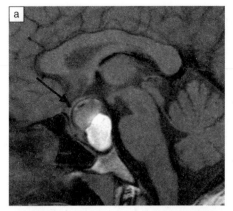 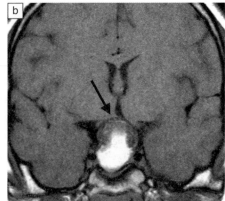

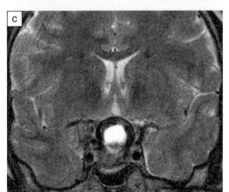

Fig. 3.51. T1W sagittal (a) and coronal (b) and T2W coronal (c) MR images illustrate an intra- and suprasellar craniopharyngioma (same patient as in Fig. 3.8). The craniopharyngioma is compressing the chiasm (arrows). The pituitary fossa is expanded and normal pituitary tissue cannot be identified. The tumour returns hyperintense signal on T1W and peripheral hypointense signal on T2W. The latter probably represents paramagnetic substances within the cyst wall.

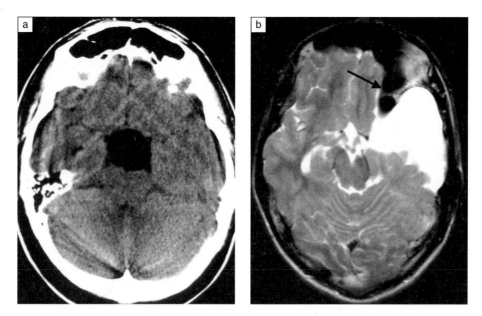

Fig. 3.52. Axial cranial CT (a) demonstrates a suprasellar mass of CSF density only. There is no solid component, no enhancement and no calcification. These are the imaging features of an arachnoid cyst. T2W axial MRI (b) in another patient demonstrates a common site – the anterior middle cranial fossa – and the appearance of an arachnoid cyst. On MRI, they are seen as extra-axial lesions returning CSF signal, without internal structure, solid elements or enhancement. They exhibit mass effect and here the temporal lobe and left midbrain are distorted. There is also excessive pneumatization of the left orbital roof (arrow), an associated phenomenon.

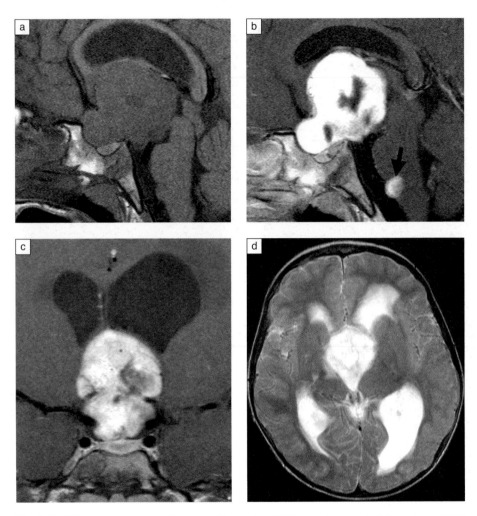

Fig. 3.53. T1W sagittal pre- (a) and post-gadolinium (b), T1W coronal post-gadolinium (c) and T2W axial (d) MR images demonstrate a large, solid brightly enhancing suprasellar mass typical of a JPA containing areas of necrosis. The tumour is compressing the third ventricle and there is obstructive hydrocephalus. Note evidence of CSF dissemination of this benign tumour (arrow – b).

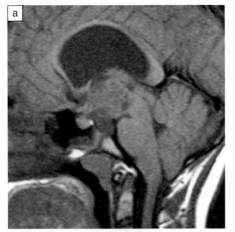

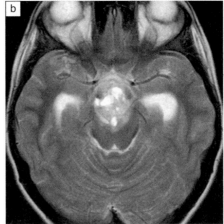

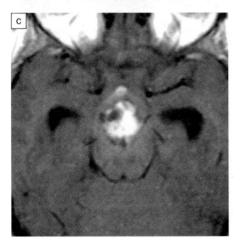

Fig. 3.54. T1W sagittal (a), T2W axial (b) and enhanced T1W axial (c) MR images in a child with a hypothalamic glioma. There are multiple small cysts. The tumour is mainly solid with marked enhancement, which is typical of a pilocytic astrocytoma. The tumour here is seen to arise in the tuber cinereum, extend upwards, and compress the 3rd ventricle. A component also extends inferiorly into the pontine cistern.

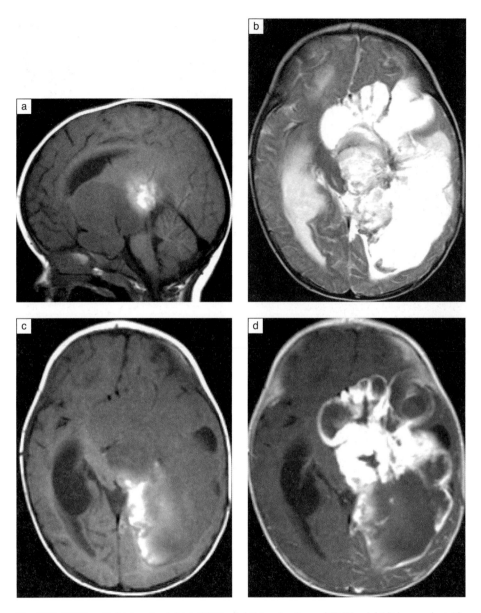

Fig. 3.55. T1W sagittal (a) and axial (c), T2W axial (b) and enhanced T1W axial (d) images in a 12-month-old girl with some developmental delay and diagnosed with cerebral palsy. She was otherwise well. Her head was growing markedly – hence the scan. The images demonstrate a cystic/solid haemorrhagic (high-signal methaemoglobin on T1W – a) hypothalamic mass extending into the left hemicranium. There is compression of the left lateral ventricle and obstructive hydrocephalus of the right lateral ventricle. This was a large hypothalamic pilocytic astrocytoma.

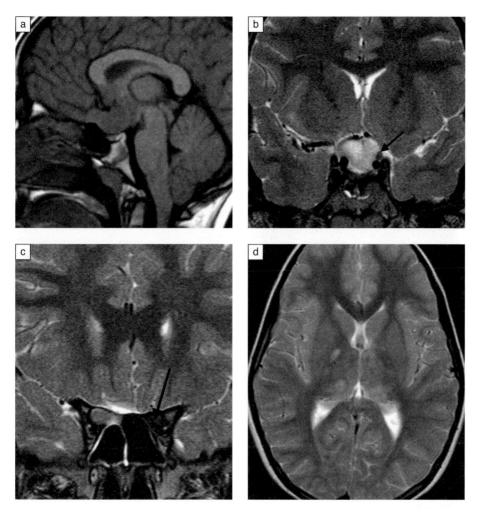

Fig. 3.56. A 9-year-old girl with no relevant past medical history or family history was scanned for progressive visual impairment. T1W sagittal (a) and T2W coronal (b,c) and axial T2W (d) MR scans demonstrate a hypothalamic/optic pathway mass, a glioma, with extension of tumour along the right optic nerve. Note the normal left optic nerve (arrow – b,c). There are multiple foci of high signal in the thalami bilaterally and right globus pallidus making the diagnosis of NF1 – a spontaneous mutation in this case.

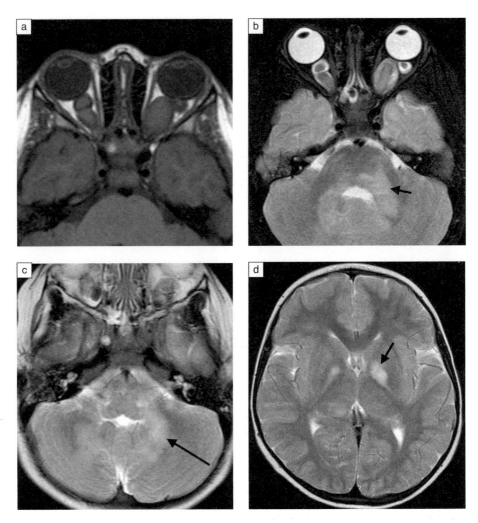

Fig. 3.57. T1W (a) and T2W (b) axial MR scans through the orbits, the latter using a fat suppression technique, demonstrate fusiform dilatation of the intraorbital optic nerves bilaterally, diagnostic of optic nerve gliomas in a small child with NF1. The tumours did not extend though the optic canals and the chiasm was normal. Note the hyperintense signal in the brainstem (b), cerebellar white matter (arrows – b,c), right thalamus and globus pallidus (d) bilaterally, seen in 75% of those with NF1.

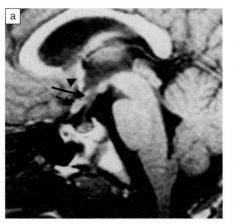
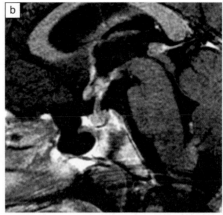

Fig. 3.58. A 6-year-old boy presented with pituitary failure and diabetes insipidus (DI). The T1W sagittal image on the first MRI examination (a) showed that the high signal of the posterior pituitary was absent, consistent with central DI and hypothalamic disturbance. There is thickening of the chiasm (short arrow), tuber cinereum (long arrow) and lamina terminalis (arrowhead) (not appreciated at the time). Gadolinium was mistakenly not given on this occasion but only at follow-up 3 months later (b) when abnormal thickening and enhancement of these structures and now the infundibulum and anterior pituitary was reported. This infiltrating process is typical of a germinoma. It is important to give gadolinium in patients with DI to pick up subtle hypothalamic pathology. A child with DI may be harbouring a very small germinoma that may at first be difficult to appreciate. In such cases it is recommended to repeat the gadolinium enhanced MRI study in 3–6 months and again in a further 3–6 months.

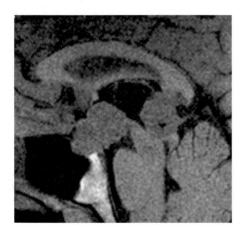

Fig. 3.59. T1W sagittal MRI demonstrates a hypo-thalamic mass in a patient with pituitary failure and diabetes insipidus, extending down into the pituitary fossa and a pineal suprasellar mass with a small area of necrosis. It is not known whether this represents multifocal disease or leptomeningeal dissemination of a pineal germinoma.

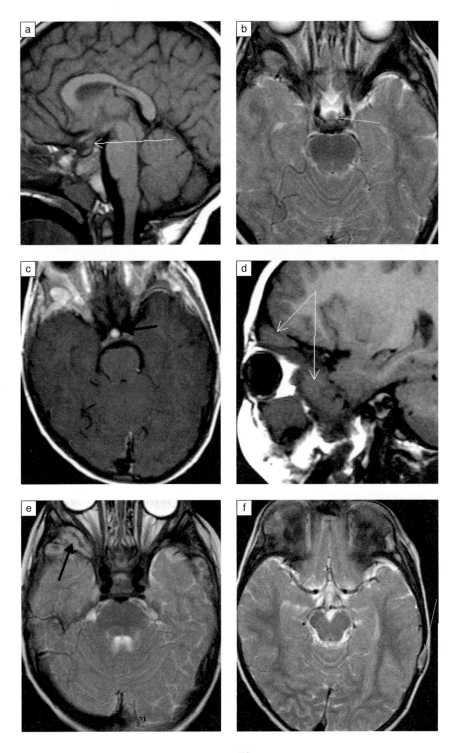

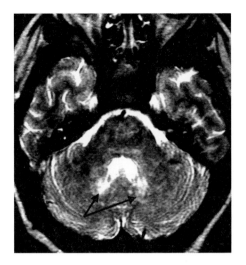

Fig. 3.61. T2W axial MRI in another patient with Langerhans cell histiocytosis demonstrates high signal in the cerebellar white matter due to gliosis and demyelination (arrows).

Fig. 3.60 *(opposite)*. T1W sagittal (a) and parasagittal (d), T2W axial (b,e,f) and T1W axial (c) MR scans post-gadolinium in a 4-year-old boy with diabetes insipidus demonstrate absence of the high signal posterior pituitary gland indicating central diabetes insipidus and the responsible lesion, an enhancing infundibular mass (arrows – a,b,c). Note also the bony destructive masses involving the orbital walls and floor of the middle cranial fossa (arrows – d,e) and the lytic calvarial deposit (arrow – f). The bone involvement makes the diagnosis of Langerhans cell histiocytosis most likely.

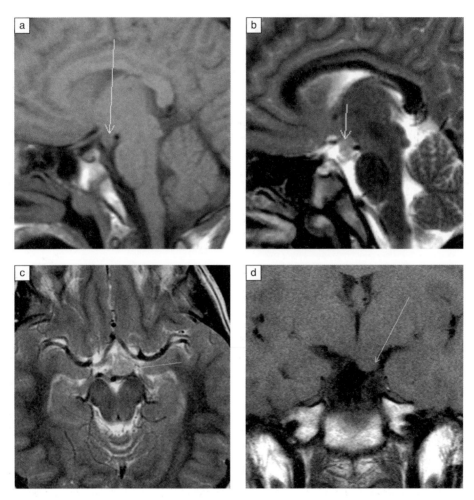

Fig. 3.62. T1W (a) and T2W (b) parasagittal, T2W axial (c) and T1W coronal (d) MR images demonstrate a well defined mass attached to the hypothalamus on the left (arrows). It returns similar signal to grey matter, did not enhance and was non-progressive, favouring the diagnosis of a hamartoma of the tuber cinereum.

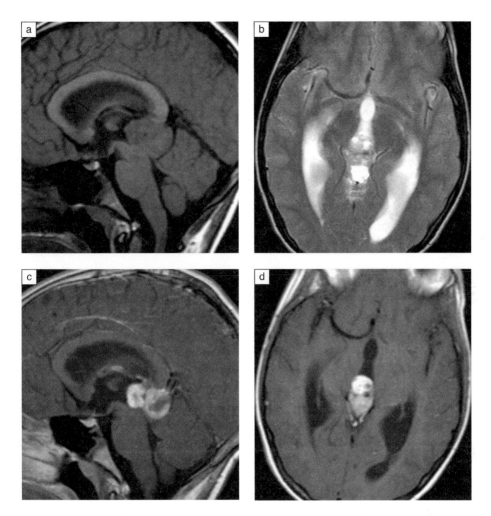

Fig. 3.63. T1W sagittal pre- (a) and post- (c) gadolinium, T1W axial post-gadolinium (d) and T2W axial (b) MR images in a 12-year-old boy demonstrate a heterogeneous pineal mass containing small cysts or areas of necrosis and a hypointense focus on T2W consistent with a small area of calcification or haemorrhage. There is marked contrast enhancement of the solid tissue. This was a germinoma. Note compression of the quadrigeminal plate and aqueduct and obstructive hydrocephalus.

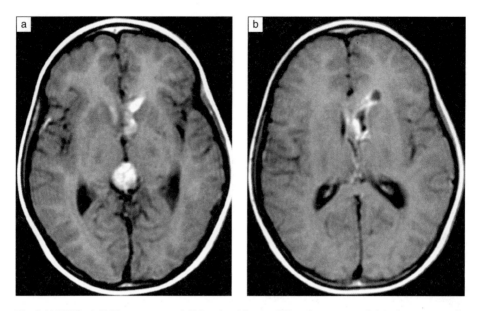

Fig. 3.64. T1W axial MR scans post-gadolinium in a 14-year-old boy demonstrate a bright, homogeneously enhancing pineal mass, typical of a germinoma. There is ependymal thickening and enhancement in the frontal horns indicating CSF dissemination of the germinoma.

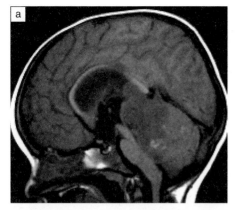

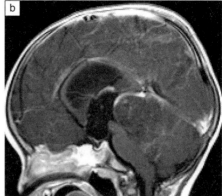

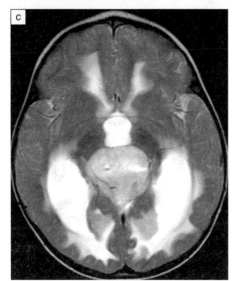

Fig. 3.65. A 4-year-old boy presented with signs of acute hydrocephalus. T1W sagittal pre- (a) and post-gadolinium (b) and T2W axial (c) MR images demonstrate a large pineal mass, hypointense on T1W with a little hyperintense signal inferiorly suggesting haemorrhagic change. There is no contrast enhancement, unusual in this case. The mass is hyperintense on T2W and compresses the tectal plate and aqueduct. This was a pinealoblastoma causing acute obstructive hydrocephalus. Note the periventricular oedema (arrow).

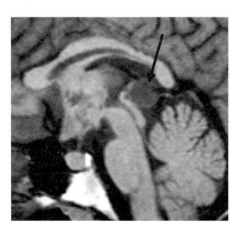

Fig. 3.66. T1W sagittal MRI demonstrates a hypothalamic glioma and an incidental pineal cyst (arrow). The signal is a little higher than that of CSF as a result of high protein content. There is no mass effect – the quadrigeminal plate is not distorted and the aqueduct is not compressed.

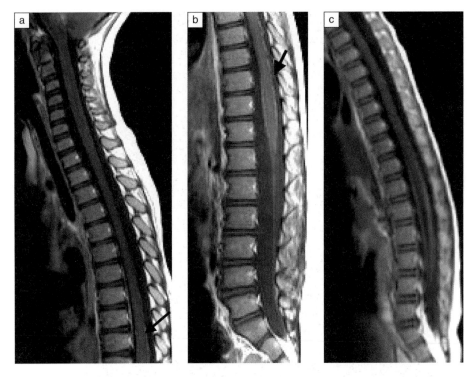

Fig. 3.67. T1W gadolinium enhanced sagittal spinal MR images (a – cervicothoracic; b – lumbosacral) demonstrate normal enhancement of the coronal venous plexus on the surface of the cord (arrow) and normal enhancement of lumbosacral nerves roots – not to be confused with leptomeningeal spread of tumour.

84

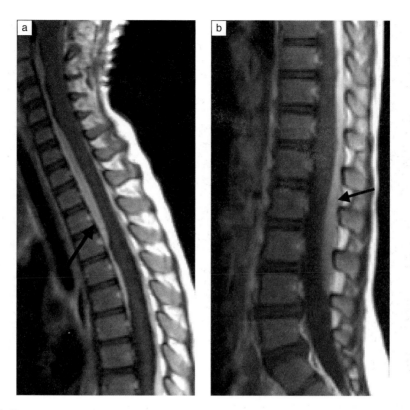

Fig. 3.68. T1W sagittal gadolinium enhanced spinal MR images (a – cervicothoracic; b – lumbosacral) obtained 2 days postoperatively demonstrate hyperintense subdural haemorrhagic fluid (arrows). The assessment of leptomeningeal disease is not reliable by MRI in the early postoperative period. It is easy to see how leptomeningeal disease could be concealed by these haemmorhagic effusions, particularly in the cervical and thoracic regions.

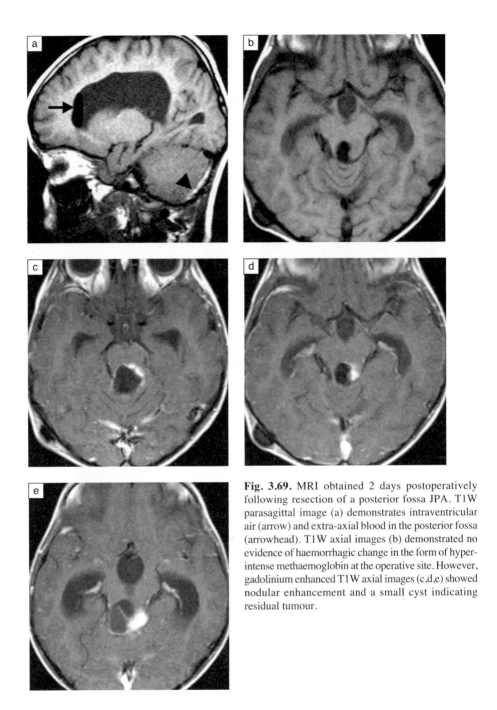

Fig. 3.69. MRI obtained 2 days postoperatively following resection of a posterior fossa JPA. T1W parasagittal image (a) demonstrates intraventricular air (arrow) and extra-axial blood in the posterior fossa (arrowhead). T1W axial images (b) demonstrated no evidence of haemorrhagic change in the form of hyperintense methaemoglobin at the operative site. However, gadolinium enhanced T1W axial images (c,d,e) showed nodular enhancement and a small cyst indicating residual tumour.

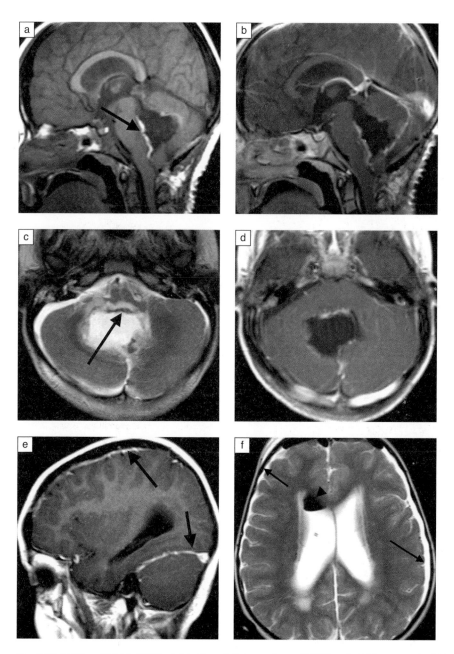

Fig. 3.70. T1W sagittal (a), T2W axial (c, f), gadolinium enhanced T1W sagittal (b), parasagittal (e) and axial (d) MR images obtained 3 days postoperatively following resection of a medulloblastoma demonstrate a CSF cavity at the site of the resected tumour with intracellular methaemoglobin related to the operative site on non-contrast T1W images (arrow – a). This is hypointense on T2W (arrow – c). There is no evidence of enhancing residual tumour. Small subdural effusions are present bilaterally (arrows – f), and there is intraventricular air (arrowhead – f) and postoperative dural enhancement (arrows – e).

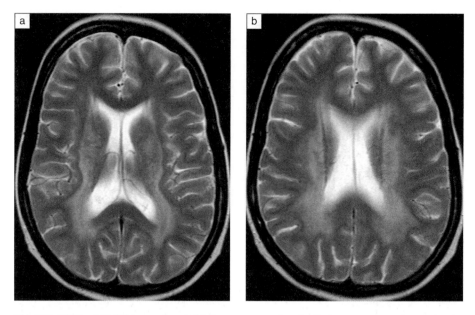

Fig. 3.71. T2W axial MRI in a patient following some months of radiotherapy as part of treatment for a medulloblastoma. There is extensive signal in the deep white matter signifying diffuse white matter damage (late radiation damage).

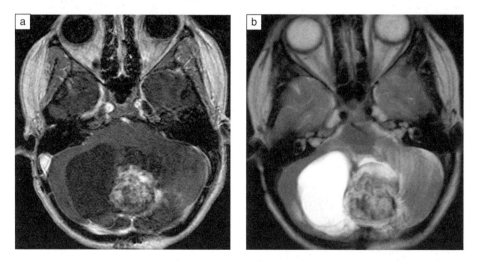

Fig. 3.72. Gadolinium enhanced T1W (a) and T2W (b) axial MR images demonstrate an enhancing heterogeneous midline posterior fossa mass with a cyst and oedema. There are areas of necrosis seen as non-enhancing areas on T1W and haemorrhagic foci seen as hypointense areas on T2W. Surgical excision showed radionecrosis. There was no evidence of tumour.

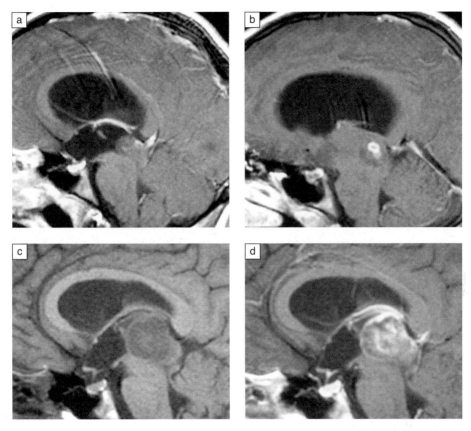

Fig. 3.73. This patient has a pilocytic astrocytoma of the tectal plate. T1W gadolinium enhanced sagittal scans (a,b) demonstrate a tectal plate mass with a focus of intense enhancement, causing hydrocephalus. Radiotherapy was given. T1W sagittal (c) and gadolinium enhanced T1W sagittal (d) images were obtained 3 months later after clinical deterioration. Biopsy revealed radiation necrosis.

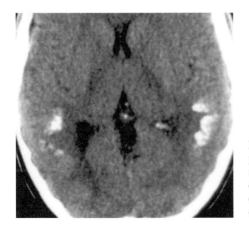

Fig. 3.74. Axial cranial CT in a patient several years after excision of a posterior fossa tumour and subsequent radiotherapy demonstrates subcortical calcification in the parietal lobes typical of a mineralizing angiopathy. The patient was experiencing complex partial seizures.

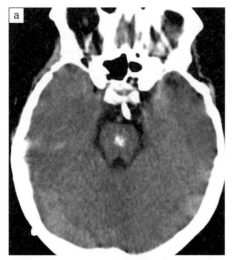
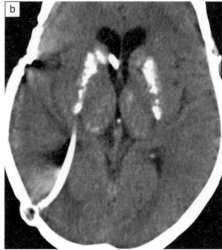
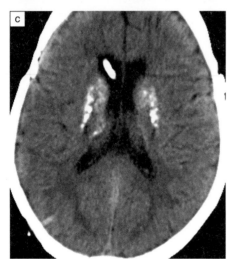

Fig. 3.75. Axial cranial CT in a patient several years after surgery for a craniopharyngioma and subsequent radiotherapy demonstrates basal ganglia and pons typical of mineralizing angiopathy. A right ventricular shunt has successfully treated the patient's hydrocephalus. A right frontal drain is also present.

Tectal plate glioma

These are usually non-progressive lesions with an excellent prognosis. Most are low-grade astrocytomas but anaplastic lesions have been reported. Patients present with hydrocephalus, and, not infrequently, small tumours are missed on CT, the ventricular dilatation being mistaken for benign aqueductal stenosis. This patient group should rather be imaged using MRI where the tumours are better delineated. A distorted expanded tectal plate, returning hypointense signal on T1W (Figs. 3.27, 3.28) and hyperintense signal on T2W, is seen (Bowers et al. 2000). Tumour may extend to involve the thalamus. There is either no or minimal gadolinium enhancement. Occasionally exophytic growth, cyst formation and calcification are noted, but these factors do not correlate well with histologic grade.

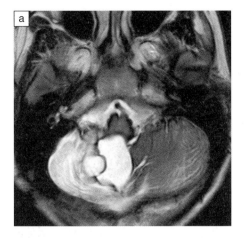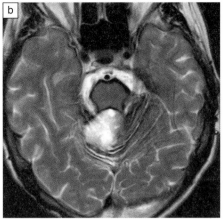

Fig. 3.76. T2W axial MRI showing superficial siderosis, some years after excision of a posterior fossa pilocytic astrocytoma. The patient developed symptoms and signs of progressive ataxia and sensorineural hearing loss. These images demonstrate postoperative changes and striking hypointense signal representing a rim of iron coating the cerebellum and brainstem.

Treatment consists of neuroendoscopic third ventriculostomy, alleviating the hydrocephalus (Fig. 3.28).

A small number of tumours may progress on MRI. Such progression is often asymptomatic over several years follow-up (Bowers et al. 2000). In these the timing of treatment is controversial.

Occasionally a tumour will be large, spanning the pineal region, and in these, biopsy may be required to obtain a diagnosis, ideally at the time of neuroendoscopic third ventriculostomy.

Malignant atypical teratoid rhabdoid tumour
This highly malignant tumour is rare and carries a bleak prognosis. It is usually found in young children (mean age 16.8 months). CSF dissemination is common and death is usual within 12 months of diagnosis. Supratentorial (Figs. 3.38, 3.39) and posterior fossa lesions occur.

The tumour is often large at presentation and imaging demonstrates a heterogeneous mass with cysts and necrosis (Fig. 3.29). There is marked enhancement and extensive oedema. CT may show flecks of calcification. The imaging appearance is therefore that of a malignant lesion, and a similar appearance may be seen with medulloblastoma, ependymoma, glioblastoma, PNET and malignant germ cell tumour.

Haemangioblastoma
These are rare benign tumours of vascular origin and approximately 10–20% occur in association with von Hippel–Lindau syndrome, usually in young/middle-aged adults but occasionally in children. They are mostly located in the cerebellar hemisphere, occasionally

the brainstem and cerebral hemisphere. They originate from the surface of the brain, and a portion of the tumour is always connected to a pial surface. Classically they are cystic tumours with a mural nodule (Fig. 3.30) but 30–40% are solid (Figs. 3.31, 3.32). Imaging demonstrates a solid, intensely enhancing mass or a solid, enhancing nodule associated with a cyst. The cyst may be haemorrhagic. With larger solid lesions, prominent vascular flow voids (Fig. 3.32) may be readily seen on MRI, clinching the diagnosis.

Dermoids and epidermoids
These are extra-axial lesions arising outside the brain parenchyma, and such lesions displace rather than invade brain. They are congenital tumours arising from intracranial rests remaining as a result of incomplete separation of the neuroectoderm from cutaneous ectoderm at the time of closure of the neural tube.

Epidermoids occur most commonly in the CPA but also in the pineal and suprasellar regions. They contain desquamated keratin and cholesterol. Slow growth insinuates between cranial nerves and blood vessels, and so complete surgical excision may not be possible. On CT, they are lobulated masses of CSF density and do not enhance or calcify. On MRI, they also return signal similar to CSF (Fig. 3.33) on all sequences but are often slightly hyperintense on proton density and FLAIR (fluid attenuated inversion recovery) and demonstrate internal structure. They characteristically show restricted diffusion on diffusion-weighted MRI.

Dermoids are seen as fatty extra-axial masses usually located in the midline. They displace blood vessels and nerves, whereas lipomas engulf them. Dermoids may also have solid or cystic components and calcification (Fig. 3.7).

SUPRATENTORIAL TUMOURS
Of those involving the cerebral hemispheres, astrocytomas are by far the most common. These are usually low grade (Figs. 3.2, 3.34), but aggressive lesions also occur (Fig. 3.35). Other benign parenchymal neoplasms include gangliogliomas, dysembryoplastic neuro-epithelial tumours, oligodendrogliomas and the desmoplastic infantile gangliogliomas. Malignant tumours include ependymomas, atypical teratoid rhabdoid tumours, PNETs and germinomas.

Astrocytoma
These are the most common, comprising nearly half of the supratentorial tumours in children. A little over half are JPAs. Thirty per cent are fibrillary astrocytomas (Figs. 3.2, 3.34) and 10% are mixed tumours.

The pilocytic astrocytoma produces a well demarcated large cyst, which unlike many of the posterior fossa tumours contains neoplastic cells within the wall. There is also a solid, slightly hypodense nodule on CT, a mural plaque or multiple mural masses that enhance. There is no oedema. Calcification in childhood astrocytomas is unusual, more often suggesting oligodendroglioma, ganglioglioma or PNET.

On MRI, pilocytic astrocytomas demonstrate the well defined cystic and solid components. The latter are low signal on T1W, high signal on T2W, and densely enhance.

Low-grade fibrillary astrocytomas infiltrate the white matter, and on CT are homogeneous, low density, poorly defined and non-enhancing. On MRI, they are also demonstrated as homogeneous infiltrative lesions, hypointense on T1W and hyperintense on T2W, occasionally with irregular enhancement.

Glioblastoma multiforme (GBM) represents 7–11% of primary brain tumours in children, with a median age of 13 years, and is associated with a poor prognosis. CSF dissemination may be seen in nearly one third of cases. Tumour haemorrhage is present in 18%. CT and MRI demonstrate an irregular heterogeneous enhancing mass which may be necrotic and is associated with marked oedema. The appearance of GBM on imaging overlaps with that of other malignant tumours.

Pleomorphic xanthoastrocytoma
This is a rare tumour probably arising from subpial astrocytes, hence its superficial location. It presents below 30 years of age, with a mean age of 14 years at presentation, and is usually benign despite its marked cellularity and pleomorphism histologically. Malignant transformation may occur (Tonn et al. 1997). It is a well circumscribed astrocytic neoplasm, occurring in the cortex most often in the temporal lobe, classically with a large cystic component and a superficial mural nodule attached to and sometimes infiltrating the leptomeninges (Kleihues et al. 1993, Tonn et al. 1997). Focal infiltration of brain parenchyma may also occur. The imaging appearances once again are nonspecific.

CT and MRI demonstrate a proteinaceous cystic lesion involving the surface of the brain with an inhomogeneous enhancing solid component. Cyst wall enhancement is variably reported (Bucciero et al. 1997). Occasionally there is dural enhancement reflecting its leptomeningeal involvement (also seen with meningiomas and malignant tumours located superficially, indicating either neoplastic dural involvement or reactive meningeal changes). Occasionally, solid tumours mimicking meningiomas have been described (Pierallini et al. 1999). Calcification may be seen on CT (Buccerio et al. 1997) but is unusual. Oedema is usually mild or absent, and its presence may correlate with more aggressive tumours.

Ependymoma
Thirty to 40 per cent of ependymomas occur in the supratentorial compartment (Vinchon et al. 2001), and they predominate in boys and in children under 5 years. They may develop in connection with the ventricular lining or at a distance from it, from ependymyocytes that are found in the ventricular ependymal and normal brain parenchyma. They are therefore located adjacent to the ventricular surface often at ends of lateral ventricles where ependymal rests are frequently found.

These tumours are usually large, invasive and necrotic (Figs. 3.36, 3.37) with calcification in one third to one half (Lefton et al. 1998). Imaging therefore shows a heterogeneous mass with enhancement of the solid component. Oedema is present in at least 50%. Haemorrhage is unusual. CSF dissemination is uncommon.

Primitive neuroectodermal tumours (PNETs)
These are primitive, embryonal, highly malignant tumours sharing common neuroepithelial

precursors. They comprise 1–5% of all paediatric brain tumours. There may be leptomeningeal dissemination (Figs. 3.38, 3.39) and occasionally metastasis outside the CNS.

These tumours commonly contain foci of calcification and cysts. Tumour haemorrhage occurs in about 10%. Imaging therefore demonstrates a heterogeneous mass. The solid portions are usually dense on CT, and these areas enhance after contrast on both CT and MRI (Fig. 3.1).

Germinomas

Most germinomas arise in the pineal region: about 10% arise in the basal ganglia and thalamus, the likely result of migration of pluripotential cells deviated off the midline by the developing third ventricle. Patients are typically male, in the second decade of life, and may present with focal neurological deficits and progressive dementia. Ipsilateral cerebral atrophy at presentation is common, due to involvement of the adjacent white matter tracts by the tumour (Fig. 3.40).

CT may demonstrate a slightly hyperdense irregular lesion with little mass effect, although these tumours may be several centimetres in diameter at presentation. Calcification and cysts are common, and there is mild to moderate heterogeneous enhancement. On MRI, they are heterogeneous enhancing masses with cysts and haemorrhagic foci. Oedema is present in one third.

Desmoplastic infantile ganglioglioma

This uncommon embryonal tumour comprises fibroblasts, astrocytes and neuronal elements, presenting within the first 18 months of life (Craver et al. 1999, Mallucci et al. 2000). The tumour is located superficially, is usually massive, partially cystic and contrast enhancing. The frontal, parietal, and to a lesser extent the temporal cortex are the most common sites of presentation. They are firmly attached to the dura and may extensively infiltrate the sub-arachnoid space. The solid component is iso- to hyperdense with respect to grey matter on CT and isointense to cortex on T1W and T2W MRI. There is marked enhancement of the solid component of the tumour (Figs. 3. 41, 3.42). Although the tumour may appear aggressive on imaging, surgery is often curative.

Oligodendroglioma

This is an infiltrating, slow growing tumour comprising 1–3% of paediatric brain tumours. It occurs most frequently in the frontal lobes followed by the temporal and parietal. It is necessary for at least 75% of the tumour to be composed of neoplastic oligodendrocytes for it to be classified as an oligodendroglioma; if less than 75%, it is termed a 'mixed glioma'.

Their density on CT is very variable and may be heterogeneous due to calcification (50–90%), cysts (in up to 20%) and haemorrhagic foci (20%). Enhancement, usually faint, is present in 50–60%. On MRI, they look well-defined (although they are infiltrative), involving the cortex and subcortical white matter (Fig. 3.5). They may appear homogeneous with low signal on T1W and high on T2W, or appear heterogeneous due to cysts, haemorrhage, etc. Most will show enhancement. Oedema is rare. The presence of calcium and lack of enhancement are associated with a better prognosis (Shaw et al. 1992, Rizk et al. 1996).

Any low-grade tumour may cause refractory seizures. Those not yet discussed include ganglioglioma/gangliocytomas and dysembryoplastic neuroepithelial tumours.

Ganglioglioma/gangliocytoma
These comprise approximately 1–8% of all paediatric brain tumours. The temporal lobe is the most common location but they may be found almost anywhere in the CNS. Both neoplastic glial and neuronal elements are present, with the neuronal element predominating in the gangliocytoma and the glial elements (usually astrocytic and low grade) in the ganglioglioma. They are indolent, mostly solid tumours but often contain cystic components. They grow slowly and exert little mass effect.

They usually show low density on CT but occasionally may be iso- or hyperdense. Contrast enhancement is seemingly variable (Matsumoto et al. 1999, Ildan et al. 2001, Nishio et al. 2001). Oedema is rare and, when present, is mild. Calcification, either flecks or large calcified masses, is present in at least 50% (Ildan et al. 2001, Nishio et al. 2001).

CT may occasionally fail to demonstrate the tumour (Matsumoto et al. 1999), and it is well accepted that MRI is the preferred imaging modality for those with refractory seizures.

On MRI, they are well defined (Fig. 3.43), cortically based and return variable signal intensity (Nishio et al. 2001) and variably enhance with gadolinium. Occasionally, solid tumours may appear 'cyst-like' with similar signal to CSF on proton density but higher signal than CSF on T2W (Matsumoto et al. 1999).

Dysembryoplastic neuroepithelial tumour (DNET)
This is a benign, non-progressive developmental tumour usually presenting in children and young adults with complex partial seizures, usually without focal deficit. They comprise about 0.4–1.3% of all primary brain tumours but 13% of tumours resected in an epilepsy series (Ostertun et al. 1996). Sixty per cent are located within the temporal lobe, and some are adjacent to areas of cortical dysplasia. They have a heterogeneous cellular composition with oligodendrocyte-like cells, astrocytes and neurons in a mucoid matrix and hence their imaging appearance is variable. They are usually well defined, lobulated cortically based masses and may be solid or cystic (Figs. 3.44, 3.45). About 20% show enhancement, and calcification is present in 20–30% (Raymond et al. 1994). There is usually no oedema.

Giant cell astrocytomas, choroid plexus papillomas (Fig. 3.46) and ependymomas are probably the most common ventricular tumours in childhood. Central neurocytomas are described below. Oligodendrogliomas may also occur within the ventricular system.

Giant cell astrocytoma
These are seen in about 15% of children with tuberous sclerosis, with an average age at

diagnosis of 13 years. They are well defined, indolent, predominantly intraventricular masses classically located in the region of the foramen of Munro. Other recognized sites include the atrium of the lateral ventricle and the temporal horn. Their growth is slow but they can obstruct the foramen of Munro with resultant hydrocephalus. They are usually non-invasive (malignant change is very rare) and probably arise from subependymal nodules that have formed secondary to the arrest of migration of dysgenetic cells.

Giant cell astrocytomas are hypo- or isointense on T1W MRI, hyperintense on T2W, and often show diffuse gadolinium enhancement (Fig. 3.47). They are histologically identical to subependymal nodules, and it is primarily their size that distinguishes them, being larger than 12 mm.

Subependymal nodules are iso- to hyperintense on T1W, iso- to hypointense on T2W, with variable contrast enhancement. They often appear calcified on CT.

Cortical hamartomas expand the gyrus. They contain giant cells with abnormal astrocytic and neuronal elements and lack a normal 6-layered cortex. These may also calcify and may enhance. Early in life, they may appear hyperintense to white matter on T1W and hypointense on T2W. As the brain myelinates they return high signal on T2W and low on T1W.

Neurocytoma

This benign tumour, carrying a good prognosis, arises in the septum pellucidum or third ventricle, usually resulting in hydrocephalus; it occurs in older children. It has been suggested that either the septum pellucidum or the subependymal layer covering the medial caudate nucleus is the site of origin, possibly from a neuroectodermal precursor cell. They are well circumscribed, usually large at presentation (Fig. 3.48), show variable contrast enhancement, and 50% appear calcified on CT. Cysts are present in 60%. As expected, they return hetero-geneous signal on MRI due to the calcification and cysts and, sometimes, vascular flow voids.

PARASELLAR TUMOURS

These constitute about 15–20% of all intracranial tumours in children. By far the most common is the craniopharyngioma. Other parasellar lesions illustrated below are the hypo-thalamic/optic pathway glioma, Rathke cleft cyst, arachnoid cyst, hamartoma of the tuber cinereum, germinoma and histiocytosis.

Craniopharyngioma

The craniopharyngioma is the most common parasellar tumour of childhood (15% of supra-tentorial tumours) and comprises half of these. They are slow growing and arise from the epithelial remnants of the craniopharyngeal duct which is the path taken by Rathke's pouch, from the oropharynx to the floor of the third ventricle. Seventy per cent are intrasellar and suprasellar, 20% are purely suprasellar and 10% purely intrasellar. Peak incidence is at 10–14 years of age.

The adamantinous type most commonly occurs in childhood. They vary in size but are often large lobulated cystic masses, rich in cholesterol, usually suprasellar encasing the circle of Willis, commonly (90%) with a thin circumferential rim of calcification in the wall or more solid chunks in the solid nodular component. There is usually enhancement of the wall and solid tissue on CT and MRI. On MRI, the signal returned by the cystic fluid is usually high on T2W (Figs. 3.49, 3.50, 3.51) but variable on T1W (low, iso- or hyperintense) depending upon protein content or methaemoglobin from haemorrhage. They may induce an intense glial reaction in the adjacent brain, becoming adherent to the hypothalamus and adjacent structures. Brain invasion is more frequent in children and in the adamantinous subtype.

The squamopapillary type is largely solid, non-calcified mass more often seen in adults and will not be discussed further.

MRS demonstrates no normal metabolites in the cystic component, just a lipid peak.

Rathke's cleft cyst

This is a benign, congenital lesion arising from failure of obliteration of the lumen of Rathke's pouch and is often an incidental finding at 13–22% of autopsies (Shanklin 1949). The cyst is lined by well-differentiated columnar ciliated epithelium with goblet cells, sometimes with squamous metaplasia. These goblet cells secrete serous or mucoid fluid. They may be intra- or suprasellar and, although usually asymptomatic because they are small (often less than 3mm), sometimes they become large enough to compress the pituitary, hypothalamus and optic chiasm. Large cysts may be difficult to differentiate from cranio-pharyngiomas or pituitary adenomas.

On CT, they are cystic, low density, non-calcified parasellar lesions.

On MRI, the signal is variable being either hypo- or hyperintense on T1W depending upon the protein content. Hyperintensity on T1W may also be due to haemorrhage.

Intracystic nodules (high signal on T1W and low on T2W) are frequently seen in Rathke's cleft cysts (Byun et al. 2000).

Arachnoid cysts and epidermoid cysts

These are extra-axial lesions that can also be found in this location.

Arachnoid cysts are congenital extra-axial lesions; they are thin walled cysts comprising flattened arachnoid cells and arising from maldeveloped leptomeninges. They return CSF signal/density only without internal structure (Fig. 3.52), enhancement or calcification. Diffusion-weighted MRI may also readily differentiate between these lesions.

Other common sites for arachnoid cysts include the anterior middle cranial fossa, posterior fossa and pineal region.

Hypothalamic glioma

Optic chiasm/hypothalamic gliomas comprise 10–15% of supratentorial masses in childhood and usually present at around 2–4 years of age. A significant number of patients will have a family history or clinical evidence of type 1 neurofibromatosis (NF1).

These tumours are commonly pilocytic astrocytomas (80%) and are usually large at the time of diagnosis. MRI optimally demonstrates the extent of the tumour along the optic pathways. Most are solid, lobulated, well defined, hypointense on T1W and hyperintense on T2W, and brightly enhancing sometimes with areas of cyst formation or necrosis (Figs.

3.53, 3.54, 3.55). They made invade the third ventricle and hydrocephalus is commonly seen.

CSF dissemination of low-grade astrocytomas in childhood is rare, estimated at 4% (Perilongo et al. 1997) and seems to occur preferentially with tumour located at this site.

Optic pathway gliomas and NF1
Twenty-five to 50 per cent of patients with optic pathway gliomas will have NF1 (Figs. 3.56, 3.57). They are usually low-grade pilocytic astrocytomas, although more aggressive lesions are known to occur. Spontaneous regression in patients with NF1 may also be seen.

The optic nerves only are most commonly involved, and on imaging there is fusiform enlargement of the nerves seen on both CT and MRI. The orbital lesion is demonstrated by CT but this modality may not reliably distinguish dural ectasia of the optic nerve sheath complex from tumour, and full delineation of any intracranial extension requires MRI. Optic nerve gliomas return similar signal to brain on T1W and T2W MRI. Chiasmatic and retrochiasmatic lesions give low signal on T1W, high on T2W, with variable enhancement. Extension beyond the lateral geniculate bodies is rare, but may extend to the occipital cortex.

The most common MRI finding in the brain in NF1 is foci of high signal on T2W, usually in the brainstem, cerebellum, basal ganglia and thalamus, seen in 75% patients (Figs. 3.56, 3.57). They may also be found in the corpus callosum, periventricular white matter and spinal cord. They are not usually seen on T1W (except for globus pallidus lesions, which may be slightly hyperintense), show no mass effect and do not enhance. They start at about 3 years, increase in size and number until 10–12 years and then decrease. Spongiotic change, gliosis and microcalcifications are the likely underling substrate. On MRI, differentiation from small low-grade glioma is impossible and follow up-imaging is therefore recommended. Alternatively, MRS may be useful because these lesions demonstrate different spectra from low-grade gliomas (Castillo et al. 1995, Gonen et al. 1999).

Gliomas, ependymomas, gangliogliomas and meningiomas also rarely occur in NF1.

Parasellar germinoma
Thirty per cent of germinomas are suprasellar and without sex predominance. Germinomas are the second most common parasellar region mass in a child, presenting usually with diabetes insipidus and pituitary failure. Central diabetes insipidus may be confirmed on MRI by noting absence of the normal high signal returned by the posterior pituitary gland on a midline sagittal T1W scan. The high signal reflects the lipid content of neurosecretory granules which store the posterior pituitary hormones.

Germinomas are infiltrating lesions involving the hypothalamus (Fig. 3.58) often extending up the lamina terminalis (anterior end of the 3rd ventricle). On CT, they are iso- or slightly hyperdense diffusely enhancing masses. The hyperdense appearance may prove a useful discriminatory feature. Calcification, haemorrhage and cysts are uncommon.

On MRI, they are round, nodular iso- or slightly hypointense on T1W (Fig. 3.59), slightly hyperintense on T2W and enhance with contrast. Tumour dissemination within the CSF may occur.

Langerhans cell histiocytosis

This is usually a multisystem disease, and isolated involvement of the CNS is rare. When CNS involvement occurs, granulomas form in the subarachnoid space and invade the hypothalamus. T1W gadolinium enhanced MRI is optimal in demonstrating the thickened enhancing infundibulum (Fig. 3.60), the most common neuroimaging finding. There is also loss of the hyperintense signal of the posterior pituitary when the patient develops diabetes insipidus. The imaging differential diagnosis of a thickened enhancing infundibulum would include germ cell tumours, lymphoma, leukaemia, tuberculosis, sarcoid, and lymphocytic hypophysitis. Other imaging features that would support the diagnosis of Langerhans cell histiocytosis rather than these others include enhancing masses involving the calvarium, orbit or skull base and areas of high signal on T2W MRI in the brainstem and cerebellum, reflecting probable myelin damage and gliosis (Fig. 3.61). The cause for these latter changes has yet to be elucidated.

Hamartoma tuber cinereum

This is a rare congenital mass lesion comprising heterotopic neuroepithelial tissue (neurons, astrocytes, oligodendrocytes) located usually in and attached to the tuber cinereum. They are usually well defined, non-invasive oval pedunculated masses, occasionally sessile, returning similar signal to grey matter on T1W and often on T2W sequences (Fig. 3.62). Sometimes, they return higher signal than grey matter on T2W scans (Boyko et al. 1991). They do not calcify nor enhance with contrast. Rarely they have been reported as cystic. Their morphology and the clinical presentation (precocious puberty, gelastic seizures, developmental delay) should facilitate the diagnosis, and on interval scanning they are non-progressive.

PINEAL TUMOURS

The pineal gland is found at the posterior aspect of the third ventricle within the quadrigeminal cistern, closely related to the tectal plate and aqueduct, the proximity of these structures explaining the presentation of pineal region tumours.

Pineal neoplasms are rare, constituting 1–3% of all intracranial neoplasms and 3–8% of intracranial tumours in children. Most common are germ cell tumours (choriocarcinoma, endodermal sinus tumour and embryonal cell carcinoma are all very rare), pineal region astrocytomas and pineal parenchymal tumours. Although the classical appearances are described below, in reality the radiological appearances lack specificity. In patients with tumours that do not secrete markers (AFP, bHCG, PLAP), biopsy is necessary for precise diagnosis and optimal management.

Germ cell tumours

• *Germinoma.* Germinomas comprise approximately two thirds of germ cell tumours, with a strong (10:1) male predominance. Most present between 10 and 30 years of age. They are generally midline tumours, the pineal and parasellar regions being the preferred locations. They are thought to arise from ectopic multipotential fragments of the embryonic primitive streak.

On imaging, germinomas are well defined, lobulated lesions, iso- or hyperdense on CT, with moderate to marked contrast enhancement. Although invasive, they generate little oedema. Calcification may be seen in 50%.

On MRI, they are also well defined, iso- or hypointense on T1W (Figs. 3.59, 3.63) and iso- or slightly hyperintense to normal brain on T2W, the latter reflecting the usually high nuclear cytoplasmic ration and decreased free water. There is marked contrast enhancement which is usually homogeneous except when foci of necrosis are present. CSF dissemination may occur (Fig. 3.64).

• *Teratoma*. Fifteen per cent of pineal tumours are teratomas, occurring most frequently in the first four years of life, almost exclusively in males. The tumour contains tissue from two or three of the three embryonic germ cell layers. Mature tumours contain fully differentiated tissues, whereas the more common immature tumours are composed of fetal appearing tissue.

On CT, they are well defined, non-invasive, heterogeneous, lobulated lesions with cysts, calcification, hair and fat. Although enhancement is not usually seen on CT, it may be seen on MRI.

Malignant lesions are infiltrative and generate surrounding oedema. Paradoxically, they are more homogeneous than their benign counterparts, with less tissue differentiation. They may enhance.

• *Pinealcytoma/blastoma*. Fifteen per cent of pineal based masses arise from pinealocytes and comprise a spectrum from well differentiated pinealocytomas to poorly differentiated pinealoblastomas.

Pinealocytomas are often very big, slow growing, unencapsulated but well defined and non-invasive lesions. On CT, they are iso- or hypodense masses with calcification within them, and only the occasionally hyperdense pinealocytoma may be seen. Heterogeneous contrast enhancement occurs in most cases. On MRI, they are hypo- or iso-intense on T1W and hyperintense on T2W with heterogeneous contrast enhancement.

Pinealoblastomas are malignant, rapidly disseminating PNETs. They tend to occur within the first decade of life. They may extend anteriorly into the 3rd ventricle, and frequently extend into the posterior fossa invading the vermis. On CT, they are dense, enhance, and may calcify. On MRI, they are generally iso- or hypointense on T1W and iso- or hyperintense on T2W (Fig. 3.65), may contain foci of necrosis, usually enhance, and may show CSF dissemination.

Pineal cysts

Normally the pineal gland appears as a 4 mm nodule but non-neoplastic cysts are found in approximately 40% of autopsies. Typically, they are asymptomatic and have thin, smooth walls (Fig. 3.66) with moderate enhancement, but nodular or irregular enhancement may also be seen reflecting enhancement of asymmetric normal pineal tissue. The cyst contents are iso- or hyperintense to CSF on T1W and T2W MRI. The hyperintense signal is due to high protein content and absence of cardiac pulsation. Very occasionally, cyst related haemorrhage has been reported. Differentiation from cystic pinealocytoma may be difficult by imaging (Engel et al. 2000), and wall thickness greater than 2 mm is suggestive (Engel et al. 2000).

SPINAL LEPTOMENINGEAL DISEASE

Leptomeningeal disease occurs in up to 32% of children with primary CNS tumours at diagnosis (Packer et al. 1985) and has been reported in virtually all types of CNS tumour, most often in embryonal tumours, medulloblastoma, PNET and malignant glioma. It implies a worse prognosis and requires more aggressive therapy.

MRI is currently the investigation of choice, and T1W gadolinium enhanced images (Fig. 3.67), which are more sensitive than T2W images, should be obtained preoperatively, optimally at the time of the diagnostic cranial study. Postoperatively, debris and blood in the CSF, subdural effusions and extradural haemorrhage (Fig. 3.68) may produce a confusing appearance and spinal MRI postoperatively may not be reliable for at least 2 weeks. Although larger deposits may be seen on T2W images, detection of small 1–2 mm nodules requires gadolinium enhancement. It was suggested that triple dose gadolinium may be more sensitive, but gadolinium only serves to increase the conspicuity of the venous plexus on the cord surface and enhances normal nerve roots resulting in false positives without an increase in sensitivity (Tam et al. 1996). The true sensitivity of MRI has not yet been determined and would obviously necessitate autopsy studies, but it is considered by most to be superior to CSF cytology and has been shown to be more sensitive than CT myelography (Kramer et al. 1991, Chamberlain et al. 1995, Heinz et al. 1995).

One study has suggested, however, that neither MRI nor CSF cytology is sufficient alone, and both may be necessary to maximize the potential identification of leptomeningeal disease (Fouladi et al. 1999). This group examined CSF samples 2–3 weeks post-surgery in 106 patients. If CSF alone had been relied upon, 14.4% of patients with leptomeningeal disease would have been missed, and with spinal MRI alone, 17.7% of patients would have been missed.

Unfortunately, CSF sampling does have drawbacks. Autopsy studies (in adults) have shown that 41% of patients with leptomeningeal disease had normal CSF cytology ante-mortem (Glass et al. 1979), and multiple CSF samples are required to increase sensitivity.

Additionally, it is not possible to sample CSF preoperatively with the risk of coning in the presence of a brain tumour. Intra-operatively and immediately postoperatively CSF cytology will be frequently positive because of tumour dispersal during handling (Batzdorf and Gold 1974), At operation, tumour cells are inevitably shed into the CSF, and these no not necessarily seed forming leptomeningeal deposits. The optimal time to sample CSF is reportedly 21 days postoperatively to avoid false positives from tumour handling at operation (Chang et al. 1969, Deutsch et al. 1985, Edwards et al. 1985).

Postoperative imaging

Postoperative MRI is recommended within 72 hours of surgery to evaluate residual disease (Fig. 3.69) and plan either further resection or adjuvant therapy, and should include T2W axial scans and T1W scans both pre- and post-gadolinium. The uncontrasted T1W images are important to delineate subacute haemorrhage in the form of methaemoglobin, which shows high signal on T1W images (Fig. 3.70).

Enhancement of granulation tissue at the operative site starts within 24 hours when it is smooth and thin. It then increases and becomes thicker and more nodular, hence scanning is recommended within 72 hours. The enhancing granulation tissue begins to diminish at about 6 weeks, with resolution at about 1 year. An increase after 8 weeks would suggest tumour progression and an increase after 4–6 months also would raise the possibility of radiation necrosis. MRS here might be helpful.

Normal dura lacks a blood–brain barrier but is relatively avascular, and normal findings post-craniotomy (or ventriculostomy or shunt insertion) commonly vary from no dural enhancement to smooth thin (up to 2 mm thick) linear enhancement (Fig. 3.70) either immediately at the operative site or diffusely over the convexities and tentorium. These may persist for 10–20 years (Hudgins et al. 1991). Conversely, leptomeningeal enhancement is always abnormal. Benign subdural effusions are also common after craniotomy (Fig. 3.70) and these may also demonstrate peripheral enhancement.

POSTOPERATIVE SURVEILLANCE IMAGING

The purpose of surveillance imaging is to detect tumour recurrence as early as possible, before it becomes symptomatic and when it is more amenable to treatment. To prove beneficial, surveillance imaging must detect tumour recurrence significantly earlier than clinical history or examination and there must be an effective treatment available once recurrence is detected. One would suspect that MRI would be more sensitive than CT but as yet this is unproven. The value of surveillance imaging has been discussed only in a few selected tumour types (Steinbok et al. 1996) and is recommended in children with 4th ventricular ependymoma, optic pathway/hypothalamic gliomas and supratentorial PNETs. The place of surveillance imaging is at present debatable for medulloblastomas (Steinbok et al. 1996, Bouffet et al. 1998, Roebuck et al. 2000, Minn et al. 2001, Yalcin et al. 2002). Imaging picks up only a small number of asymptomatic relapses, and there is no evidence of long-term benefit from treatment in relapsing patients. Its potential value may lie in the assessment of new treatment options.

As yet, there is no standard accepted surveillance protocol for tumours unless the children are enrolled in a specific study. Suggested approaches are, for high-grade gliomas, ependymomas and PNETs, to scan at 3, 6 and 12 months and yearly thereafter (Steinbok et al. 1996), and for low-grade gliomas, to scan at 3 and 12 months postoperatively, yearly thereafter for 5 years and then every 3–5 years.

For totally resected juvenile cerebellar astrocytoma, surveillance imaging does not appear to be beneficial because the completely resected tumour does not recur (Abdollahzadeh et al. 1994, Steinbok et al. 1996, Sutton et al. 1996). If postoperative imaging demonstrates residual tumour, there is a high likelihood of tumour progression requiring surgery, and either surveillance imaging or repeat surgery to achieve complete resection would be appropriate. Postoperative imaging may sometimes prove equivocal – small foci of enhancement may represent postoperative scar or tumour, haemorrhage into the tumour bed may obscure enhancing tumour, and non-enhancing portions of the tumour may be difficult to detect and may be suspected only by distortion of the 4th ventricle. In these, follow-up at 12, 18, 30, 42, 66 and 78 months is suggested (Sutton et al. 1996).

Surveillance imaging is also considered unnecessary for completely resected supratentorial ganglioglioma as recurrence would be unusual. Even with incomplete resection, surveillance imaging may not be appropriate because it is probable that a favourable outcome would result regardless of recurrent tumour size, and early detection when the tumour is asymptomatic may not necessarily improve outcome.

Iatrogenic problems

Complications relating to treatment have become important, the downside of prolonged survival as a result of advances in multidisciplinary treatment in children with brain tumours. Clinically, these manifest as cognitive problems, hypopituitary dysfunction and development of a second neoplasm.

Cerebral radiation changes may be acute, early, delayed or late (Valk and Dillon 1991). Acute injury occurs during treatment with transient worsening of symptoms without accompanying corresponding MRI changes (Jena et al. 1991). Early delayed changes seen up to 3 months after treatment may be manifest on imaging as areas of transient altered signal or density. Delayed radiation injury presents from a few months to 10 years or more later and is both progressive and irreversible. Fibrinoid necrosis of small arteries and arterioles is present with focal or diffuse white matter damage (Fig. 3.71). Focal radiation necrosis may be seen as an enhancing mass with oedema indistinguishable from tumour (Figs. 3.72, 3.73) on routine MRI. Diffuse white matter changes of variable extent (more extensive with whole brain rather than local radiotherapy) may also be seen, more reliably on MRI. Typically, the brainstem, cerebellum, internal capsule, basal ganglia and corpus callosum are spared (Tsuruda et al. 1987). Atrophy (with sulcal and ventricular enlargement), presumably related to the white matter damage, may also be present.

Parasellar radiation is known to induce a moya-moya like effect in children, and other radiation induced vasculopathies include the formation of telangectasias.

Mineralizing angiopathy with dystrophic calcification may be seen in nearly one third of children treated with intrathecal methotrexate and cranial irradiation or cranial irradiation alone (Davis et al. 1986). The calcification is seen in the basal ganglia and subcortical white matter (Figs. 3.74, 3.75) and there may be associated areas of white matter damage. Calcium is deposited in small blood vessels, which are surrounded by necrotic mineralized brain. It is uncertain as to whether these lesions produce symptoms.

Superficial siderosis can occur up to 22 years after successful excision of a brain tumour and is clinically manifest by slowly progressive neurological dysfunction (Anderson et al. 1999). Bilateral sensorineural hearing loss and cerebellar ataxia are the main clinical features but there is also cognitive impairment, dysarthria, nystagmus, visual loss radiculopathies, upper motor neuron signs and anosmia. It is caused by repeated subarachnoid bleeding, and CSF examination reveals red blood cells, high levels of iron and ferritin, high protein and a lymphocytic pleocytosis. Chronic exposure to haemoglobin and its breakdown deposits in the CSF results in accumulation of ferritin and haemosiderin in subpial microglia and cerebellar Bergmann glia accompanied by proliferation of microglia and astrocytes and axonal

103

spheroid swelling. The cerebellum, brainstem, vestibulocochlear nerves, spinal cord, spinal nerve roots, basal frontal lobes, olfactory bulbs and temporal cortex are the most severely affected. There is no effective treatment. The precise underlying cause is not usually identified, and angiography and technetium-labelled red blood cell scans rarely demonstrate a bleeding source. It has been suggested that radiotherapy may have a causative role in the formation of telangectasias and cavernous angiomas, or alternatively, the post-resection cavity may have multiple small bleeding sites.

With MRI, a hypointense rim of iron coating the cerebellum, brainstem, cranial nerves, optic chiasm and spinal cord is seen on T2W sequences (Fig. 3.76).

ACKNOWLEDGEMENT

I would like to thank the MR radiographers at Frenchay Hospital, not only for doing most of the scans but also for retrieving them from the many optical discs to enable my illustrations.

REFERENCES

Abdollahzadeh M, Hoffman HJ, Blazer SI, Becker LE, Humphreys RP, Drake JM, Rutka JT (1994) Benign cerebellar astrocytoma in childhood: experience at the Hospital for Sick Children 1980–1992. *Child's Nerv Syst* **10**: 380–383.

Anderson NE, Sheffield S, Hope JK (1999) Superficial siderosis of the central nervous system: a late complication of cerebellar tumors. *Neurology* **52**: 163–169.

Batzdorf U, Gold V (1974) Dispersion of central nervous system tumours. Correlation between clinical aspects and tissue culture studies. *J Neurosurg* **41**: 691–698.

Bouffet E, Doz F, Demaille MC (1998) Improving survival in recurrent medulloblastoma: earlier detection, better treatment or still an impasse? *Br J Cancer* **77**: 1321–1326.

Bowers DC, Georgiades C, Aronson LJ, Carson BS, Weingart JD, Wharam MD, Melhem ER, Burger PC, Cohen KJ (2000) Tectal gliomas: natural history of an indolent lesion in pediatric patients. *Pediatr Neurosurg* **32**: 24–29.

Boyko OB, Curnes JT, Oakes WJ, Burger PC (1991) Hamartomas of the tuber cinereum: CT, MR and pathologic findings. *AJNR* **12**: 309–314.

Bucciero A, De Caro M, De Stefano V, Tedeschi E, Monticelli A, Siciliano A, Cappabianca P, Vizioli L, Cerillo A (1997) Pleomorphic xanthoastrocytoma: clinical, imaging and pathological features of four cases. *Clin Neurol Neurosurg* **99**: 40–45.

Burtscher IM, Holtas S (1999) In vivo proton MR spectroscopy of untreated and treated brain abscesses. *AJNR* **20**: 1049–1053.

Byrd SE, Tomita T, Palka PS, Darling CF, Norfray JP, Fan J (1996) Magnetic resonance spectroscopy (MRS) in the evaluation of pediatric brain tumors. Part II: Clinical analysis. *J Nat Med Assoc* **88**: 717–723.

Byun WM, Kim OL, Kim DS (2000) MR imaging findings of Rathke's cleft cysts: significance of intracystic nodules. *AJNR* **21**: 485–488.

Castillo M, Green C, Kwock L, Smith K, Wilson D, Schiro S, Greenwood R (1995) Proton MR spectroscopy in patients with neurofibromatosis type 1: Evaluation of hamartomas and clinical correlation. *AJNR* **16**: 141–147.

Chamberlain MC (1995) Comparative spine imaging in leptomeningeal metasteses. *J Neurooncol* **23**: 233–238.

Chang CH, Housepian EM, Herbert C (1969) An operative staging system and a megavoltage radiotherapeutic technique for cerebellar medulloblastoma. *Radiology* **93**: 1351–1355.

Comi AM, Backstrom JW, Burger PC, Duffner PK (1998) Clinical and neuroradiological findings in infants with intracranial ependymomas. *Pediatr Neurol* **18**: 23–29.

Craver RD, Nadell J, Nelson JS (1999) Desmoplastic infantile ganglioglioma. *Pediatr Dev Pathol* **2**: 582–587.

Davis PC, Hoffman JC, Pearl GS, Braun IF (1986) CT evaluation of effects of cranial irradiation in children. *AJR* **147**: 587–592.

Deutsch M, Laurent JP, Cohan ME (1985) Myelography for staging medulloblastoma. *Cancer* **56**: 1763–1766.

Dev R, Gupta RK, Poptani H, Rog R, Sharma S, Husain M (1998) Role of in vivo proton magnetic resonance spectroscopy in the diagnosis and management of brain abscesses. *Neurosurgery* **42**: 37–43.

Edwards MS, Davis RL, Laurent JP (1985) Tumour markers and cytologic features of cerebrospinal fluid. *Cancer* **56**: 1773–1777.

Engel U, Gottschalk S, Niehaus L, Lehmann R, May C, Vogel S, Janisch W (2000) Cystic lesions of the pineal region – MRI and pathology. *Neuroradiology* **42**: 399–402.

Farmer J-P, Montes JL, Freeman CR (2001) Brainstem gliomas. *Pediatr Neurosurg* **34**: 206–214.

Fouladi M, Gajjar A, Boyett JM, Walter AW, Thompson SJ, Merchant TE, Jenkins JJ, Langston JW, Liu A, Kun LE, Heideman RL (1999) Comparison of CSF cytology and spinal magnetic resonance imaging in the detection of leptomeningeal disease in pediatric medulloblastoma or primitive neuroectodermal tumour. *J Clin Oncol* **17**: 3234–3237.

Girard N, Wang ZJ, Erbetta A, Sutton LN, Phillips PC, Rorke LB, Zimmerman RA (1998) Prognostic value of proton MR spectroscopy of cerebral hemisphere tumours in children. *Neuroradiology* **40**: 121–125.

Glass JP, Melamed M, Chernik NL, Posner JB (1979) Malignant cells in cerebrospinal fluid (CSF): the meaning of a positive CSF cytology. *Neurology* **29**: 1369–1375.

Gonen O, Zhiyue J, Wang A, Viswanathan K, Molloy PT, Zimmerman RA (1999) Three-dimensional multi-voxel spectroscopy of the brain in children with neurofibromatosis type 1. *AJNR* **20**: 1333–1341.

Griffiths, PD (1999) A protocol for imaging paediatric brain tumours. United Kingdom Children's Cancer Study Group and Societe Francaise d'Oncologie Pediatrique Panelists. *Clin Radiol* **54**: 558–562.

Heinz R, Wiener D, Friedman H, Tien R (1995) Detection of cerebrospinal fluid metastasis: CT myelography or MR? *AJNR* **16**: 1147–1151.

Hudgins PA, Davis PC, Hoffman JC (1991) Gadopentate dimeglumine-enhnaced MR imaging in children following surgery for brain tumour: spectrum of meningeal findings. *AJNR* **12**: 301–307.

Hwang J-H, Egnaczyk GF, Ballard E, Dunn RS, Holland SK, Ball WS (1998) Proton MR spectroscopic characteristics of pediatric pilocytic astrocytomas. *AJNR* **19**: 535–540

Ildan F, Tuna M, Gocer IA, Erman T, Cetinalp E (2001) Intracerebral ganglioglioma: clinical and radiological study of eleven surgically treated cases with follow up. *Neurosurg Rev* **24**: 114–118.

Jena A, Rath GK, Ravichandran R, Sahi UP, Khushu S (1991) Effects of radiation therapy on the normal human brain (white matter) visualized by MR imaging. *Magn Reson Imaging* **9**: 959–961.

Kleihues P, Burger PC, Scheithauer BW (1993) 'Histological typing of tumours of the central nervous system.' In: *WHO International Histological Classification of Tumours, 2nd edn*. Berlin: Springer, p. 15.

Kramer ED, Rafto S, Packer RJ, Zimmerman RA (1991) Comparison of myelography with CT follow-up versus gadolinium MRI for subarachnoid metastatic disease in children. *Neurology* **41**: 46–50.

Lefton DL, Pinto RS, Martin SW (1998) MRI features of intracranial and spinal ependymomas. *Pediatr Neurosurg* **28**: 97–105.

Levy RA, Blaivas M, Muraszko K, Robertson PL (1997) Desmoplastic medulloblastoma: MR findings. *AJNR* **18**: 1364–1366.

Mallucci C, Lellouch-Tubiana A, Salazar C, Cinalli G, Renier D, Sainte-Rose C, Pierre-Kahn A, Zerah M (2000) The management of desmoplastic neuroepithelial tumours in childhood. *Child's Nerv Syst* **16**: 8–14.

Matsumoto K, Tamiya T, Furuta OT, Asari S, Ohmoto T (1999) Cerebral gangliogliomas: clinical characteristics, CT and MRI. *Acta Neurochirur* **141**: 135–141.

McEvoy AW, Harding BN, Phipps KP, Ellison DW, Elsmore AJ, Thompson D, Harkness W, Hayward RD (2000) Management of choroid plexus tumours in children: 20 years experience at a single neurosurgical centre. *Pediatr Neurosurg* **32**: 192–199.

Minn AY, Pollock BH, Garzarella L, Dahl GV, Kun LE, Ducore JM, Shibita A, Kepner J, Fisher PG (2001) Surveillance neuroimaging to detect relapse in childhood brain tumors: a Pediatric Oncology Group study. *J Clin Oncol* **19**: 4135–4140.

Nishio S, Morioka T, Mihara F, Gondo K, Fukui M (2001) Cerebral ganglioglioma with epilepsy: neuroimaging features and treatment. *Neurosurg Rev* **24**: 14–19.

Ostertun B, Wolf HK, Campos MG (1996) Dysembryoplastic neuroepithelial tumours: MR and CT evaluation. *AJNR* **17**: 419–430.

Packer RJ, Siegel KR, Sutton LN, Litmann P, Bruce DA, Schut L (1985) Leptomeningeal dissemination of primary central nervous system tumors of childhood. *Ann Neurol* **18**: 217–221.

Perilongo G, Carollo C, Salvati L, Murgia A, Pillon M, Basso G, Gardiman M, Laverda A (1997) Diencephalic syndrome and disseminated juvenile pilocytic astrocytomas of the hypothalamic–optic chiasm region. *Cancer* **80**: 142–146.

Pierallini A, Bonamini M, Di Stefano D, Siciliano P, Bozzao L (1999) Pleomorphic xanthoastrocytoma with CT and MRI appearance of meningioma. *Neuroradiology* **41**: 30–34.

Raymond AA, Halpin SF, Alsanjari N, Cook MJ, Kitchen ND, Fish DR, Stevens JM, Harding BN, Scaravilli F, Kendall B, et al. (1994) Dysembryoplastic neuroepithelial tumour. Features in 16 patients. *Brain* **117**: 461–475.

Rizk T, Mottolese C, Bouffet E, Jouvet A, Guyotat J, Bret P, Lapras C (1996) Cerebral oligodendrogliomas in children: an analysis of 15 cases. *Child's Nerv Syst* **12**: 527–529.

Roebuck DJ, Villablanca JG, Nelson MD (2000) Surveillance imaging in children with medulloblastoma (posterior fossa PNET). *Pediatr Radiol* **30**: 447–450.

Sarkar C, Sharma MC, Shilesh G, Sharma C, Singh VP (1999) Choroid plexus papilloma: a clinicopathological study of 23 cases. *Surg Neurol* **52**: 37–39.

Selvapandian S, Rajshekar V, Chandy MJ (1999) Brainstem glioma: comparative study of clinico-radiological presentation, pathology and outcome in children and adults. *Acta Neurochir* **141**: 721–727.

Shankin WM (1949) On the presence of cysts in the human pituitary. *Anat Rec* **104**: 399–407.

Shaw EG, Scheithauer BW, Fallon JR, Tazelaar HD, Davis DH (1992) Oligidendrogliomas: the Mayo experience. *J Neurosurg* **76**: 428–434.

Sijens PE, van den Bent MJ, Nowak JCM, van Dijk P, Oudkerk M (1997) 1H chemical shift imaging reveals loss of brain tumor choline signal after administration of Gd-contrast. *Magn Reson Med* **37**: 222–225.

Steinbok P, Hentschel S, Cochrane DD, Kestle JRW (1996) Value of postoperative surveillance imaging in the management of children with some common brain tumours. *J Neurosurg* **84**: 726–732.

Sutton LN, Cnaan A, Klatt L, Zhao H, Zimmerman R, Needle M, Molloy P, Phillips P (1996) Postoperative surveillance imaging in children with cerebellar astrocytomas. *J Neurosurg* **84**: 721–725.

Tam JK, Bradley WG, Goergen SK, Chen DY, Pema PJ, Dubin MD, Teresi LM, Jordan JE (1996) Patterns of contrast enhancement in the pediatric spine at MR imaging with single- and triple-dose gadolinium. *Radiology* **198**: 273–278.

Tonn JC, Paulus W, Warmuth-Metz M, Schachenmayr W, Sorensen N, Roosen K (1997) Pleomorphic xantho-astrocytoma: report of six cases with special consideration of diagnostic and therapeutic pitfalls. *Surg Neurol* **47**: 162–169.

Tsuruda JS, Kortman KE, Bradley WG, Wheeler DC, Van Dalsem W, Bradley TP (1987) Radiation effects on cerebral white matter: MR evaluation. *AJR* **149**: 165–171.

Tzika AA, Vajapeyam S, Barnes PD (1997) Multivoxel proton MR spectroscopy and hemodymanic MR imaging of childhood brain tumours: preliminary observations. *AJNR* **18**: 203–218.

Valk PE, Dillon WP (1991) Radiation injury and the brain. *AJNR* **12**: 45–62.

Vinchon M, Soto-Ares G, Riffaud L, Ruchoux M-M, Dhellemmes P (2001) Supratentorial ependymoma in children. *Paediatr Neusosurg* **34**: 77–87.

Warren KE, Frank JA, Black JL, Hill RS, Duyn JH, Aikin AA, Lewis BK, Adamson PC, Balis FM (2000) Proton magnetic spectroscopic imaging in children with recurrent primary brain tumors. *J Clin Oncol* **18**: 1020–1026.

Yalcin B, Buyukpamukcu M, Akalan N, Cila A, Kutluk MT, Akyuz C (2002) Value of surveillance imaging in the management of medulloblastoma. *Med Pediatr Oncol* **38**: 91–97.

4
PATHOLOGY AND MOLECULAR ONCOLOGY OF CHILDHOOD CNS TUMOURS

Lucy B Rorke-Adams and Jaclyn A Biegel

The use of classical histological techniques remains the cornerstone for diagnosis of tumours regardless of their site of origin. However, use of ancillary diagnostic tools such as electron microscopy and immunohistochemistry has allowed greater understanding of their basic nature and led to more precise classification schemes. Studies of genetic footprints controlling their biology are now providing insight relative to the interrelationship of histologic, cytogenetic and prognostic features.

This chapter will focus upon histologic and cytogenetic features of CNS tumours in children and their relevance to prognosis. It is generally agreed that CNS tumours in children differ in many respects from those in adults, hence a modified classification is employed in the younger age group. The current classification scheme for childhood CNS tumours is provided in Table 4.1.

The a priori assumption that there are unique cytogenetic abnormalities for each histological type of tumour has not proven valid. For example, established histologic criteria are used to make a diagnosis of glioblastoma multiforme, but molecular genetic studies have demonstrated two subtypes, namely a de novo glioblastoma and a secondary glioblastoma. Although they are indistinguishable histologically, the genetic profiles are different (Kleihues et al. 2000).

Moreover, a molecular genetic study of tumours with mixed morphology, i.e. combined tumours, suggests that cells with different phenotypes within the same tumour share a similar genotype, although in a minority they differ (Huang et al. 2002). Whereas any histological type of CNS tumour can theoretically occur at any age, certain groups are more common in children than in adults, namely embryonal tumours, mixed neuronal–glial tumours, germ cell tumours, craniopharyngiomas, and specific subtypes of astrocytomas, such as pilocytic and desmoplastic.

Beyond histologic features per se, tumour location cannot be ignored, as the biology and hence prognosis are sometimes governed by site of origin of the neoplasm. This is particularly striking in the case of brainstem gliomas, which are primarily childhood tumours and most commonly arise in the pons. The majority of brainstem tumours at the outset are formed by histologically benign astrocytes. When located in the midbrain or medulla, they tend to be indolent growths and retain their original histological features for several years. Those in the pons, on the other hand, characteristically evolve into glioblastoma multiforme,

TABLE 4.1
Classification of brain tumours in children

I. Tumours of neuroepithelial tissues
  A. Glial tumours
    1. Astrocytic tumours
      a. Astrocytoma (fibrillary, protoplasmic,
         gemistocytic, pilocytic)
      b. Anaplastic astrocytoma
      c. Gigantocellular glioma
    2. Oligodendroglial tumours
      a. Oligodendroglioma
      b. Anaplastic oligodendroglioma
    3. Ependymal tumours
      a. Ependymoma
      b. Anaplastic ependymoma
      c. Myxopapillary ependymoma
    4. Choroid plexus tumours
      a. Papilloma
        i. Oncocytic papilloma
      b. Adenoma
      c. Carcinoma
    5. Mixed gliomas
      a. Oligoastrocytoma
        i. Anaplastic oligoastrocytoma
      b. Astroependymoma
        i. Anaplastic astroependymoma
      c. Oligoastroependymoma
        i. Anaplastic oligoastroependymoma
      d. Oligoependymoma
        i. Anaplastic oligoependymoma
      e. Subependymoma – subependymal glomerate
         astrocytoma
      f. Gliofibroma
    6. Glioblastomatous tumours
      a. Glioblastoma multiforme
      b. Giant cell glioblastoma
      c. Gliosarcoma
    7. Gliomatosis cerebri
  B. Neuronal tumours
    1. Gangliocytoma
      a. Anaplastic gangliocytoma
      b. Cerebellar gangliocytoma –
         Lhermitte–Duclos
    2. Central neurocytoma
  C. Mixed neuronal–glial tumours
    1. Ganglioglioma
      a. Anaplastic ganglioglioma
      b. Dysembryoplastic neuroepithelial tumour
         (DNET)
    2. Desmoplastic astrocytoma/ganglioglioma
    3. Pleomorphic xanthoastrocytoma
    4. Subependymal giant cell tumour
  D. Embryonal tumours
    1. Medulloepithelioma
    2. Primitive neuroectodermal tumours (PNET)
      a. Medulloblastoma
    3. Atypical teratoid/rhabdoid tumour
  E. Pineal cell tumours
    1. PNET (pineoblastoma)
    2. Pineocytoma

II. Tumours of meningeal and related tissues
  A. Meningiomas
    1. Meningioma, not otherwise specified (NOS)

    2. Papillary meningioma
    3. Anaplastic meningioma
  B. Meningeal sarcomatous tumours
    1. Meningeal sarcoma, NOS
    2. Rhabdomyosarcoma or leiomyosarcoma
    3. Fibrosarcoma
    4. Others
  C. Primary melanocytic tumours
    1. Malignant melanoma
    2. Melanomatosis
    3. Melanocytic tumours, miscellaneous

III. Tumours of nerve sheath cells
  A. Schwannoma
  B. Neurofibroma
  C. Perineurinoma
  D. Malignant peripheral nerve sheath tumour
     (MPNST)

IV. Primary tumours of the haematopoietic system
  A. Malignant lymphoma
  B. Histiocytic tumours

V. Vascular tumours
  A. Haemangioblastoma
  B. Haemangiopericytoma
  C. Epithelial haemangioendothelioma

VI. Germ cell tumours
  A. Germinoma
  B. Embryonal carcinoma
  C. Choriocarcinoma
  D. Endodermal sinus tumours
  E. Teratomatous tumours
    1. Immature teratoma
    2. Mature teratoma
    3. Teratocarcinoma
  F. Mixed

VII. Malformative tumours
  A. Craniopharyngioma
  B. Rathke's cleft cyst
  C. Epidermal cyst
  D. Dermoid cyst
  E. Colloid cyst of third ventricle
  F. Enterogenous or bronchial cyst
  G. Cyst, NOS
  H. Lipoma
  I. Granular cell tumour (choristoma)
  J. Hamartoma
    1. Neuronal
    2. Glial
    3. Neuronoglial
    4. Meningioangioneurinomatosis

VIII. Tumours of neuroendocrine origin
  A. Tumours of anterior pituitary
    1. Adenoma
    2. Carcinoma
  B. Paraganglioma

IX. **Local extension from regional tumours**
  Type to be specified according to primary
  diagnosis

X. **Metastatic tumours**

XI. **Unclassified tumours**

TABLE 4.2

Types of neuroepithelial tumours diagnosed in children 0–18 years of age at the Children's Hospital of Philadelphia, 1979–2002 (N=1195)

Histologic type	N	%
Gliomas	718	59.3
Astrocytoma		
Fibrillary, NOS	260	(36.2)
Pilocytic	194	(27.0)
Anaplastic/glioblastoma	81	(11.6)
Gliomatosis cerebri	14	(1.9)
Mixed glioma	34	(4.7)
Ependymoma	81	(11.6)
Choroid plexus papilloma/carcinoma	40	(5.5)
Oligodendroglioma	14	(1.9)
Gangion cell tumours	193	16.1
Ganglioglioma/DNET	152	(78.2)
Subependymal giant cell tumour	21	(10.8)
Dural astrocytoma/ganglioglioma	13	(6.7)
Pleomorphic xanthoastrocytoma	7	(3.6)
Embryonal tumours	277	23.2
PNET	232	(83.7)
Atypical teratoid/rhabdoid tumour	36	(13.0)
Medulloepithelioma	9	(3.2)
Pineocytoma	7	0.5

Abbreviations: NOS = not otherwise specified; DNET = dysembryoplastic neuroepithelial tumour; PNET = primitive neuroepithelial tumour.

usually within two years after onset of clinical symptoms. Why neoplastic astrocytes in the pons are biologically different from those in other brainstem levels remains an intriguing question for oncologists. It is therefore important to include site of origin of the tumour, along with the histological diagnosis when diagnosing CNS tumours in children, a practice recommended by Rorke et al. (1985).

As an indication of the relative frequency of occurrence of the differing types of childhood CNS tumour, a survey of 1436 CNS tumours in children from 0 to 18 years of age who were treated at The Children's Hospital of Philadelphia from 1979 to 2002 is presented. The survey revealed that approximately 80% of tumours were of neuroepithelial origin, whereas the remainder consisted of a heterogeneous group including craniopharyngiomas, germ cell tumours, meningiomas, pituitary tumours, etc. (Tables 4.2, 4.3). This information will be used to underpin the clinicopathological descriptions of the individual tumour types below. The histologic and cytogenetic features of the large group of neuroepithelial tumours will be presented first, followed by a brief discussion of the smaller group of common non-neuroepithelial tumours.

As noted above the application of immunohistochemical techniques utilizing selected antibodies has led to a better understanding and a more precise classification of nervous system tumours. Most commonly utilized are glial fibrillate acidic protein (GFAP) which is expressed by astrocytes, ependymal cells, and occasionally by oligodendrocytes and

TABLE 4.3
Types of non-neuroepithelial tumours diagnosed in children 0–18 years of age at the Children's Hospital of Philadelphia, 1979–2002 (N=241)

Histologic type	N	%
Craniopharyngiomas	75	31.1
Germ cell tumours	55	22.8
Meningiomas	29	12.0
Cysts	21	8.7
Pituitary tumours	14	5.8
Lymphomas	10	4.1
Hamartomas	9	3.7
Sarcomas	8	3.3
Meningo-encephalo-angio-neurinomatosis (MEAN)	7	2.4
Vascular	4	1.6
Other	9	3.7

choroid plexus epithelium, and neurofilament protein (NFP), the intermediate filament of neurons. Vimentin, the most primitive intermediate filament, is also commonly used and is especially helpful in diagnosing meningiomas, atypical teratoid/rhabdoid tumours (AT/RTs), desmoplastic tumours of various types and subependymal giant cell tumours.

Other commonly used antibodies include epithelial membrane antigen (EMA), smooth muscle actin (SMA), keratin and desmin. A variety of markers are applied to tissues thought to belong to the group of germ cell tumours such as human chorionic gonadotropin (HCG), placental alkaline phosphatase (PLAP) and alpha fetoprotein (AFP).

Neuroepithelial tumours
Neuroepithelial tumours may be divided into four major diagnostic groups, the most common being gliomas (almost 60%), and the rarest, pineal parenchymal tumours (less than 1%). The glioma group contains four general types, although astrocytomas are further divided into four subcategories, and choroid plexus tumours are here considered a subtype of ependymoma, although this is not strictly true.

GLIOMAS
Conspicuous by their absence in this classification scheme of astrocytic tumours is subependymal giant cell tumours, typically found in individuals with tuberous sclerosis, and pleomorphic xanthoastrocytoma. It is currently more appropriate to include them with the mixed glial–neuronal group, for several reasons. Studies of subependymal giant cell tumours for antigen expression and at the ultrastructural level have demonstrated little or no evidence of an astrocytic component in many of them. Rather, the predominant intermediate filament in these tumours is vimentin. Cells exhibiting ganglion cell features, both ultrastructurally and by expression of NFP, are frequently found (Nakamura and Becker 1983, Lantos et al. 1996, Lopes et al. 1996). On the other hand, expression of GFAP is common in pleomorphic xanthoastrocytomas, but a proportion also have a ganglion cell component (Powell et al. 1996, Perry et al. 1997).

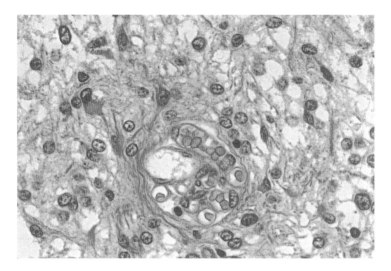

Fig. 4.1. Pilocytic astrocytoma showing fibre-forming astrocytes around a vascular wickerwork and adjacent microcystic field. Haematoxylin–eosin, ×400.

Astrocytomas

Astrocytomas are separated into four histological subtypes, namely fibrillary (47.3%), pilocytic (35.3%), anaplastic/glioblastoma (14.7%) and gliomatosis cerebri (2.5%). Most common is the fibrillary type; although included in this group are a few gigantocellular astrocytomas. Thirty-seven per cent originate in the cerebrum, whereas an equal number (21.5% each) are found in the cerebellum and brainstem. However, the figure for the brainstem is spuriously low, given that tumours in the pons, in particular, are currently rarely biopsied. Other common sites are the spinal cord (8.8%) and optic nerve (7.7%). Basically, these are infiltrating tumours composed of a population of generally small, pleomorphic, fibre-forming astrocytes. They may contain granular bodies and Rosenthal fibres. These cells typically express GFAP and often vimentin as well.

Slightly over one-third of astrocytic tumours display the unique histological features that define the pilocytic type. This consists of a biphasic pattern in which the fibre-forming astrocytes that make up the tumour are arranged in a dense meshwork around blood vessels, alternating with fields in which the delicate cellular processes form a 'chicken-wire' pattern (Fig. 4.1). Granular bodies and/or Rosenthal fibres may be prominent but are not always present. Nuclei are typically mature, but in some may be pleomorphic and hyperchromatic. In the absence of mitoses this is not a feature of concern. Occasionally, there is striking nuclear clustering. These tumours often contain unusual vessels that have been described as 'wicker-works' (Sato and Rorke 1990). They may contain one or more cysts, evidence of haemorrhage, and growth in the subarachnoid space, a feature not generally associated with a poor prognosis. The majority of pilocytic astrocytomas arise in the cerebellum (70%), while the hypothalamic/chiasmatic region accounts for 15%, and 10% arise in the cerebrum. They are rare in the optic nerve (2.5%) and spinal cord (1%).

Histological features of anaplastic astrocytomas/glioblastomas differ in no way from those in adults. These are densely cellular growths composed of pleomorphic glial cells with anaplastic nuclei, a variable number of mitotic figures, neovascularization and necrosis. This is of the pseudo-palisading type in the glioblastomas, which also contain multinucleated giant cells and bizarre nuclei.

Malignant astrocytic tumours are relatively uncommon in children; they make up 11.6% of the astrocytoma group, but comprise only 6.7% of the entire group of neuroepithelial tumours. Three-quarters arise in the cerebrum, the remainder occurring in other sites, such as the cerebellum (12.3%) and spinal cord (5.0%). Five of 81 tumours in this group were found in two sites, namely brainstem/cerebrum, brainstem/cerebellum, and pineal/cerebrum.

The entity known as gliomatosis cerebri is a rare neoplasm consisting of a widespread, diffuse growth of small, apparently mature astrocytes, which generally do not display anaplastic features or mitotic activity. Although the majority are located in the cerebrum, they may also involve cerebellum, brainstem, and/or spinal cord. Rarely, the primary site is the cerebellum.

Histological features of these tumours are unique, as they are characterized by a diffuse growth of generally smaller than normal astrocytes that may simply appear as bare nuclei or may have a small perikaryon with or without delicate short processes. Rarely, the glial cells resemble oligodendroglia. In the cortex the tumour cells are often arranged around neurons (satellitosis) or blood vessels, similar to Scherer's secondary structures (Scherer 1940). Somewhere in this diffuse growth there may be a focus of more obviously anaplastic tumour. All 14 tumours of this type in this group were located in the cerebrum, five of which primarily involved the thalamus and basal ganglia bilaterally.

Cytogenetic studies of pilocytic astrocytomas have revealed normal karyotypes. A variety of numerical abnormalities have been reported in small series of fibrillary astrocytomas, including trisomy 5, 6, 7, 8, 11 and/or 12. TP53 mutations are not seen (Biegel et al. 1999). Genetic alterations in anaplastic astrocytomas are similar to those found in adult malignant astrocytomas. Cytogenetic studies have demonstrated trisomy 7, as well as alterations of 1, 6, 9, 10, 17 and the sex chromosomes. Loss of 17p with mutation of TP53 is present in approximately 35% of anaplastic astrocytomas, although the frequency is lower in patients who are less than 3 years of age at diagnosis (Raffel et al. 1999, Pollack et al. 2002). Alterations identified by comparative genomic hybridization (CGH) include gain of 1q, which may be associated with a worse prognosis (Rickert et al. 2001b), as well as gain of 5q, and loss of 6q, 9q, 12q and 22q.

The karyotypic findings for paediatric glioblastoma are similar to those found for adult glioblastoma, and include trisomy 7, loss of 9p, 10q, 17, 22, and X and Y. Double minute chromosomes reflective of epidermal growth factor receptor (EGFR) amplification are much less common in childhood tumours compared to those in adults. Overexpression of EGFR, however, appears to be a consistent finding in paediatric malignant astrocytomas (Bredel et al. 1999), and may represent a biologic target for therapy. Overexpression and/or mutation of TP53 are present in approximately 30–50% of paediatric glioblastomas, and may be associated with decreased survival compared with patients who have tumours with normal TP53 (Pollack et al. 2002). High proliferation index, as assessed by MIB1 labelling,

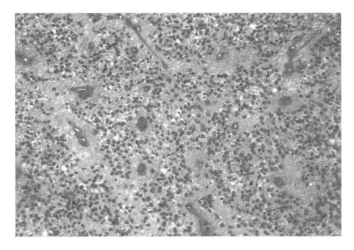

Fig. 4.2. A field containing typical pseudo-rosettes in ependymoma. Haematoxylin–eosin, ×250.

high expression of basic fibroblast growth factor (Pollack et al. 2002), and loss of 10q with mutation of the PTEN gene (Raffel et al. 1999) also appear to be associated with a worse outcome for children with malignant gliomas. Loss of 9p21 and the cell cycle regulatory genes CDKN2A/ARF are seen more commonly in glioblastoma, as compared to anaplastic astrocytoma, although there is no independent association with prognosis (Raffel et al. 1999).

Mixed gliomas
Almost 5% of glial tumours are composed of a mixed population of glial cells: astrocytes–oligodendroglia (15/34), astrocytes–ependymal cells (15/34), astrocytes–oligodendrocytes–ganglion cells (3/34), astrocytes–oligodendrocytes–ependymal cells–ganglion cells (1/34); two were gliofibromas. These tumours are located almost equally in the cerebrum (12/34) and cerebellum (11/34); one-quarter are ventricular.

The histological features of mixed gliomas are obviously a function of the cell types forming them. Whereas the 34 tumours in this group were histologically benign, they may certainly be anaplastic. The rare gliofibromas are different from superficial desmoplastic astrocytoma/ganglioglioma, as they can occur anywhere, are not typically associated with a cyst, and tend to occur in children older than 2 years.

Ependymomas
Almost 12% of glial tumours are ependymomas. Slightly greater than half (54%) arise within the fourth ventricle, whereas 30% are supratentorial and 17% are spinal. The majority (83%) are histologically benign. However, there is little relationship between histological features and the biology of this tumour (Barker et al. 1999). About two-thirds display characteristic pseudo-rosettes with intervening sheets of cells with round to oval, mature nuclei that may display considerable mitotic activity (Fig. 4.2). Necrosis, haemorrhage and

113

neovascularization are common, and calcific deposits or even frank bone formation may be seen.

Aside from those ependymomas comprised of frankly anaplastic cells, the other histologic types consist of myxopapillary, papillary and clear cell forms. A small number (6.2%) are formed by a combination of ependymal and astrocytic cells in a pattern characteristic of what is traditionally called a subependymoma. Strictly speaking, this is a mixed glial tumour and should more correctly be classified in the mixed glioma group.

Monosomy or deletion of chromosome 22 is the most frequent finding in ependymoma (for a review, see Hamilton and Pollack 1997), and is preferentially observed in adult spinal cord tumours and intracranial neoplasms in children. Mutation of the NF2 gene, which maps to 22q12, is rare in sporadic childhood tumours (Slavc et al. 1995). Furthermore, although loss of alleles in the region that contains the hSNF5/INI1 locus is commonly seen in paediatric ependymomas, mutations of the INI1 gene have not been identified (Kraus et al. 2001). Thus, a novel tumour suppresser gene must be involved in the development or progression of paediatric ependymoma.

In addition to loss of chromosome 22, common genetic changes in primary paediatric ependymomas include loss of chromosome 6 (Kramer et al. 1998) and gain of the long arm of chromosome 1 (Hirose et al. 2001, Ward et al. 2001). Deletions of chromosome band 13q14 and 17 have also been noted, although mutations in the tumour suppresser retinoblastoma gene (RB-1) in 13q14 or TP53 gene are extremely rare. The lack of these abnormalities, in particular, suggests that the genetic basis for ependymoma is distinct from astrocytic neoplasms, which are frequently associated with loss and mutation of the RB-1 or TP53 genes.

Choroid plexus tumours
Choroid plexus tumours are basically childhood lesions. They are generally divided into two major groups – papillomas and carcinomas. However, a small number are more accurately regarded as adenomas, while a few choroid plexus lesions are simply cysts.

Forty of the 718 glial tumours (5.5%) fell into this category. Twenty-nine of these were simple papillomas, and there were equal numbers (4/40) of carcinomas and adenomas, one of which was an oncocytoma. Three of the forty plexus lesions were cysts. The majority of these tumours arose in the lateral ventricles or third ventricle (27/40 and 5/40 respectively). Seven were located in the fourth ventricle, and one remarkable tumour arose in the spinal cord.

Histological features of papillomas are relatively straightforward. The tumour cells are typically cuboid and rest on a basement membrane below which the papillary core is composed of a delicate fibrovascular stroma. Nuclei are round and exhibit a speckled chromatin pattern. Mitoses are uncommon. These cells typically express keratin, less often EMA, and uncommonly GFAP. Some histologically benign tumours have an inconspicuous papillary configuration but are more solid glandular growths resembling adenomas arising in other types of epithelial tissues. Rarely, the tumour cells display features of oncocytes. These are cells with prominent eosinophilic cytoplasm and a central nucleus. At the ultrastructural level the perikaryon is filled with mitochondria.

The plexus carcinomas are characterized by a cell population in which there is obvious pleomorphism and nuclear anaplasia. Papillary features are obscured, and the cells grow in a haphazard, sheet-like arrangement. Mitotic activity is usually striking, and foci of necrosis, with or without haemorrhage, may be seen. The transformed cells may lose their ability to express antigen.

Little is known about the genetics of choroid plexus tumours, and much of the recent data has been generated through chromosomal genomic hybridization analysis (CGH). Karyotypes from choroid plexus papillomas are either normal or demonstrate a non-random pattern of trisomies, including extra copies of chromosomes 7, 12 and 20, especially in atypical cases (Bhattacharjee et al. 1997). Grill et al. (2002) confirmed the gain of chromosomes 7 and 12 in choroid plexus papillomas using CGH. Rickert et al. (2002) analysed a series of 14 paediatric choroid plexus carcinomas using CGH. Common gains included chromosomes 1, 4q, 10, 14q, 20q and 21q. The tumours had frequent losses of 5q, 9p, 11, 15q, and 18q. Deletion of 22q was noted in 10/14 cases.

The loss of 22q in choroid plexus carcinomas raised the possibility that mutations of the INI1 gene might contribute to their development. Although mutations of INI1 in a small number of choroid plexus carcinomas have been reported (Sevenet et al. 1999), the possibility exists that these tumours may be AT/RTs that were misclassified. Further studies of a larger number of choroid plexus carcinomas are required to determine if INI1 mutations are specific for AT/RT.

A viral aetiology for choroid plexus tumours has been suggested by the finding of SV40 sequences in primary choroid plexus tumours (Bergsagel et al. 1992). However, this continues to be debated, based on conflicting reports from a variety of investigators who have not ruled out contamination with the reagents used for study. Choroid plexus tumours may be seen in the setting of Li–Fraumeni syndrome. Such patients have germline mutations in the TP53 gene. Deletions of 17p and TP53 mutations are uncommon in sporadic choroid plexus tumours.

Oligodendroglioma
Oligodendrogliomas are rare childhood tumours comprising 1% of the group of neuroepithelial tumours and 2% of the gliomas. Almost three-quarters of them arise in the cerebrum, and about two-thirds are histologically benign.

Histological features are relatively easy to recognize, although some may offer challenges to the diagnostician. The tumour cells tend to grow in sheets separated into poorly defined lobules by compressed, linear capillaries with delicate walls and flattened endothelial cells. Nuclei are small and round and have a variable complement of chromatin, although it is typically dense. The perikaryon is usually 'empty', but cell borders are distinct, hence the cell assumes the typical 'fried egg' look. On the other hand, the neoplastic cells may have a pink, homogeneous cytoplasm and a small plump cell body that is generally described as a minigemistocyte.

The malignant forms display a disordered architecture, pleomorphism with nuclear anaplasia, mitotic activity and neovascularization, with or without necrosis.

Adult oligodendrogliomas are often characterized by deletions of the short arm of

115

chromosome 1 and the long arm of chromosome 19, which appear to be associated with improved responsiveness to specific chemotherapeutic approaches (Cairncross et al. 1998). A study of pediatric oligodendrogliomas by Raghavan et al. (2003) found that alterations on 1p or 19q are infrequent in children, and are virtually absent in children whose tumours present during the first decade of life. This suggests that different genetic pathways are involved in the pathogenesis of pediatric oligodendrogliomas.

GANGLION CELL TUMOURS

These tumours, almost entirely composed of neurons, are uncommon and, although they tend to occur in children and young adults, only one was found among the group of 1195 neuroepithelial tumours seen at the Children's Hospital over a 23 year period.

There are two major types in this category, namely gangliocytomas and neurocytomas. Both are largely composed of cells committed to a neuronal phenotype, although they may contain a variable glial population. The cells forming the gangliocytoma are medium to large and have a plump cell body, a round nucleus and a prominent nucleolus; they basically look like ganglion cells. Both histologically benign and anaplastic forms exist.

The rare cerebellar gangliocytoma or Lhermitte–Duclos disease is a peculiar lesion that more correctly belongs in the category of a cortical dysplasia or malformation (primarily of granular neurons) but which may behave clinically as a space occupying lesion.

In contrast to the gangliocytomas, the central neurocytoma is composed of cells with little or no resemblance to neurons at the light microscopic level. In fact, for many years these tumours were placed in the oligodendroglioma category. Ultrastructural study unmasked their true nature, and immunohistochemical techniques, utilizing neuronal markers, simplified the diagnostic problem (Hassoun et al. 1982, Hassoun et al. 1993).

In addition to individuals with Cowden syndrome, germline mutation of the PTEN gene in 10q23 has been described in at least one patient with apparently sporadic Lhermitte–Duclos disease (Iida et al. 1998).

MIXED NEURONAL–GLIAL TUMOURS

These tumours, composed of a mixture of neurons and glial cells, are relatively common in children and comprise 16% of all neuroepithelial tumours.

Ganglioglioma/dysembryoplastic neuroepithelial tumour (DNET)

Three-quarters of the neuronal–glial tumours fall into this category, 85% of which are found in the cerebrum, the temporal lobe being the favoured site. They may be associated with cortical dysplasia, and many behave more like hamartomas than neoplasms. This is especially characteristic of the lesions that have been separated into a subgroup of ganglioglioma, namely the dysembryoplastic neuroepithelial tumours (DNETs) (Daumas-Duport et al. 1988). On the other hand, about 10% of gangliogliomas may undergo anaplastic transformation, usually of the glial component, although the ganglion cells may rarely be targets of this change.

Like the majority of gliomas, these are poorly defined tumours that infiltrate and replace the normal architecture in which they arise. The most common type of glial cell forming

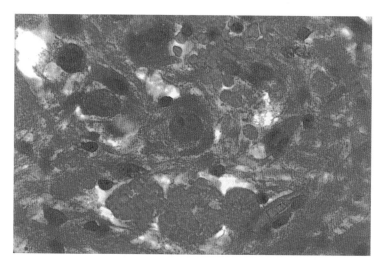

Fig. 4.3. Large neoplastic ganglion cells in cerebral ganglioglioma. Haematoxylin–eosin, ×400.

this tumour is fibre-forming astrocytes. The ganglion cells are randomly distributed and may be more abundant in some regions than in others. They may exhibit morphological abnormalities, most easily identified with an NFP preparation, but only rarely do they have more than one nucleus (Fig. 4.3). If these tumours involve cortex or a deep nucleus it may be difficult to determine whether the neurons are residual or neoplastic. The distinction may be especially difficult, as cortical neurons may undergo grotesque morphological changes in the presence of an infiltrating neoplasm. Gangliogliomas often contain abundant thin-walled vessels that may bleed slowly or massively; calcification is common.

The DNETs exhibit a unique histology. They tend to be demarcated intracortical lesions that expand the cortical ribbon. They have a loose, hypocellular, microcystic character. The predominant cell has a small, round nucleus with relatively dense chromatin and an appearance not unlike an oligodendrocyte. Small astrocytes with or without processes are often present, and the ganglion cells are randomly distributed within this network, often appearing like a bug caught in a web. Use of antibodies for GFAP and NFP are helpful in defining the feature of these tumours.

Cytogenetic studies of ganglioglioma have been limited. A recent study using CGH (Yin et al. 2002) demonstrated loss of 9p and trisomy 7 in a small series of cases. Platten et al. (1997) suggested that a variant splice site polymorphism in the tuberous sclerosis 2 gene might predispose to sporadic ganglioglioma.

Subependymal giant cell tumours
As noted above, these tumours have traditionally been classified as a subtype of astrocytoma, but the pattern of antigen expression and ultrastructural features clearly establish them as mixed neuronal–glial neoplasms. In fact, some of them exhibit little or no evidence of glial differentiation (Fig. 4.4). They comprise almost 11% of the mixed ganglion cell tumours.

117

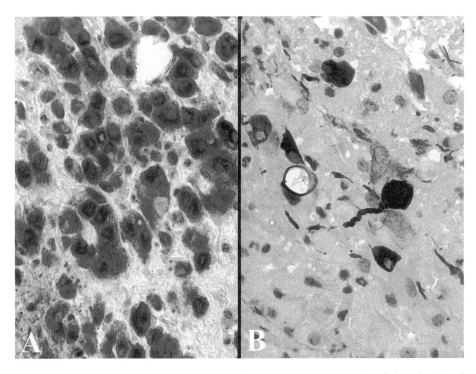

Fig. 4.4. Giant cells in subependymal giant cell tumour ,showing strong expression of vimentin (A) and of neurofilament protein (B). Immunoperoxidase preparations, ×400.

All are located in the region of the foramina of Monro. They are firm, nodular masses that may contain cysts, calcific deposits or, in some circumstances, haemorrhage.

The tumour cells are medium to large. Nuclei are mildly pleomorphic and often contain a nucleolus, and may be globular or spindle-shaped. The cell body has a finely granular homogeneous character, mitotic figures are rare, and anaplastic transformation does not occur. They rarely contain a vascular malformation, which may bleed (Ecklund et al. 1993) (Fig. 4.4).

Dural astrocytoma/ganglioglioma
Evolution of these tumours as an entity dates back to 1945, when Bailey and Ingraham reported a rare dural lesion of childhood, which they called a fibrosarcoma, but which did not behave aggressively. Taratuto et al. (1984) studied a group of these tumours and found that many of the cells expressed GFAP; they called them 'desmoplastic infantile astrocytomas'. Three years later, VandenBerg et al. (1987) described a similar tumour that contained a neuronal component, calling that tumour 'desmoplastic infantile ganglioglioma'. These two tumour types are now regarded as variations of a single entity. They characteristically have a large cystic component, arise in infants 2 years of age or less, and, if completely removed, do not recur. They consist of an intermixture of astrocytes and mesenchymal cells with or without

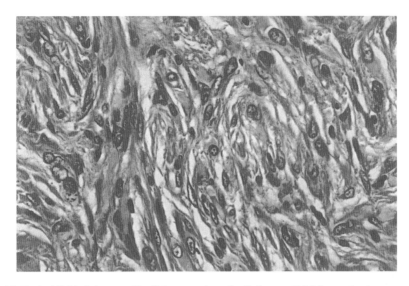

Fig. 4.5. Typical field of pleomorphic glial–mesenchymal cells in superficial desmoplastic astrocytoma. Haematoxylin–eosin, ×400.

ganglion cells; they may contain nests of poorly differentiated neuroepithelial cells, which, if present, do not carry an ominous prognosis (Fig. 4.5). They typically express GFAP and vimentin, plus or minus NFP. On the other hand, when tumours with these histological features (but generally not associated with a cyst) occur in older children, they tend to pursue a more aggressive course.

Pleomorphic xanthoastrocytoma
This tumour, initially defined as a unique entity by Kepes et al. (1979), is usually classified as a subtype of astrocytoma; however, as noted above, many contain ganglion cells, so it seems more correct to regard them as mixed neuronal–glial tumours.

These tend to be superficially located primarily in the cerebrum, and may also have a cystic component. As the name implies, the cells are pleomorphic, many being large with irregular cell borders and bizarre single or multiple nuclei, despite which the tumour does not ordinarily behave in an aggressive manner. Cytoplasm of a variable number of cells is vacuolated (representing fat removed in processing). A connective tissue component and infiltrates of mononuclear cells are common features. The neuronal population is most easily identifiable by use of antibodies for NFP. Many cells express GFAP and there is usually abundant reticulin.

Single case reports of pleomorphic xanthoastrocytoma have not yet revealed any specific genetic alterations. Kaulich et al. (2002) examined a large series of 62 tumours for abnormalities of CDKN2A, CDK4, MDM2, TP53 and EGFR. Only three tumours had a mutation of TP53, whereas the other genes did not appear to be altered. These studies suggest a mechanism of tumour development distinct from other mixed glial–neuronal tumours.

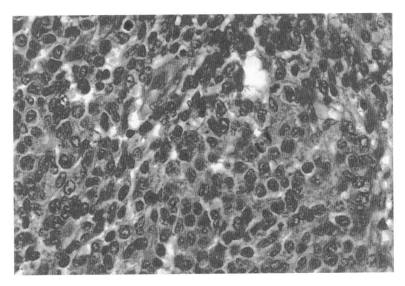

Fig. 4.6. Primitive neuroectodermal tumour–medulloblastoma composed of poorly differentiated neuroepithelial cells. Haematoxylin–eosin, ×400.

EMBRYONAL TUMOURS

Tumours composed of primitive neuroepithelial cells are largely found in infants and children, and comprise almost one-quarter of the primary CNS neoplasms. There are three major subtypes, namely PNET (83.7%), AT/RT (13%) and medulloepithelioma (3.2%).

Primitive neuroectodermal tumour (PNET)

This is the most common type of embryonal tumour. Eighty per cent are located in the cerebellum, in which site they are called medulloblastomas (MBs). An almost equal number arise in the pineal (8.6%), where they are known as pineoblastomas, and cerebrum (8.1%). The remainder are located in the cerebellopontine angle, suprasellar region, brainstem and spinal cord.

PNETs, regardless of where they arise in the CNS, are basically phenotypically similar, with the exception of the desmoplastic subtype, which occurs only in the cerebellum. The genotypes, on the other hand, differ depending upon whether they arise in the cerebellum or cerebrum.

Although many PNETs are composed of a monotonous population of small, closely packed cells with basophilic round nuclei that have little surrounding cytoplasm, the histological features may be quite variable (Fig. 4.6).

Rosettes of the Homer Wright variety are sometimes found, or the tumours rarely contain ependymal canals. A subgroup that only occurs in the cerebellum is the desmoplastic type, which contains nodules of more loosely arranged cells in a background of neuropil and with a surrounding network of reticulin. A second nodular pattern is characteristic of some PNETs that exhibit advanced neuronal differentiation, a type sometimes referred to as 'cerebellar neuroblastoma.' Tumour cells in both histological subtypes of PNET-MBs may form linear arrays. In the desmoplastic variety, the neoplastic cells form along a delicate connective tissue process, whereas those in the neuroblastic tumours look like migrating post-mitotic neuronal precursors within a neuropil-type background.

A small number of these tumours are composed of bizarre large cells, some of which may have more than one nucleus. They may also contain nucleoli. These are called large cell medulloblastomas and are associated with a grim prognosis (Giangaspero et al. 1992).

Utilization of a panel of monoclonal antibodies often indicates differentiation along neuronal, or less often glial, lines. Much less frequently, the cells may express desmin, keratin or retinal S antigen. Studies have indicated dual or triple expression in some of these tumour cells (Gould et al. 1990, Molenaar and Trojanowski 1994).

The most common molecular genetic alteration in PNET-MB is an isochromosome 17q (Biegel et al. 1989). The deletion of 17p that arises as a result is present in approximately 40% of tumours. TP53 mutations are extremely rare. In addition to the isochromosome 17q, trisomy 7, loss of an X or Y chromosome, and deletions of 9, 10, 11 and 16 are common. Structural abnormalities of chromosome 1 are frequent but nonspecific. Deletion of 9q may be accompanied by mutations of the PTCH gene, seen most often in the desmoplastic subtype of PNET (Raffel et al. 1997). The SUFU gene that maps to 10q24 is mutated in the germline and somatic tissues of patients with medulloblastoma, further implicating the sonic hedgehog-patched pathway in the development of a subset of tumours (Taylor et al. 2002).

The expression of several developmentally related and oncogenic proteins has been used to identify prognostic factors for children with medulloblastoma. High expression of MYCC (Grotzer et al. 2001) and erbB-2 (Gilbertson et al. 1995) appears to be associated with a poor prognosis, whereas high expression of TrkC predicts a favourable outcome (Segal et al. 1994, Grotzer et al. 2000). Microarray analysis of a large series of pediatric brain tumours has shown that expression profiles may be used to distinguish specific subsets of malignant brain tumours, such as medulloblastoma, PNET and AT/RT (Pomeroy et al. 2002). Furthermore, a novel multigene predictor model was superior to clinical parameters, including presence of metastatic disease, in predicting outcome for children with medulloblastoma. Gene expression profiling has also implicated the PDGFR alpha and Ras-MAP kinase pathways in metastatic disease (MacDonald et al. 2001).

Cytogenetic studies of supratentorial PNETs have demonstrated a variety of abnormalities. The presence of an isochromosome 17q has been noted in only a few tumours. Deletion of chromosome 22 and mutation analysis of INI1 are used to distinguish PNET from AT/RT (Rorke et al. 1996, Biegel et al. 1999). Comparative genomic hybridization was employed to compare the chromosomal gains and losses in a series of infratentorial and supratentorial PNETs (Russo et al. 1999). Isochromosome 17q, and deletions of 9, 10, 11, 16 and the sex chromosomes were common in the infratentorial tumours, whereas supratentorial PNETs had losses of 4q, 9, 13q, 14q, 18q and 19q.

Atypical teratoid/rhabdoid tumour (AT/RT)
This embryonal tumour was separated from the general group of PNETs less than 10 years

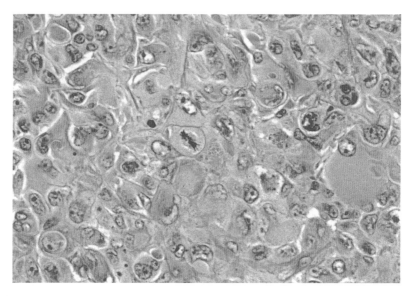

Fig. 4.7. Field of rhabdoid cells in cerebral atypical teratoid/rhabdoid tumour. Note large cell body, eccentrically placed nucleus and prominent nucleolus. Haematoxylin–eosin, ×400.

ago (Rorke et al. 1996). It had been included with PNET-MBs as about 65% of them contain fields of primitive neuroepithelial cells. However, it was recognized that they also contained a population of rhabdoid cells similar to those found in renal rhabdoid tumours of infants. Thirteen per cent of the embryonal tumours are of this type.

In contrast to the PNET-MBs, only about one-third are found within cerebellar parenchyma. One-quarter are located in the cerebrum, one-fifth in the cerebello-pontine angle, and 14% in the pineal. The majority occur in infants 2 years of age or less, and prognosis for these patients is poor.

The histological features of these tumours are complex. They most frequently consist of fields resembling PNET while other areas are composed of rhabdoid cells. These are larger than the embryonic neuroepithelial cells, have a plump cell body, and an eccentrically placed nucleus with a prominent nucleolus (Fig. 4.7). In addition, there may be an epithelial component, glandular or squamous, and/or fields of neoplastic mesenchymal tissue. Necrosis and mitotic activity are typically striking. These tumours commonly express a variety of antigens, the most frequent being EMA, vimentin and smooth muscle actin (SMA). They may also express keratin, NFP and GFAP.

AT/RT is characterized by deletion of one or both copies of the hSNF/INI1 gene in chromosome band 22q11.2 (Biegel et al. 1999). The remaining allele contains a coding sequence mutation, or another inactivating alteration that results in loss of expression at the RNA and protein level (Biegel et al. 2000). The INI1 gene functions as a classic tumour suppressor gene such that germline mutations predispose infants to the development of brain, renal and/or extrarenal rhabdoid tumours.

Medulloepithelioma

Medulloepitheliomas are the most infrequent type of embryonal tumour, comprising only 3.2% of the total of 277. Like the AT/RTs, they are also most common in infants 2 years of age or less. The three sites of origin among this group were cerebrum (4/9), cerebellum (2/9) and pons (2/9).

This tumour primarily consists of tubular structures that resemble the primitive neural tube (Karch and Urich 1972). There is both an internal and an external limiting membrane, although the latter is not always distinct. Cells forming the tubes are pseudostratified, and mitotic activity is typical near the luminal border. Intervening tissues contain neurons and glia exhibiting varying degrees of maturity, best recognized with NFP and GFAP antibodies. Rarely, mesenchymal components are also present (Auer and Becker 1983). Cells forming the tubular structures typically express vimentin (Caccamo et al. 1989).

PINEAL TUMOURS

Traditionally, pineal parenchymal tumours have been separated into two major groups, namely pineocytoma and pineoblastoma. In view of the fact that pineoblastomas are phenotypically similar to PNETs, they more appropriately belong in that diagnostic niche.

Pineocytomas are rare; only seven were found among the 1195 childhood neuroepithelial tumours diagnosed at The Children's Hospital of Philadelphia during a 23 year period.

Diagnosis may be difficult, especially if the biopsy is small, as these tumours look like the pineal itself. A histological variant described by Trojanowski et al. (1982) exhibits a papillary architecture (Vaquero et al. 1990). These neoplastic cells express NFP and retinal S antigen. Fleurettes are rare among this group but are occasionally found in the PNET–pineo-blastoma group.

There is very little known regarding the genetics of pineoblastoma. Deletion of chromo-some band 22q11.2 and mutation analysis of the INI1 rhabdoid tumour gene are helpful in distinguishing supratentorial PNETs, including pineoblastoma, from AT/RT.

Comparative genomic hybridization analysis of a small number of pineal tumours demonstrated a variety of abnormalities in pineoblastomas, compared to balanced genomes in pineocytomas (Rickert et al. 2001a).

Non-neuroepithelial tumours

Tumours originating from tissues within the cranium and spinal cord are considerably less common in children than the primary neuroepithelial tumours. They made up 16.7% of the total (241/1436) and consisted of a wide variety of lesions (see Table 4.2). Only the three most common types will be mentioned, namely craniopharyngiomas (31.1%), germ cell tumours (22.8%) and meningiomas (12.0%).

CRANIOPHARYNGIOMA

Although these tumours are presumed to arise from residual embryonic epithelium of Rathke's pouch, they rarely present before 3 years of age (3/75); the youngest patient in this group was 13 months old. They arise in the region of the sella and produce symptoms consequent to compression of adjacent structures, most importantly, the optic chiasm,

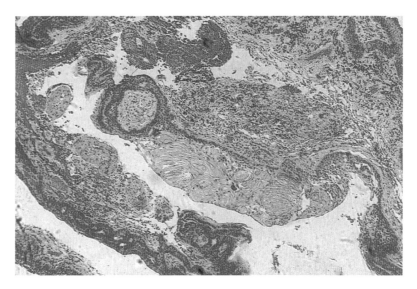

Fig. 4.8. Typical field of craniopharyngioma showing bands of epithelium, keratin and inflammatory cells. Haematoxylin–eosin, ×250.

posterior pituitary and hypothalamus. Although for practical purposes these are histologically benign tumours, they produce considerable morbidity because of their location.

Two histological subtypes have been described, adamantinomatous and papillary, the former being more common in children. The squamous epithelium is arranged in strands and cords and produces keratin, which often undergoes calcification. Cells may be loosely arranged, and inflammation, with or without giant cells and cholesterol clefts, may be seen (Fig. 4.8).

GERM CELL TUMOURS

These tumours arise in the supratentorial space, most commonly in the pineal (56.3%) or the sellar/suprasellar regions (25.4%). There is a striking preponderance in boys (2.6:1).

In general, the diverse histological types that occur in reproductive organs are also found in the intracranial cavity; over half (56.3%) are germinomas. Malignant teratomas are next in frequency (14.5%), followed by embryonal carcinoma (10.9%).

Gain of the X chromosome is the most common alteration in intracranial germ cell tumours, regardless of the histologic subtype (Okada et al. 2002). Isochromosome 12p, a frequent structural abnormality in testicular germ tumours, is seen infrequently in CNS germ cell tumours (Rickert et al. 2000). Gain of whole chromosome 12, structural abnormalities of chromosome 1, and loss of 13q are also seen less frequently in CNS, as compared to testicular or mediastinal, germ cell tumours. Loss of CKDN2A or 9p21 is rare.

MENINGIOMA

Whereas meningiomas are among the most common CNS tumours in adults, they comprise only 2% of the entire group in children. The majority arise somewhere in the intracranial cavity (21/29); 6/29 were found in the optic canal; and only 2/29 arise in the spinal region. The majority are histologically benign (27/29). Moreover, histological features are basically similar to those that occur in older individuals. Although histologically benign, these tumours may recur and produce significant morbidity.

Although meningioma is rare in children, the cytogenetic abnormalities among the pediatric tumours are similar to those reported in their adult counterparts (for a review, see Zang 2001). Monosomy 22 or deletion of the long arm of chromosome 22 is the most common alteration. Deletion of the short arm of chromosome 1 is the most common secondary cytogenetic change in meningioma. A non-random pattern of chromosome loss involves monosomy 14, 6, 18, 10, and X or Y. Similar losses are seen in the childhood meningiomas, although the pediatric cases may present initially with more complex karyotypes, frequently involving structural changes of chromosomes 1, 6 and 14. Meningiomas seen in association with NF2 have mutations of the NF2 gene in chromosome 22q12, although these are rare in sporadic tumours. At present, there are no new candidate tumour suppressor genes for meningioma.

REFERENCES

Auer RM, Becker LE (1983) Cerebral medulloepithelioma with bone, cartilage and striated muscle. Light microscopic and immunohistochemical study. *J Neuropathol Exp Neurol* **42**: 256–267.

Bailey OT, Ingraham FD (1945) Intracranial fibrosarcoma of the dura mater in childhood: pathological characteristics and surgical management. *J Neurosurg* **2**: 1–15.

Barker FG, Huhn SL, Prados MD (1999) Clinical characteristics of long-term glioma survivors. In: Berger MS, Wilson CB, eds. *The Gliomas*. Philadelphia: WB Saunders, pp. 718–179.

Bergsagel DJ, Finegold MJ, Butel JS, Kupsky WJ, Garcea RL (1992) DNA sequences similar to those of simian virus 40 in ependymomas and choroid plexus tumors of childhood. *N Engl J Med* **326**: 988–993.

Bhattacharjee MB, Armstrong DD, Vogel H, Cooley LD (1997) Cytogenetic analysis of 120 primary pediatric brain tumors and literature review. *Cancer Genet Cytogenet* **97**: 39–53.

Biegel JA (1999) Cytogenetics and molecular genetics of childhood brain tumors. *Neuro-Oncology* **1**: 139–151.

Biegel JA, Rorke LB, Packer RJ, Sutton LN, Schut L, Bonner K, Emanuel BS (1989) Isochromosome 17q in primitive neuroectodermal tumors of the central nervous system. *Genes Chrom Cancer* **1**: 139–147.

Biegel JA, Zhou JY, Rorke LB, Stenstrom C, Wainwright LM, Fogelgren B (1999) Germ-line and acquired mutations of INI1 in atypical teratoid and rhabdoid tumors. *Cancer Res* **59**: 74–79.

Biegel JA, Tan L, Zhang F, Wainwright L, Russo P, Rorke LB (2002) Alterations of the hSNF5/INI1 gene in central nervous system atypical teratoid/rhabdoid tumors and renal and extrarenal rhabdoid tumors. *Clin Cancer Res* **8**: 3461–3467.

Bredel M, Pollack IF, Hamilton RI, James CD (1999) Epidermal growth factor receptor expression and gene amplification in high-grade non-brainstem gliomas of childhood. *Clin Cancer Res* **7**: 1786–1792.

Caccamo DV, Herman MM, Rubinstein LJ (1989) An immunohistochemical study of the primitive and maturing elements of human cerebral medulloepithelioma. *Acta Neuropathol* **79**: 248–254.

Daumas-Duport C, Scheithauer BW, Chodkiewicz JP, Laws ER, Vedrenne C (1988) Dysembryoplastic neuroepithelial tumor: a surgically curable tumor of young patients with intractable partial seizures. Report of thirty-nine cases. *Neurosurgery* **23**: 545–556.

Ecklund J, Schut L, Rorke L (1993) Associated vascular malformations and neoplasms in children. *Pediatr Neurosurg* **19**: 196–201.

Giangaspero F, Rigobello L, Badioli M, Loda M, Andreini L, Basso G, Zorzi F, Montaldi A (1992) Large cell medulloblastoma. A distinct variant with highly aggressive behavior. *Am J Surg Pathol* **16**: 687–693.

Gilbertson RJ, Pearson AD, Perry RH, Jaros E, Kelly PJ (1995) Prognostic significance of the c-erB-2 oncogene product in childhood medulloblastoma. *Brit J Cancer* **71**: 473–477.

Gould VE, Jansson DS, Molenaar WM, Rorke LB, Trojanowski JQ, Lee VM, Packer RJ, Franke WW (1990)

Primitive neuroectodermal tumor of the central nervous system. Patterns of expression of neuroendocrine markers, and all classes of intermediate filament protein. *Lab Invest* **62**: 498–509.

Grill J, Avet-Loiseau H, Lellouch-Tubiana A, Sevenet N, Terrier-Lacombe M-J, Venuat A-M, Doz F, Sainte-Rose C, Kalifa C, Vassal G (2002) Comparative genomic hybridization detects specific cytogenetic abnormalities in pediatric ependymomas and choroid plexus papillomas. *Cancer Genet Cytogenet* **136**: 121–125.

Grotzer MA, Janss AJ, Fung K, Biegel JA, Sutton LN, Rorke LB, Zhao H, Cnaan A, Phillips PC, Lee VM, Trojanowski JQ (2000) TrkC expression predicts good clinical outcome in primitive neuroectodermal brain tumors. *J Clin Oncol* **5**: 1027–1035.

Grotzer MA, Hogarty MD, Janss AJ, Liu X, Zhao H, Eggert A, Sutton LN, Rorke LB, Brodeur GM, Phillips PC (2001) MYC messenger RNA expression predicts survival outcome in childhood primitive neuroectodermal tumor/medulloblastoma. *Clin Cancer Res* **7**: 2425–2433.

Hamilton RL, Pollack IF (1997) The molecular biology of ependymomas. *Brain Pathol* **7**: 807–822.

Hassoun J, Giambarelli D, Grisoli F, Pellet W, Salamon G, Pellisier JF, Toga M (1982) Central neurocytoma. An electron microscopic study of two cases. *Acta Neuropathol* **56**: 151–156.

Hassoun J, Soylemezoglu F, Gambarelli D, Figarella B, von Ammon K, Kleihues P (1993) Central neurocytoma: a synopsis of clinical and histological features. *Brain Pathol* **3**: 297–306.

Hirose T, Aldape K, Bollen A, James CD, Brat D, Lamborn K, Berger M, Feuerstein BG (2001) Chromosomal abnormalities subdivide ependymal tumors into clinically relevant groups. *Am J Pathol* **158**: 1137–1143.

Huang J, Behrens C, Wistuba II, Gazdar AF, Jagirdar J (2002) Clonality of combined tumors. A molecular genetic study. *Arch Pathol Lab Med* **126**: 437–441.

Iida S, Tanaka Y, Fujii H, Hayashi S, Kimura M, Nagareda T, Moriwaki K (1998) A heterozygous flameshift mutation of the PTEN/MMAC1 gene in a patient with Lhermitte–Duclos disease – only the mutated allele was expressed in the cerebellar tumor. *Int J Molec Med* **6**: 925–929.

Karch SB, Urich H (1972) Medulloblastoma: definition of an entity. *J Neuropathol Exp Neurol* **31**: 27–53.

Kaulich K, Blaschke B, Numann A, von Deimling A, Wiestler OD, Weber RG, Reifenberger G (2002) Genetic alterations commonly found in diffusely infiltrating gliomas are rare or absent pleomorphic xanthoastrocytomas. *J Neuropathol Exp Neurol* **12**: 1092–1099.

Kepes JJ, Rubinstein LJ, Eng LF (1979) Pleomorphic xanthoastrocytoma: a distinct meningocerebral glioma of young subjects with relatively favorable prognosis: a study of 12 cases. *Cancer* **44**: 1839–1852.

Kleihues P, Burger PC, Collins VP, Newcomb EW, Ohzaki H, Cavenee WK (2000) Glioblastoma. In: Kleihues P, Cavanee WK, eds. *Pathology and Genetics. Tumors of the Nervous System*. Lyon: IARC Press, pp. 36–38.

Kramer DL, Parmiter AH, Rorke LB, Sutton LN, Biegel JA (1998) Molecular cytogenetic studies of pediatric ependymomas. *J Neuro-Oncol* **37**: 25–33.

Kraus JA, de Millas W. Sorensen N, Herbold C, Scichor C, Tonn JC, Wiestler OT, von Deimling A, Pietsch T (2001) Indications for a tumor suppressor gene at 22q11 involved in the pathogenesis of ependymal tumors and distinct from hSNF5/INI1. *Acta Neuropathol* **102**: 69–74.

Lantos PL, VandenBerg SH, Kleihues P (1996) Tumors of the nervous system. In: Graham DI, Lantos PL, eds. *Greenfield's Neuropathology. 6th edn.* London: Arnold, pp. 583–879.

Lopes MBS, Altermatt HJ, Scheithauer BW, VandenBerg SR (1996) Immunohistochemical characterization of subependymal giant cell astrocytoma. *Acta Neuropathol* **91**: 368–375.

MacDonald TJ, Brown KM, LaFleur B, Peterson K, Lawlor C, Chen Y, Packer RJ, Cogen P, Stephen DA (2001) Expression profiling of medulloblastoma: PDGFRA and the RAS/MAPK pathway as therapeutic targets for metastatic disease. *Nat Genet* **29**: 143–152.

Molenaar WM, Trojanowski JQ (1994) Primitive neuroectodermal tumors of the central nervous system in childhood: tumor biological aspects. *Crit Rev Oncol Hematol* **17**: 1–25.

Nakamura Y, Becker LE (1983) Subependymal giant cell tumor: Astrocytic or neuronal? *Acta Neuropathol* **60**: 270–277.

Okada Y, Nishikawa R, Matsutani M, Louis DN (2002) Hypomethylated X chromosome gain and rare isochromosome 12p in diverse intracranial germ cell tumors. *J Neuropathol Exp Neurol* **61**: 531–538.

Perry A, Giannini C, Scheithauer BW, Rojiani AM, Yachnis AT, Seo IS, Johnson P, Kho J, Shapiro S (1997) Composite pleomorphic xanthoastrocytoma and ganglioglioma: report of four cases and review of the literature. *Am J Surg Pathol* **21**: 763–771.

Platten M, Meyer-Puttlitz B, Blumcke I, Waha A, Wolf HK, Nothen MM, Louis DN, Sampson JR, von Deimling A (1997) A novel splice site associated polymorphism in the tuberous sclerosis 2 (TSC2) gene may predispose to the development of sporadic gangliogliomas. *J Neuropathol Exp Neurol* **56**: 806–810.

Pollack IF, Biegel JA, Yates AJ, Hamilton RL, Finkelstein SD (2002) Risk assignment in childhood brain tumors: The emerging role of molecular and biological classification. *Curr Biol Rep* **4**: 114–122.

Pomeroy SK, Tamayo P, Gaasenbeek M, Sturla LM, Angelo M, McLaughlin ME, Kim JY, Goumnerova LC, Black PM, Lau C, Allen JC, Zagzag D, Olson JM, Curran T, Wetmore C, Biegel JA, Poggio T, Mukherjee S, Rifkin R, Califano A, Stolovitzky G, Louis DN, Mesirov JP, Lander ES, Golub TR (2002) Prediction of central nervous system embryonal tumor outcome based on gene expression. *Nature* **415**: 436–442.

Powell SZ, Yachnis AT, Rorke LB, Rojiani AM, Eskin TA (1996) Divergent differentiation in pleomorphic xanthoastrocytoma. Evidence for a neuronal element and possible relationship to ganglion cell tumors. *Am J Surg Pathol* **20**: 80–85.

Raffel C, Jenkins RB, Frederick L, Hebrink D, Alderete B, Fults DW, James CD (1997) Sporadic medulloblastomas contain PTCH mutations. *Cancer Res* **57**: 842–845.

Raffel C, Frederick L, O'Fallon JR, Atherton-Skaff P, Perry A, Jenkins RB, James CD (1999) Analysis of oncogene and tumor suppressor gene alterations in pediatric malignant astrocytomas reveals reduced survival for patients with PTEN mutations. *Clin Cancer Res* **5**: 4085–4090.

Raghavan R, Balani J, Perry A, Margraf L, Vono M, Cai DX, Wyatt RE, Rushing EJ, Bowen DC, Hyman LS, White CL (2003) Pediatric oligodendrogliomas: A study of molecular alterations on 1p and 19q using fluorescence in situ hybridization. *J Neuropath Exp Neurol* **62**: 530–537.

Rickert CH, Simon R, Bergmann M, Dockhorn-Dworniczak B, Paulus W (2000) Comparative genomic hybridization in pineal germ cell tumors. *J Neuropathol Exp Neurol* **59**: 815–821.

Rickert CH, Simon R, Bergmann M, Dockhorn-Dworniczak B, Paulus W (2001a) Comparative genomic hybridization in pineal parenchymal tumors. *Genes Chromosomes Cancer* **30**: 99–104.

Rickert CH, Strater R, Kaatsch P, Wassmann H, Jurgens H, Dockhorn-Dworniczak B, Paulus W (2001b) Pediatric high-grade astrocytomas show chromosomal imbalances distinct from adult cases. *Am J Pathol* **158**: 1525–1532.

Rickert CH, Wiestler OT, Paulus W (2002) Chromosomal imbalances in choroid plexus tumors. *Am J Pathol* **160**: 1105–1113.

Rorke LB, Gilles FH, Davis RL, Becker LE (1985) Revision of the World Health Organization classification of brain tumors for childhood brain tumors. *Cancer* **56** (Suppl.): 1869–1886.

Rorke LB, Packer RJ, Biegel JA (1996) Central nervous system atypical teratoid/rhabdoid tumors of infancy and childhood: definition of an entity. *J Neurosurg* **85**: 56–65.

Russo C, Pellarin M, Tingby O, Bollen AW, Lamborn KR, Mohapatra G, Collins VP, Feuerstein BG (1999) Comparative genomic hybridization in patients with supratentorial and infratentorial primitive neuroectodermal tumors. *Cancer* **86**: 331–339.

Sato K, Rorke LB (1990) Vascular bundles and wickerworks in childhood brain tumors. *Pediatr Neurosci* **73**: 710–714.

Scherer HJ (1940) The forms of growth in gliomas and their practical significance. *Brain* **63**: 1–35.

Segal RA, Goumnerova LC, Kwon YK, Stiles CD, Pomeroy SL (1994) Expression of the neurotrophin receptor TrkC is linked to a favorable outcome in medulloblastoma. *Proc Natl Acad Sci USA* **91**: 12867–12871.

Sevenet N, Lellouch-Tubiana A, Schofield D, Hoang-Xuan K, Gessler M, Birnbaum D, Jeanpierre C, Jouvet A, Delattre O (1999) Spectrum of hSNF5/INI1 somatic mutations in cancer and genotype–phenotype correlations. *Hum Molec Genet* **8**: 2359–2368.

Slavc I, MacCollin MM, Dunn M, Jones S, Sutton L, Gusella JF, Biegel JA (1995) Exon scanning for mutations of the NF2 gene in pediatric ependymomas, rhabdoid tumors and meningiomas. *Int J Cancer* **64**: 243–247.

Taratuto AL, Menges J, Lylyk P, Leiguarda R (1984) Superficial cerebral astrocytoma attached to the dura. Report of six cases in infants. *Cancer* **54**: 2505–2512.

Taylor MD, Liu L, Raffel C, Hui C-C, Mainprize TG, Zhang X, Agatep R, Chiappa S, Gao L, Lowrance A, Hao A, Goldstein AM, Stavrou T, Scherer SW, Dura WT, Wainwright B, Squire JA, Rutka JT, Hogg D (2002) Mutations in SUFU predispose to medulloblastoma. *Nature Genet* **31**: 306–310.

Trojanowski JQ, Tascos NA, Rorke LB (1982) Malignant pineocytoma. Case report. *J Neurosurg* **73**: 135–137.

VandenBerg SR, May EE, Rubinstein LJ, Herman MM, Perenbes E, Vinores SA, Collins VP, Park TS (1987) Desmoplastic supratentorial neuroepithelial tumors of infancy with divergent differentiation potential ("desmoplastic infantile gangliogliomas"). Report of 11 cases of a distinctive embryonal tumor with favorable prognosis. *J Neurosurg* **66**: 58–71.

Vaquero J, Coca S, Martinez R, Escandon J (1990) Papillary pineocytoma. Case report. *J Neurosurg* **73**: 135–137.

Versteege I, Sevenet N, Lange J, Rousseau-Merck M-F, Ambros P, Handgretinger R, Aurias A, Delattre O (1998) Truncating mutations of Hsnf5/INI1 in aggressive paediatric cancer. *Nature* **394**: 203–206.

Ward S, Harding B, Wilkins P, Harkness W, Hayward R, Darling JL, Thomas DGT, Warr T (2001) Gain of 1q and loss of 22 are the most common changes detected by comparative genomic hybridization in paediatric ependymoma. *Genes Chromosome Cancer* **32**: 59–66.

Yin X-L, Hui B-Y, Pang JC-S, Poon WB, Ng H-K (2002) Genome-wide survey for chromosomal imbalances in ganglioglioma using comparative genomic hybridization. *Cancer Genet Cytogenet* **134**: 71–76.

Zang KD (2001) Meningioma: a cytogenetic model of a complex benign human tumor, including data on 394 karyotyped cases. *Cytogenet Cell Genet* **93**: 207–220.

5
MOLECULAR APPROACHES TO THE UNDERSTANDING AND TREATMENT OF CHILDHOOD CNS TUMOURS

Richard J Gilbertson

A complete and accurate diagnosis is crucial for the optimum management of cancer. Without this, it is impossible for clinicians to inform patients of disease prognosis, instigate appropriate therapy or accurately assess the efficacy of new treatments. The contemporary classification of tumours derived from cells of the central nervous system (CNS) is largely based on morphological and immunohistochemical criteria (Kleihues et al. 2002). While this approach has proven useful for guiding the treatment and predicting the prognosis of certain childhood brain tumours, it lacks the precision required for accurately managing many of these diseases. A poor understanding of the molecular abnormalities that are causative in childhood brain tumours has compounded this situation and hindered the development of new treatments. Consequently, the outlook for children with brain tumours has remained largely unchanged in recent years (Legler et al. 1999). In contrast, considerably more is known regarding the molecular genetics of adult cancers, including CNS tumours; this knowledge is now leading to the development of molecular based disease staging systems and treatments (Cairncross et al. 1998, Ichimura et al. 2000, Takeshima et al. 2000, Holland 2001, Cavenee 2002, Zhu and Parada 2002). Further, large government supported initiatives are underway in the USA that are aiming to provide a comprehensive map of the molecular alterations in adult glioma (http://home.ccr.cancer.gov/nob/mds/research.asp). This chapter will review recent advances in molecular biology and discuss how these approaches are being applied to the study and clinical management of childhood CNS tumours.

Advances in molecular biology techniques
The development of cancer is a multistep process in which diseased cells acquire a series of genetic insults that disrupt normal proliferation, apoptosis, angiogenesis and migration (Hanahan and Weinberg 2000, Vogelstein and Kinzler 2004). These abnormalities impact the function of oncogenes, tumour suppressor genes and stability genes (Vogelstein and Kinzler 2004). Knowledge of the sequence of the human genome (Lander et al. 2001) and genome-wide approaches for studying tumour cytogenetics (see below) are being used to identify further cancer genes (Futreal et al. 2001).

The structure and expression of oncogenes, tumour suppressor genes and stability genes within cancer cells can be altered by structural abnormalities in the DNA sequence or

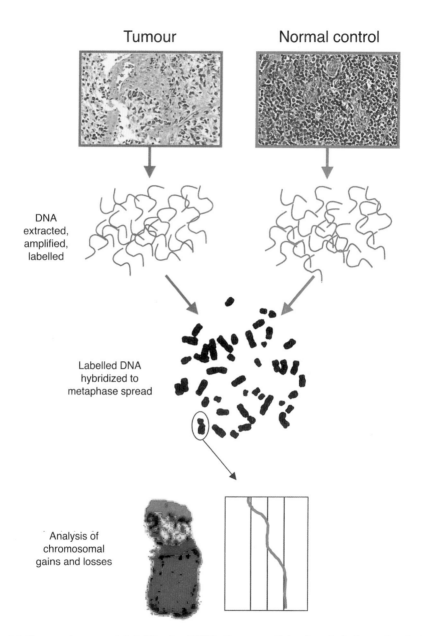

Tumour

Normal control

DNA extracted, amplified, labelled

Labelled DNA hybridized to metaphase spread

Analysis of chromosomal gains and losses

Fig. 5.1. Comparative genomic hybridization (CGH). Cartoon outlining the principal steps involved in CGH analysis of tumour DNA. Equal amounts of DNA extracted from tumour and normal control tissue are amplified and differentially labeled with green and red fluorochromes, respectively, and then hybridized in a competitive manner to preparations of normal metaphase chromosomes. Array CGH involves a similar procedure, although the labeled DNA sequences are hybridized to BAC arrays. Areas on each chromosome that are greener than average exist as extra copies in the tumour sample, while more red areas highlight regions of loss. Representative analysis of one chromosome is depicted at the bottom of the figure and illustrates loss of the short arm and gain of the long arm.

130

through epigenetic changes, e.g. methylation (Jones and Takai 2001, Smiraglia and Plass 2002, Zardo et al. 2002). A variety of cytogenetic tools capable of characterizing chromosomal alterations in detail are now available (Trask 2002). A full discussion of these methodologies is beyond the scope of this chapter. However, a number of recent advances and their application to the investigation of paediatric brain tumours will be discussed.

GLOBAL ANALYSES OF THE STRUCTURE AND EXPRESSION OF THE CANCER GENOME
The most recent significant advances in cancer research include the development of techniques that allow the analysis of the structure and expression of the entire genome. The cost efficiency, both in terms of financial and tissue costs, and the resolution of these methodologies, has increased dramatically over the last few years. As a consequence we now have access to extremely powerful tools that are enabling the identification of causative molecular alterations in paediatric brain tumours.

Genomic gains and losses
Comparative genomic hybridization (CGH) is a genome-wide technique that can detect chromosomal gains and losses (Trask 2002). Conventional or chromosome CGH (cCGH) employs an equal mix of tumour and normal control tissue-derived DNA that is differentially labeled green and red, respectively, and then hybridized in a competitive manner to preparations of normal metaphase chromosomes (Fig. 5.1). This technique is capable of scanning the entire genome for chromosomal imbalance, and can be applied to both fixed and fresh tumour material. CGH analyses of ependymomas (Reardon et al. 1999, Granzow et al. 2001, Scheil et al. 2001, Ward et al. 2001, Carter et al. 2002, Dyer et al. 2002, Grill et al. 2002, Jeuken et al. 2002), medulloblastomas (Bayani et al. 1995, 2000; Reardon et al. 1997; Avet-Loiseau et al. 1999; Nicholson et al. 1999; Gilhuis et al. 2000) and gliomas (Nishizaki et al. 1998, Bigner et al. 1999, Kubota et al. 2001, Koschny et al. 2002) have confirmed the presence and incidence of known chromosomal abnormalities and identified new alterations.

While cCGH has proved useful for detecting gross chromosomal changes, it lacks the resolution required to identify specific genes that are targeted by genomic alterations. Array CGH (aCGH) is a recently developed and significantly more powerful variant of CGH (Pinkel et al. 1998). In aCGH the genome is represented by thousands of short segments of DNA [e.g. within bacterial artificial chromosome (BAC) clones], that are arrayed on a solid surface (usually a glass slide). Depending on the density of the array, this system can provide the researcher with details of chromosome gains and losses at <1 Mb intervals across the genome (Mantripragada et al. 2004). Fluorescently labelled tumour and normal DNA is competitively hybridized to these BACs and analysed in a manner similar to that of cCGH. aCGH holds great promise for high-resolution, rapid throughput study of chromosome alterations in large numbers of tumours. This technology is now being used to study adult glioma (Zardo et al. 2002), and is currently being used in a prospective clinical trial of medulloblastoma that is ongoing in North America.

Single nucleotide polymorphism (SNP) oligonucleotide arrays are a more recently developed tool for studying genomic gains and losses. These array systems have exploited

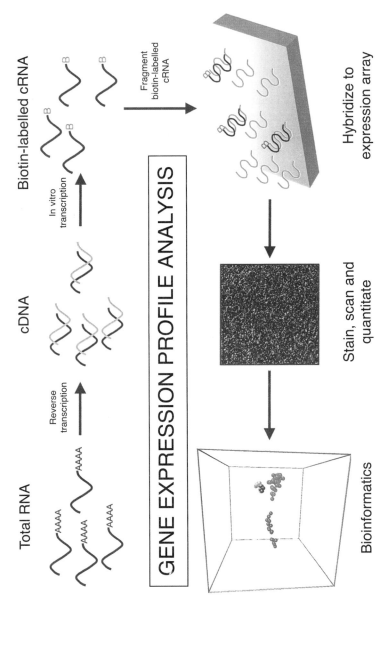

Total RNA   cDNA   Biotin-labelled cRNA

Reverse transcription

In vitro transcription

Fragment biotin-labelled cRNA

GENE EXPRESSION PROFILE ANALYSIS

Hybridize to expression array

Stain, scan and quantitate

Bioinformatics

Fig. 5.2. Gene expression profile analysis using oligonucleotide GeneChip® arrays. Total RNA is extracted from tumour samples and reverse transcribed into cDNA. Biotinylated cRNA is then generated and hybridized to short oligonucleotide probes arrayed onto a solid support. The arrays are then stained, e.g. with phycoerythrein conjugated streptavidin, and the fluorescence intensities determined using a laser confocal scanner. By monitoring the amount of label associated with each DNA location, it is possible to infer the abundance of each mRNA species represented. Analyzing the huge amounts of data generated by microarray analysis is proving to be one of the most challenging aspects of expression profiling and requires considerable expertise in bioinformatics. Bottom middle panel shows a single stained GeneChip® probe array. (Image courtesy of Affymetrix.)

the technologies developed for oligonucleotide based expression arrays (described below) to detect and quantify the copy number of thousands of SNPs across the genome. Commercial arrays are now available that can determine the copy number and loss of heterozygosity of 100,000 SNPs (Huang et al. 2004). These will soon be expanded to arrays that included over 500,000 SNPs, providing unprecedented data, pinpointing genetic alterations in cancers at the level of individual genes.

Genome-wide expression

Array based systems have also been developed that can determine genome-wide expression patterns (Liotta and Petricoin 2000). Microarray methods employ either full-length cDNAs or multiple short oligonucleotide sequences representing different regions of a gene, spotted onto glass slides (Fig. 5.2). In olignonucleotide based arrays (e.g. Affymetrix) each gene is represented by 15 to 20 perfect match (PM) oligonucleotides (or probes) of around 24 base pairs long each. Labeled copy RNA generated from tumour mRNA are then hybridized to the microarray. Measuring the amount of label associated with each PM probe location provides a measure of abundance of each mRNA species represented. To control for non-specific hybridization, each PM probe has a paired control mismatch (MM) probe that is identical to the PM probe except for a single base mismatch in its sequence. Subtraction analysis of the amount of label at PM relative to MM locations provides the final measure of specific hybridization.

A number of groups have employed oligonucleotide microarrays to investigate the biology of paediatric brain tumours. Recent analyses of medulloblastoma have demonstrated platelet-derived growth factor receptor (PDGFR) and members of the RAS/MAP kinase pathway are significantly up regulated in metastatic tumours (MacDonald et al. 2001, Gilbertson and Clifford 2003). Microarray analysis has also been used to identify differences in gene expression patterns between clinicopathological subgroups of medulloblastoma (Pomeroy et al. 2002) and to identify pro-metastatic genes that are upregulated by ERBB2 signaling in aggressive medulloblastomas (Hernan et al. 2003).

Proteins carry out the biological functions encoded by genes. Therefore, understanding the impact of gene sequence abnormalities on cell biology requires analysis of the encoded protein. *Proteomics* refers to the study of protein abundance, distribution, modification, function and interaction with other macromolecules (MacBeath 2002; Petricoin et al. 2002a,b). A number of advances in proteomics in recent years have exciting applications to the study of malignant disease, including array-based analyses of protein expression and phosphorylation similar to those already employed for measuring mRNA. Recent studies of human glioma suggest proteome analysis might be used in the future to identify biologically and clinically distinct subsets of astrocytoma (Iwadate et al. 2004).

STUDYING SPECIFIC CHROMOSOMAL REGIONS

Genome-wide approaches to studying genetic alterations have dramatically accelerated the identification of genomic regions that are likely to harbour cancer genes. Once these regions are located it is important to identify the gene(s) within these regions that are involved in the malignant process.

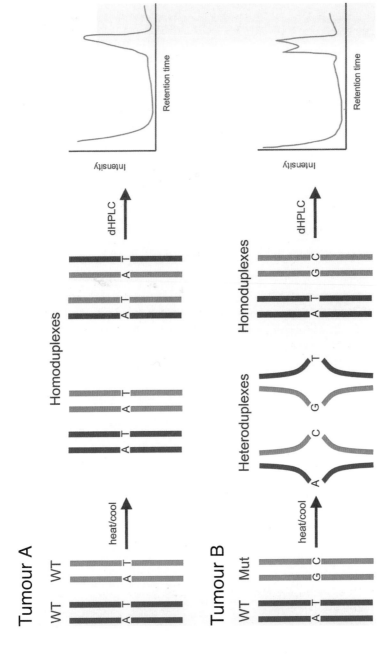

Fig. 5.3. Mutation scanning using denaturing high-performance liquid chromatography (dHPLC). Genomic DNA is extracted from tumour samples and the DNA sequence of interest amplified by PCR. Tumour A represents samples that are homozygous for the wild-type allele; Tumour B illustrates a tumour that is heterozygous, containing both wild-type and mutant (A>G) alleles. PCR products generated from tumour samples are heated and cooled. During cooling Tumour A PCR products form homoduplexes, while Tumour B derived PCR products form both homo- and heteroduplexes. Samples are then run through a dHPLC system, and OD260 peaks are resolved as they are eluted from the column under gradient conditions. The dual peak from the analysis of Tumour B indicates the presence of homo- and heteroduplex PCR products.

Mutation scanning

Until recently it was not feasible to directly sequence the entire coding region of oncogenes and tumour suppressor genes in large cohorts of tumour samples. Therefore, mutation scanning methods have been developed that can reliably detect single nucleotide abnormalities in tumour DNA. Denaturing high-performance liquid chromatography (dHPLC) allows the identification of DNA mutations (with a sensitivity of around 90%) in tumour samples by detecting heteroduplex formation between mismatched nucleotides in double stranded polymerase chain reaction (PCR) amplified DNA (Xiao and Oefner 2001) (Fig. 5.3). Using this technology, specific regions of DNA from large numbers of tumour samples can be rapidly screened for mutations. Tumours yielding heteroduplex PCR products can then be selected for analysis by direct sequencing (Liu et al. 1998). Inactivating mutations have been identified in a number of tumour suppressor genes in a variety of paediatric brain tumours (Raffel et al. 1999, Ellison 2002, Gilbertson 2002, Goussia et al. 2000, Lusher et al. 2002). The application of mutation scanning techniques such as dHPLC is likely to prove invaluable in determining the incidence and clinical significance of these abnormalities in future studies.

Fluorescent in situ hybridization

Fluorescent in situ hybridization (FISH) allows the visualization of specific DNA sequences in interphase cells, enabling the detection of deletions, amplifications and translocations within fresh frozen and fixed tumour samples (Fig. 5.4).

FISH is now proving a highly useful diagnostic tool for brain tumours. For example, atypical teratoid/rhabdoid tumours (AT/RTs) are characterized histologically by a mix of rhabdoid, classical primitive neuroectodermal, epithelial and neoplastic mesenchymal cells (Ellison 2002, Gilbertson 2002). This complex morphology can make it difficult to definitively diagnose this aggressive posterior fossa tumour. However, FISH detection of deletion of 22q11.2, the locus of the hSNF5/INI1 gene that is deleted or mutated in AT/RT (Versteege et al. 1998, Biegel et al. 2002), can assist the diagnosis of this disease (Fig. 5.4D). In addition to deletions, FISH is also being used to detect oncogene amplification in childhood brain tumours, e.g. MYCC and MYCN in medulloblastoma (Fig. 5.4C) (Gilbertson et al. 2001, Aldosari et al. 2002).

Detection of epigenetic modifications

Epigenetic modifications of the genome affect the expression but not the sequence of genes. DNA methylation, the addition of a methyl group to the 5′-carbon of cytosine, is the best characterized epigenetic modification of DNA (Plass 2002). Cytosine groups within CG-rich sequences (e.g. CpG islands) are the major target for methylation. CpG islands are typically sited in the promoter region and first exon of most genes, including known tumour suppressor genes; methylation of these regions can result in transcriptional silencing (Fig. 5.5).

The introduction of sodium bisulfite treatment as a means of selectively converting unmethylated cytosines to uracils has enabled the development of PCR-based assays for the detection of methylated DNA regions (Fig. 5.5). Methylated tumour suppressor genes have since been identified in almost all tumour types including paediatric brain tumours, e.g. methylation of RASSF1A in >80% of medulloblastomas (Fruhwald et al. 2001a,b;

135

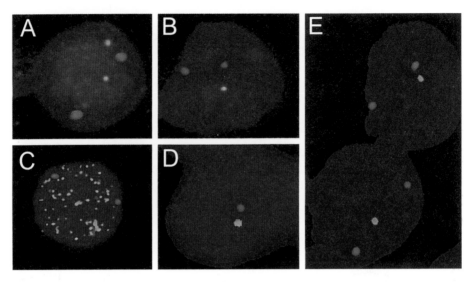

Fig. 5.4. Fluorescent in situ hybridization (FISH) analyses of brain tumour samples. Panels A–C include the results of FISH analysis of three different paediatric medulloblastoma samples. A. 'Normal' chromosome 17 compatible pattern showing two 17p subtelomeric (green) and two 17 centromeric (red) probe signals. B, Deletion of chromosome 17p, showing a single 17p subtelomeric (green) and two 17 centromeric (red) probe signals. C, MYC amplification (green). D, deletion of 1p (green) and 19q (red) in a section of oligodendroglioma. This cytogenetic pattern has been associated with treatment sensitivity and improved clinical outcome. E, Deletion of the hSNF5/INI1 locus (22q11.2; green probe) relative to a probe directed to NF2 at 22q12 (red) in a case of infant CNS AT/RT. (Panels A–C reproduced by permission from Gilbertson et al. 2001; panels D and E courtesy of Dr C Fuller, Dept of Pathology, St Jude Children's Research Hospital, Memphis.)

Lusher 2002; Smiraglia and Plass 2002; Zuzak et al. 2002). Using these techniques, analyses of large tumour cohorts are underway to establish the incidence and clinical significance of DNA methylation in childhood CNS malignancies. Additionally, DNA methylation is currently under investigation as a target for novel therapeutic approaches (see below). Therefore, methylation-specific PCR analysis may eventually become an important means of assessing the activity of these agents or identifying patients for specific novel therapies.

Advances in pre-clinical disease models

MOUSE MODELS OF CNS TUMOURS

It is now possible to produce mice with germline alterations that generate a gain-of-function (transgenic mice) or loss-of-function (knock-out or targeted deletion mice) in specific genes. Furthermore, the use of 'conditional' technology has increased the accuracy with which these alterations can be targeted to specific tissues (Fig. 5.6). This approach has already contributed extensively to the field of cancer research (Van Dyke and Jacks 2002) and holds great promise for studying tumorigenesis in the nervous system (Holland 2001, Wechsler-Reya and Scott 2001, Weiss et al. 2002). Indeed, a number of genetic mouse models of neuroectodermal and glial malignancies are now available.

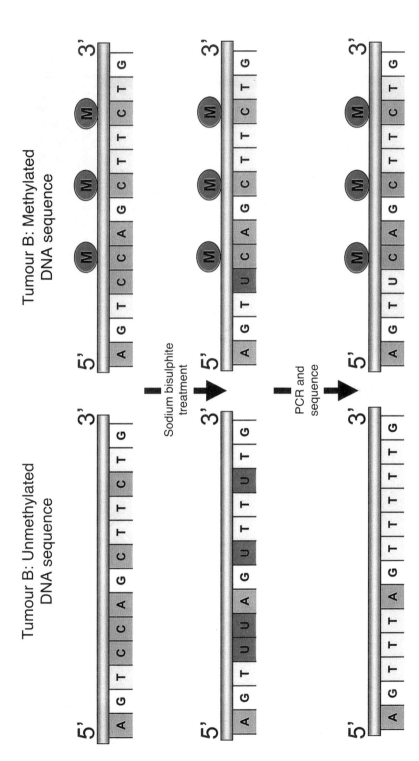

Fig. 5.5. DNA methylation and detection following sodium bisulfite modification. Cartoon depicting a portion of a CpG island within the promoter region of a tumour suppressor gene. In contrast to Tumour A, a number of the cytosine residues within this region are methylated in Tumour B, potentially silencing gene transcription. Sodium bisulfite treatment of DNA from both tumours results in the conversion of unmethylated cytosine residues to uracils. Subsequent PCR amplification and sequencing enables the differentiation of tumours containing methylated DNA sequence from those with unmethylated cytosine residues.

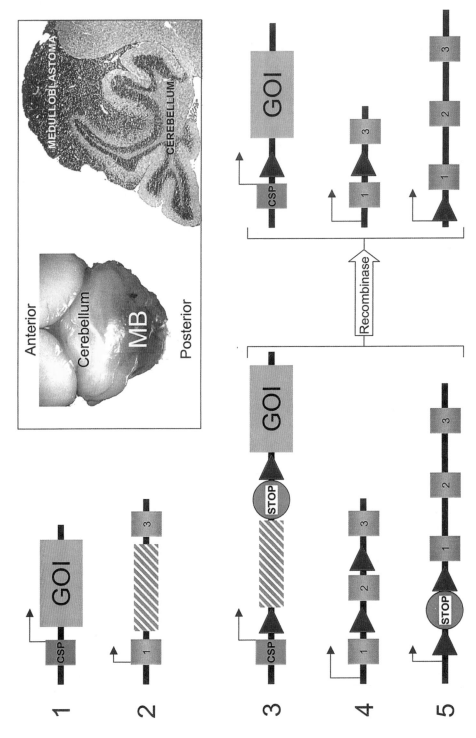

The value of genetic mouse tumour models depends upon the degree to which they mimic the human disease. Therefore, comprehensive characterization of genetic mouse CNS tumour models is crucial if they are to be used effectively. Characterization should include detailed macro- and microscopic examination of tumour pathology; a careful study of the tissue of origin of the disease; and characterization of the pattern of progression and clinical behaviour. Characterization of genetic mouse models of CNS tumours is still at an early stage; however, initial data suggest that a number of the available mouse models of medulloblastoma do mimic a subgroup of human medulloblastoma (Lee et al. 2003). Further, a recent study successfully employed the $Ptc1^{+/-}/p53^{-/-}$ mouse model of medulloblastoma to demonstrate the therapeutic efficacy of ShhAntag, an inhibitor of Ptc pathway signalling (Romer et al. 2004). Although these initial data are encouraging, the use of genetic mouse models for pre-clinical drug development is challenging and requires large cohorts of genetically manipulated mice and sophisticated imaging techniques to prospectively assess treatment responses. Further characterization studies, and in particular comparative analysis of mouse and human tumours, will be required before we can clearly determine the value and role of each tumour model.

STEM CELL BIOLOGY

Neurons, oligodendrocytes and astrocytes, the three main cell types in the mammalian CNS, are derived from multipotent neural stem cells (Temple 2001). Increasing attention is being focused on the role of neural stem cells in CNS disease and whether they may be

---

Fig. 5.6 *(opposite).* Different genetic approaches for generating cancer models in mice. Figure depicts the principal strategies available for generating mice with specific genetic lesions. In (1) the gene of interest (GOI), e.g. an oncogene, is placed under the control of a cell specific promoter (CSP). This transgene is then randomly inserted, e.g. by pronuclear DNA injection, into the mouse genome. Cell-specific expression is achieved via the CSP; however, effects may also be observed secondary to random insertion of the transgene. Alternatively (2), targeted mutations of endogenous genes can be generated via embryonic stem cells. Here the example depicts the knock-out of a gene by replacing exon 2 of the GOI with a reporter element (hatched box). In this approach the transgene integrates into the genome by homologous recombination. Cell-specific expression is therefore controlled by endogenous regulatory signals. Strategies (3)–(5) demonstrate the use of conditional genetic technology. These techniques exploit the properties of enzymes known as site-specific recombinases, e.g. Cre-recombinase. Cre-recombinase recognizes a 34 bp inverted repeat sequence separated by an asymmetric 8 bp spacer, known as a loxP site (represented in the figure as a blue triangle). If two loxP sites are located on the same DNA molecule in the same orientation, then Cre-recombinase cuts out the intervening sequence. This allows for an extra level of control, restricting the site of transgene expression or gene deletion, only to cells engineered to express Cre-recombinase. For example, in (3) and (5) activation of gene expression by a CSP or endogenous control elements, respectively, cannot occur until the intervening reporter and/or stop sequence is excised. Alternatively, knock-out of genes may also be restricted to cells expressing Cre-recombinase (4). Cre-recombinase can itself be targeted to cells using the same genetic approaches. The inset panel shows a mouse model of medulloblastoma generated by knocking-out the DNA repair gene Lig4 and p53 (Lee and McKinnon 2002). The cerebellum of a mouse-containing tumour (MB) is shown on the left, and a low power hematoxylin and eosin stained photomicrograph of the cerebellum and tumour is shown on the right. (Images courtesy of Dr Peter McKinnon, Dept of Genetics, St Jude Children's Research Hospital, Memphis.)

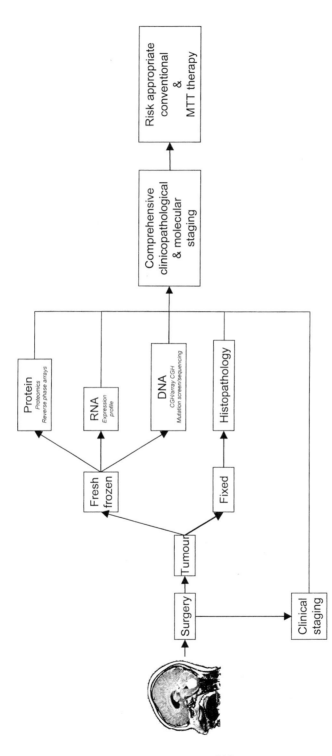

Fig. 5.7. Strategy for the future management of children with brain tumours. Clinical trials over the next few years will prospectively evaluate the prognostic significance of molecular abnormalities and tumour histopathology in children with brain tumours. It is hoped that the results of these studies will refine the way we stratify and treat patients. The figure depicts a strategy that may ultimately be used in the clinical management of paediatric brain tumours. Following surgery, patients will undergo clinical staging and their tumour will be subjected to a battery of molecular tests. These will be directed at defining the presence or absence of molecular risk factors, identifying specific targets for any available molecular targeted therapies (MTTs) and increasing knowledge of disease biology. Integration of this data with the clinical and histopathological disease features will allow comprehensive risk staging. Patients will then receive tailored conventional and MTT. Measurement of molecular end-points may also become a routine part of patient follow-up and tracking disease response to treatment.

140

exploited for therapeutic gain. Of particular note, recent evidence suggests that cancers (Lapidot et al. 1994, Al-Hajj et al. 2003, Pardal et al. 2003), including certain brain tumours (Ignatova et al. 2002, Hemmati et al. 2003, Singh et al. 2004, Yuan et al. 2004), are maintained by small populations of stem cell-like cancer cells. These cancer stem cells are thought to arise from normal stem cells that are transformed by the accumulation of genetic mutations. Considerable efforts are ongoing to determine the role that stem-cell-like cancer cells play in maintaining paediatric brain tumours. Advances in cell sorting technologies that allow the isolation of small subpopulations of tumour cells have been especially important in these studies. It is hoped that drugs that target cell signal pathways important in the self-renewal and survival of stem-cell-like cancer cells may ultimately prove to be highly effective anti-cancer therapies. Certain properties of neural stem cells, including their capacity to track migrating glioma cells, may also be exploited therapeutically. Recently, interleukin 12 secreting neural stem cells inoculated into gliomas in mice prolonged the survival of animals compared to treatment with nonsecretory stem cells (Ehtesham et al. 2002). Stem cell research is still a very young discipline; nonetheless, it is likely to play an increasing role in the analysis of paediatric CNS tumours.

Application of molecular biology to disease management
The preceding sections describe a number of new molecular biology techniques and research systems that are currently being applied to the study of childhood brain tumours. It is hoped that these methods will contribute to the development of non-toxic curative treatment regimens for all children with brain tumours. There are at least two ways in which this might be achieved. First, advances in molecular biology might assist estimation of prognosis and selection of appropriate therapy for patients. Second, the identification of molecular defects that are important for neuro-oncogenesis may serve as targets for new therapeutic approaches.

DISEASE CLASSIFICATION AND STAGING
Molecular prognostic factors are routinely used in disease staging of a number of haemato-logical and solid paediatric malignancies (Maris and Matthay 1999, Pui et al. 2001). In contrast, there are no established biological prognostic factors for childhood brain tumours. This is largely because molecular markers have been evaluated in statistically underpowered studies involving heterogeneous groups of patients. Attempts are now underway to evaluate molecular risk factors among larger numbers of homogeneously treated children with brain tumours (Gajjar et al. 2004). Completing these studies will be difficult, not least because they will require the recruitment of adequate amounts of fresh frozen tumour material; however, if successful they should lead to the development of molecular-based staging systems and identify potential targets for novel therapeutic approaches (Gilbertson 2004) (Fig. 5.7).

MOLECULAR TARGETED THERAPIES
Progress in understanding the molecular basis of malignant disease has brought about a revolution in cancer therapeutics. Molecular targeted therapies (MTTs) that inhibit the activity of aberrant signal pathways are now in the clinic (Sausville et al. 2003). Although the development of MTTs is still in its infancy, important lessons have already been learnt.

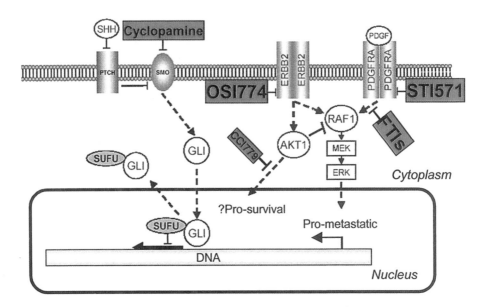

Fig. 5.8. Signal transduction pathways in medulloblastoma: an example of potential molecular targeted therapy (MTT) for childhood brain tumours. Abnormalities within the SHH/PTCH1, ERBB2 and PDGFRA signaling pathways have been implicated in medulloblastoma tumorigenesis. PTCH1 suppresses the activity of smoothened (SMO). Binding of sonic hedgehog (SHH) to PTCH releases suppression of SMO, activating GLI which in turn mediates the transcription of a number of genes, including PTCH1 itself. GLI-dependent transcription is negatively regulated by suppressor of fused (SUFU) that also exports GLI out of the nucleus. Overexpression of ERBB2 results in spontaneous homodimerization. This activates the RAF/MEK/ERK and AKT pathways driving proliferation and the expression of pro-metastatic genes. Signalling through the PDGFRA/RAS/MAPK has been implicated in medulloblastoma metastasis, possibly by upregulating pro-invasive genes. At least five MTTs that target these pathways are undergoing pre-clinical development in medulloblastoma. These include the smoothened inhibitor cyclopamine; OSI774 (Erlotinib) and STI571 (Gleevec) that inhibit the ERBB2 and PDGFR tyrosine kinases, respectively; and inhibitors of second messengers, e.g. the mTOR inhibitor CCI779 and farnesyl transferase inhibitors (FTIs).

In this regard, characterization of the molecular target and appropriate pre-clinical and clinical evaluation of MTTs are crucial for the successful development of these drugs.

Development of MTTs
• *Target identification*. The most successful MTTs target molecules that are pivotal in cancer biology, e.g. the BCR-ABL kinase inhibitor STI-571 (Gleevec, Imatinib Mesylate) and the anti-ERBB2 monoclonal antibody Herceptin (Trastuzumab) (Druker 2002, Vogel et al. 2002). The best molecular targets for paediatric CNS tumours will be those that are causative in the disease process and can be readily identified early in disease. A number of targets for MTTs have already been identified for childhood brain tumours, in particular medulloblastoma (Fig. 5.8); additional targets are likely to be discovered over the next few years. Efforts are underway to define the role that each of these molecules plays in brain

tumour biology and therefore the likely therapeutic value of pharmacological inhibition. In addition, it will also be important to identify disease subtypes that are 'target-dependent' in order to establish which patients are most likely to be sensitive to specific MTTs.

• *Pre-clinical assessment.* Pre-clinical assessment of potential MTTs should determine how they alter target function and tumour biology and the concentration and duration of drug exposure required to achieve any biological effect(s). Additionally, biochemical assays that provide an optimal assessment of biological activity should be developed in preparation for clinical trials. The increasing availability of transgenic mouse models of brain tumours may assist in this process (Weiss et al. 2002, Romer et al. 2004).

• *Clinical assessment.* The clinical phase of MTT drug development should build on pre-clinical analyses and incorporate molecular end-points into all phases of clinical trial. This requirement will significantly increase the complexity of clinical trial design by demanding tissue acquisition from all patients; the development of clinically viable molecular assays of drug activity; and the re-definition of trial end-points. Conducting such studies in the brain, which has restricted surgical and pharmacological access, adds an additional level of difficulty (Lang et al. 2002). Although the challenge of developing MTTs for brain tumours is formidable, this is far outweighed by the potential rewards for all children with brain tumours.

MTTs in development for paediatric brain tumours
• *Cell surface receptors and second messenger networks.* The ERBB family of cell surface receptor tyrosine kinases has been implicated in the biology of a number of CNS tumours. ERBB1 is amplified and overexpressed in up to one-half of adult high-grade gliomas (Wong et al. 1987, 1992; Ekstrand et al. 1991) and overexpressed, usually in the absence of gene amplification, in around 30% of paediatric non-brainstem high-grade gliomas (Sure et al. 1997, Bredel et al. 1999, Cheng et al. 1999, Sung et al. 2000). ERBB1 over expression and gene amplification is also a feature of high-grade glioma (Gilbertson et al. 2003). Furthermore, upregulation of ERBB1 cell signaling promotes gliomagenesis in mice (Holland et al. 1998, Bachoo 2002) and an invasive (Maity et al. 2000, Lal et al. 2002) and radio-resistant phenotype in human glioma cells (Chakravarti et al. 2002). Consequently, the Pediatric Brain Tumor Consortium (PBTC) in the USA is currently assessing the safety and efficacy of ZD1839 (Iressa), an inhibitor of the ERBB1 tyrosine kinase, in children with supratentorial high-grade glioma and brainstem glioma (clinical trial PBTC-007). ERBB2 and ERBB4 have also been reported to mediate aggressive disease behaviour in childhood medulloblastoma and ependymoma (Gilbertson et al. 1997, 2002; Herms et al. 1997; Hernan et al. 2003, Gajjar et al. 2004). Clinical trials of ERBB2 tyrosine kinase inhibitors in children with brain tumours are now open in the USA within both the Paediatric Brain Tumor Consortium and the Children's Oncology Group.

Evidence from a variety of different sources has implicated the PDGFR signaling system in the development of glioma and medulloblastoma. Most recently, microarray analysis of paediatric medulloblastoma identified an increase in the expression of PDGFRA and members of the MAPK cascade in primary tumours from patients with metastases at

143

diagnosis, suggesting that this signaling system may play a role in aggressive disease behaviour of primitive neuroectodermal tumours (MacDonald et al. 2001, Gilbertson and Clifford 2003). Furthermore, PDGFRA neutralizing antibodies appear to inhibit the migration of medulloblastoma cells across basement membranes in culture. The PBTC in the USA is currently conducting a phase I/II study of STI-571 in children with newly diagnosed brain-stem glioma or recurrent high-grade glioma (clinical trial PBTC-006). Further validation of PDGFR as a target in medulloblastoma is required before clinical trials in this disease can begin.

Cell surface receptors converge on common second messenger pathways including the RAS/MAPK pathway. RAS, like many cytosolic signal proteins, must locate to the cell membrane to participate in signal transduction. This is achieved through the process of prenylation in which a farnesyl group is transferred from farnesyl-pyrophosphate (FPP) to the cysteine residue of a 'CAAX' motif on the c-terminus of RAS (Ghobrial and Adjei 2002). Inhibitors of this process, termed farnesyl transferase inhibitors (FTIs), are under development as potential cancer drugs. FTIs may be divided into three groups: (a) CAAX competitive inhibitors, e.g. SCH66336 and R115777 that compete with this motif on RAS for FT; (b) FPP competitive inhibitors, e.g. PD169451; and (c) bisubstrate inhibitors, e.g. BMS-186511. A Phase I study of SCH 66336 is currently underway within the PBTC in the USA assessing the toxicity of the drug in children with recurrent or progressive brain tumours (clinical trial PBTC-003).

The SHH/PTCH1 pathway plays a significant role in the development of certain medullo-blastomas (Ruiz i Altaba et al. 2002). Consequently, efforts are underway to identify MTTs that can silence this pathway. These include cyclopamine, a plant-derived teratogen that inhibits the SHH/PTCH1 pathway by binding to, and altering the conformation of smoothened (SMO) (Taipale et al. 2000, Berman et al. 2002, Chen et al. 2002). An elegant series of studies using a mouse model of medulloblastoma have clearly demonstrated the pre-clinical efficacy of SMO inhibitors (Romer et al. 2004).

• *Inhibition of angiogenesis*. Anti-angiogenic agents include drugs that inhibit the signal pathways that stimulate angiogenesis and drugs that induce endothelial cell death (Kerbel and Folkman 2002). The first group of compounds includes inhibitors of vascular endothelial growth factor receptor-1 (VEGFR-1), e.g. SU5416, and broader acting agents that inhibit fibroblast growth factor (FGF) and PDGF receptors as well as VEGFR-1, e.g. SU6668. A large number of agents with anti-endothelial cell activity have been identified. These include inhibitors of endothelial-specific integrin/survival signals, e.g. EMD 121974. Clinical trials of anti-angiogenic compounds in children with brain tumours are underway within the PBTC. However, the potential for these compounds to induce growth related toxicity in the devel-oping child requires particular attention as these agents enter clinical paediatric practice.

• *Inhibition of brain tumour cell invasive capacity*. High-grade gliomas widely disseminate in the brain along anatomical structures, and medulloblastoma, and more rarely ependymoma, may actively metastasize through the neuraxis. The process by which malignant cells spread beyond their site of origin involves a complex series of protein–protein interactions (Liotta and Kohn 2001). For example, astrocytoma migration involves interactions between the malignant cell and extracellular matrix proteins including lamin, collagen type IV, fibronectin and vitronectin. Other secreted proteins believed to promote the proliferation and migration of glioma cells include PDGF-AA, PDGF-BB, and their receptors, as well as ERBB and FGF ligands and the matrix metalloproteinases. The complexity of cell signal and adhesion networks involved in tumour cell migration suggests that a variety of different MTTs may have anti-invasive properties. It remains to be determined whether these agents will be most effective as monotherapies or when used in combination.

• *Inhibitors of DNA methylation and histone deacetylation.* There is increasing evidence that epigenetic mechanisms are responsible for silencing tumour suppressor gene expression (see above). Of particular note, DNA methylation and histone deacetylation appear to co-operate to silence the expression of certain genes. The methylation of cysteine residues with CpG rich gene promoter regions enables the recruitment of histone deacetylase complexes (HDACs) that modify the surrounding chromatin structure resulting in repression of gene expression. Consequently, a variety of DNA methylation and histone deacetylase (HDAC) inhibitors are currently in clinical trials in adults and have demonstrated ability to alter gene expression in vivo (Szyf 2000, Yoshida et al. 2001, Karpf and Jones 2002). Given the co-operation between DNA methylation and HDAC in gene silencing, agents that target these processes may prove especially effective in combination.

Summary

In recent years significant progress has been made in our understanding of the molecular biology of human cancer. This has been achieved through the development of innovative laboratory techniques that provide focused and genome-wide information on molecular abnormalities in cancer cells. These tools are now being applied to the study of paediatric brain tumours. It is hoped that cooperation between clinical and basic science professionals will allow these skills to be used in the development of effective new treatments for all children with brain tumours.

ACKNOWLEDGEMENTS

RJG is supported by NIH grants P01CA096832 and U01CA081457, a 'Translational Grant' from the V-Foundation for Cancer Research, the 'Sontag Foundation's Distinguished Scientist Award', Musicians Against Childhood Cancer and the American Lebanese Syrian Associated Charities (ALSAC).

REFERENCES

Aldosari N, Bigner SH, Burger PC, Becker L, Kepner JL, Friedman HS, McLendon RE (2002) MYCC and MYCN oncogene amplification in medulloblastoma. A fluorescence in situ hybridization study on paraffin sections from the Children's Oncology Group. *Arch Pathol Lab Med* **126**: 540–544.
Al-Hajj M, Wicha MS, Benito-Hernandez A, Morrison SJ, Clarke MF (2003) Prospective identification of tumorigenic breast cancer cells. *Proc Natl Acad Sci USA* **100**: 3983–3988.
Avet-Loiseau H, Venuat AM, Terrier-Lacombe MJ, Lellouch-Tubiana A, Zerah M, Vassal G (1999) Comparative genomic hybridization detects many recurrent imbalances in central nervous system primitive neuroectodermal tumours in children. *Br J Cancer* **79**: 1843–1847.
Bachoo RM, Maher EA, Ligon KL, Sharpless NE, Chan SS, You MJ, Tang Y, DeFrances J, Stover E, Weissleder

R, Rowitch DH, Louis DN, DePinho RA (2002) Epidermal growth factor receptor and Ink4a/Arf: convergent mechanisms governing terminal differentiation and transformation along the neural stem cell to astrocyte axis. *Cancer Cell* **1**: 269–277.

Bayani J, Thorner P, Zielenska M, Pandita A, Beatty B, Squire JA (1995) Application of a simplified comparative genomic hybridization technique to screen for gene amplification in pediatric solid tumors. *Pediatr Pathol Lab Med* **15**: 831–844.

Bayani J, Zielenska M, Marrano P, Kwan Ng Y, Taylor MD, Jay V, Rutka JT, Squire JA (2000) Molecular cytogenetic analysis of medulloblastomas and supratentorial primitive neuroectodermal tumors by using conventional banding, comparative genomic hybridization, and spectral karyotyping. *J Neurosurg* **93**: 437–438.

Berman DM, Karhadkar SS, Hallahan AR, Pritchard JI, Eberhart CG, Watkins DN, Chen JK, Cooper MK, Taipale J, Olson JM, Beachy PA (2002) Medulloblastoma growth inhibition by hedgehog pathway blockade. *Science* **297**: 1559–1561.

Biegel JA, Kalpana G, Knudsen ES, Packer RJ, Roberts CW, Thiele CJ, Weissman B, Smith M (2002) The role of INI1 and the SWI/SNF complex in the development of rhabdoid tumors: meeting summary from the workshop on childhood atypical teratoid/rhabdoid tumors. *Cancer Res* **62**: 323–328.

Bigner SH, Matthews MR, Rasheed BK, Wiltshire RN, Friedman HS, Friedman AH, Stenzel TT, Dawes DM, McLendon RE, Bigner DD (1999) Molecular genetic aspects of oligodendrogliomas including analysis by comparative genomic hybridization. *Am J Pathol* **155**: 375–386.

Bredel M, Pollack IF, Hamilton RL, James CD (1999) Epidermal growth factor receptor expression and gene amplification in high-grade non-brainstem gliomas of childhood. *Clin Cancer Res* **5**: 1786–1792.

Cairncross JG, Ueki K, Zlatescu MC, Lisle DK, Finkelstein DM, Hammond RR, Silver JS, Stark PC, Macdonald DR, Ino Y, Ramsay DA, Louis DN (1998) Specific genetic predictors of chemotherapeutic response and survival in patients with anaplastic oligodendrogliomas. *J Natl Cancer Inst* **90**: 1473–1479.

Carter M, Nicholson J, Ross F, Crolla J, Allibone R, Balaji V, Perry R, Walker D, Gilbertson R, Ellison DW (2002) Genetic abnormalities detected in ependymomas by comparative genomic hybridisation. *Br J Cancer* **86**: 929–939.

Cavenee WK (2002) Genetics and new approaches to cancer therapy. *Carcinogenesis* **23**: 683–686.

Chakravarti A, Chakladar A, Delaney MA, Latham DE, Loeffler JS (2002) The epidermal growth factor receptor pathway mediates resistance to sequential administration of radiation and chemotherapy in primary human glioblastoma cells in a RAS-dependent manner. *Cancer Res* **62**: 4307–4315.

Chen JK, Taipale J, Cooper MK, Beachy PA (2002) Inhibition of Hedgehog signaling by direct binding of cyclopamine to Smoothened. *Genes Dev* **16**: 2743–2748.

Cheng Y, Ng HK, Zhang SF, Ding M, Pang JC, Zheng J, Poon WS (1999) Genetic alterations in pediatric high-grade astrocytomas. *Hum Pathol* **30**: 1284–1290.

Druker BJ (2002) Perspectives on the development of a molecularly targeted agent. *Cancer Cell* **1**: 31–36.

Dyer S, Prebble E, Davison V, Davies P, Ramani P, Ellison D, Grundy R (2002) Genomic imbalances in pediatric intracranial ependymomas define clinically relevant groups. *Am J Pathol* **161**: 2133–2141.

Ehtesham M, Kabos P, Kabosova A, Neuman T, Black KL, Yu JS (2002) The use of interleukin 12-secreting neural stem cells for the treatment of intracranial glioma. *Cancer Res* **62**: 5657–5663.

Ekstrand AJ, James CD, Cavenee WK, Seliger B, Pettersson RF, Collins VP (1991) Genes for epidermal growth factor receptor, transforming growth factor alpha, and epidermal growth factor and their expression in human gliomas in vivo. *Cancer Res* **51**: 2164–2172.

Ellison D (2002) Classifying the medulloblastoma: insights from morphology and molecular genetics. *Neuropathol Appl Neurobiol* **28**: 257–282.

Fruhwald MC, O'Dorisio MS, Dai Z, Rush LJ, Krahe R, Smiraglia DJ, Pietsch T, Elsea SH, Plass C (2001a) Aberrant hypermethylation of the major breakpoint cluster region in 17p11.2 in medulloblastomas but not supratentorial PNETs. *Genes Chromosomes Cancer* **30**: 38–47.

Fruhwald MC, O'Dorisio MS, Dai Z, Tanner SM, Balster DA, Gao X, Wright FA, Plass C (2001b) Aberrant promoter methylation of previously unidentified target genes is a common abnormality in medulloblastomas—implications for tumor biology and potential clinical utility. *Oncogene* **20**: 5033–5042.

Futreal PA, Kasprzyk A, Birney E, Mullikin JC, Wooster R, Stratton MR (2001) Cancer and genomics. *Nature* **409**: 850–852.

Gajjar A, Hernan R, Kocak M, Fuller C, Lee Y, McKinnon PJ, Wallace D, Lau C, Chintagumpala M, Ashley DM, Kellie SJ, Kun L, Gilbertson RJ (2004) Clinical, histopathologic, and molecular markers of prognosis: toward a new disease risk stratification system for medulloblastoma. *J Clin Oncol* **22**: 984–993.

146

Ghobrial IM, Adjei AA (2002) Inhibitors of the ras oncogene as therapeutic targets. *Hematol Oncol Clin North Am* **16**: 1065–1088.

Gilbertson R (2002) Paediatric embryonic brain tumours. biological and clinical relevance of molecular genetic abnormalities. *Eur J Cancer* **38**: 675–685.

Gilbertson RJ (2004) Medulloblastoma: signalling a change in treatment. *Lancet Oncol* **5**: 209–218.

Gilbertson RJ, Clifford SC (2003) PDGFRB is overexpressed in metastatic medulloblastoma. *Nat Genet* **35**: 197–198.

Gilbertson RJ, Perry RH, Kelly PJ, Pearson AD, Lunec J (1997) Prognostic significance of HER2 and HER4 coexpression in childhood medulloblastoma. *Cancer Res* **57**: 3272–3280.

Gilbertson R, Wickramasinghe C, Hernan R, Balaji V, Hunt D, Jones-Wallace D, Crolla J, Perry R, Lunec J, Pearson A, Ellison D (2001) Clinical and molecular stratification of disease risk in medulloblastoma. *Br J Cancer* **85**: 705–712.

Gilbertson RJ, Bentley L, Hernan R, Junttila TT, Frank AJ, Haapasalo H, Connelly M, Wetmore C, Curran T, Elenius K, Ellison DW (2002) ERBB receptor signaling promotes ependymoma cell proliferation and represents a potential novel therapeutic target for this disease. *Clin Cancer Res* **8**: 3054–3064.

Gilbertson RJ, Hill DA, Hernan R, Kocak M, Geyer R, Olson J, Gajjar A, Rush L, Hamilton RL, Finkelstein SD, Pollack IF (2003) ERBB1 is amplified and overexpressed in high-grade diffusely infiltrative pediatric brain stem glioma. *Clin Cancer Res* **9**: 3620–3624.

Gilhuis HJ, Anderl KL, Boerman RH, Jeuken JM, James CD, Raffel C, Scheithauer BW, Jenkins RB (2000) Comparative genomic hybridization of medulloblastomas and clinical relevance: eleven new cases and a review of the literature. *Clin Neurol Neurosurg* **102**: 203–209.

Goussia AC, Bruner JM, Kyritsis AP, Agnantis NJ, Fuller GN. (2000) Cytogenetic and molecular genetic abnormalities in primitive neuroectodermal tumors of the central nervous system. *Anticancer Res* **20**: 65–73.

Granzow M, Popp S, Weber S, Schoell B, Holtgreve-Grez H, Senf L, Hager D, Boschert J, Scheurlen W, Jauch A (2001) Isochromosome 1q as an early genetic event in a child with intracranial ependymoma characterized by molecular cytogenetics. *Cancer Genet Cytogenet* **130**: 79–83.

Grill J, Avet-Loiseau H, Lellouch-Tubiana A, Sevenet N, Terrier-Lacombe MJ, Venuat AM, Doz F, Sainte-Rose C, Kalifa C, Vassal G (2002) Comparative genomic hybridization detects specific cytogenetic abnormalities in pediatric ependymomas and choroid plexus papillomas. *Cancer Genet Cytogenet* **136**: 121–125.

Hanahan D, Weinberg RA (2000) The hallmarks of cancer. *Cell* **100**: 57–70.

Hemmati HD, Nakano I, Lazareff JA, Masterman-Smith M, Geschwind DH, Bronner-Fraser M, Kornblum HI (2003) Cancerous stem cells can arise from pediatric brain tumors. *Proc Natl Acad Sci USA* **100**: 15178–15183.

Herms JW, Behnke J, Bergmann M, Christen HJ, Kolb R, Wilkening M, Markakis E, Hanefeld F, Kretzschmar HA (1997) Potential prognostic value of C-erbB-2 expression in medulloblastomas in very young children. *J Pediatr Hematol Oncol* **19**: 510–515.

Hernan R, Fasheh R, Calabrese C, Frank AJ, Maclean KH, Allard D, Barraclough R, Gilbertson RJ (2003) ERBB2 up-regulates S100A4 and several other prometastatic genes in medulloblastoma. *Cancer Res* **63**: 140–148.

Holland EC (2001) Gliomagenesis: genetic alterations and mouse models. *Nat Rev Genet* **2**: 120–129.

Holland EC, Hively WP, DePinho RA, Varmus HE (1998) A constitutively active epidermal growth factor receptor cooperates with disruption of G1 cell-cycle arrest pathways to induce glioma-like lesions in mice. *Genes Dev* **12**: 3675–3685.

Huang J, Wei W, Zhang J, Liu G, Bignell GR, Stratton MR, Futreal PA, Wooster R, Jones KW, Shapero MH (2004) Whole genome DNA copy number changes identified by high density oligonucleotide arrays. *Hum Genomics* **1**: 287–299.

Ichimura K, Bolin MB, Goike HM, Schmidt EE, Moshref A, Collins VP (2000) Deregulation of the p14ARF/MDM2/p53 pathway is a prerequisite for human astrocytic gliomas with G1-S transition control gene abnormalities. *Cancer Res* **60**: 417–424.

Ignatova TN, Kukekov VG, Laywell ED, Suslov ON, Vrionis FD, Steindler DA (2002) Human cortical glial tumors contain neural stem-like cells expressing astroglial and neuronal markers in vitro. *Glia* **39**: 193–206.

Iwadate Y, Sakaida T, Hiwasa T, Nagai Y, Ishikura H, Takiguchi M, Yamaura A (2004) Molecular classification and survival prediction in human gliomas based on proteome analysis. *Cancer Res* **64**: 2496–2501.

Jeuken JW, Sprenger SH, Gilhuis J, Teepen HL, Grotenhuis AJ, Wesseling P (2002) Correlation between localization, age, and chromosomal imbalances in ependymal tumours as detected by CGH. *J Pathol* **197**: 238–244.

Jones PA, Takai D (2001) The role of DNA methylation in mammalian epigenetics. *Science* **293**: 1068–1070.

Karpf AR, Jones DA (2002) Reactivating the expression of methylation silenced genes in human cancer. *Oncogene* **21**: 5496–5503.

Kerbel R, Folkman J (2002) Clinical translation of angiogenesis inhibitors. *Nat Rev Cancer* **2**: 727–739.

Kleihues P, Louis DN, Scheithauer BW, Rorke LB, Reifenberger G, Burger PC, Cavenee WK (2002) The WHO classification of tumors of the nervous system. *J Neuropathol Exp Neurol* **61**: 215–225; discussion 226–229.

Koschny R, Koschny T, Froster UG, Krupp W, Zuber MA (2002) Comparative genomic hybridization in glioma: a meta-analysis of 509 cases. *Cancer Genet Cytogenet* **135**: 147–159.

Kubota H, Nishizaki T, Harada K, Oga A, Ito H, Suzuki M, Sasaki K (2001) Identification of recurrent chromosomal rearrangements and the unique relationship between low-level amplification and translocation in glioblastoma. *Genes Chromosomes Cancer* **31**: 125–133.

Lal A, Glazer CA, Martinson HM, Friedman HS, Archer GE, Sampson JH, Riggins GJ (2002) Mutant epidermal growth factor receptor up-regulates molecular effectors of tumor invasion. *Cancer Res* **62**: 3335–3339.

Lander ES, Linton LM, Birren B, Nusbaum C, Zody MC, Baldwin J, Devon K, Dewar K, Doyle M, FitzHugh W, Funke R, Gage D, Harris K, Heaford A, Howland J, Kann L, Lehoczky J, LeVine R, McEwan P, McKernan K, Meldrim J, Mesirov JP, Miranda C, Morris W, Naylor J, Raymond C, Rosetti M, Santos R, Sheridan A, Sougnez C, Stange-Thomann N, Stojanovic N, Subramanian A, Wyman D, Rogers J, Sulston J, Ainscough R, Beck S, Bentley D, Burton J, Clee C, Carter N, Coulson A, Deadman R, Deloukas P, Dunham A, Dunham I, Durbin R, French L, Grafham D, Gregory S, Hubbard T, Humphray S, Hunt A, Jones M, Lloyd C, McMurray A, Matthews L, Mercer S, Milne S, Mullikin JC, Mungall A, Plumb R, Ross M, Shownkeen R, Sims S, Waterston RH, Wilson RK, Hillier LW, McPherson JD, Marra MA, Mardis ER, Fulton LA, Chinwalla AT, Pepin KH, Gish WR, Chissoe SL, Wendl MC, Delehaunty KD, Miner TL, Delehaunty A, Kramer JB, Cook LL, Fulton RS, Johnson DL, Minx PJ, Clifton SW, Hawkins T, Branscomb E, Predki P, Richardson P, Wenning S, Slezak T, Doggett N, Cheng JF, Olsen A, Lucas S, Elkin C, Uberbacher E, Frazier M, Gibbs RA, Muzny DM, Scherer SE, Bouck JB, Sodergren EJ, Worley KC, Rives CM, Gorrell JH, Metzker ML, Naylor SL, Kucherlapati RS, Nelson DL, Weinstock GM, Sakaki Y, Fujiyama A, Hattori M, Yada T, Toyoda A, Itoh T, Kawagoe C, Watanabe H, Totoki Y, Taylor T, Weissenbach J, Heilig R, Saurin W, Artiguenave F, Brottier P, Bruls T, Pelletier E, Robert C, Wincker P, Smith DR, Doucette-Stamm L, Rubenfield M, Weinstock K, Lee HM, Dubois J, Rosenthal A, Platzer M, Nyakatura G, Taudien S, Rump A, Yang H, Yu J, Wang J, Huang G, Gu J, Hood L, Rowen L, Madan A, Qin S, Davis RW, Federspiel NA, Abola AP, Proctor MJ, Myers RM, Schmutz J, Dickson M, Grimwood J, Cox DR, Olson MV, Kaul R, Raymond C, Shimizu N, Kawasaki K, Minoshima S, Evans GA, Athanasiou M, Schultz R, Roe BA, Chen F, Pan H, Ramser J, Lehrach H, Reinhardt R, McCombie WR, de la Bastide M, Dedhia N, Blocker H, Hornischer K, Nordsiek G, Agarwala R, Aravind L, Bailey JA, Bateman A, Batzoglou S, Birney E, Bork P, Brown DG, Burge CB, Cerutti L, Chen HC, Church D, Clamp M, Copley RR, Doerks T, Eddy SR, Eichler EE, Furey TS, Galagan J, Gilbert JG, Harmon C, Hayashizaki Y, Haussler D, Hermjakob H, Hokamp K, Jang W, Johnson LS, Jones TA, Kasif S, Kasprzyk A, Kennedy S, Kent WJ, Kitts P, Koonin EV, Korf I, Kulp D, Lancet D, Lowe TM, McLysaght A, Mikkelsen T, Moran JV, Mulder N, Pollara VJ, Ponting CP, Schuler G, Schultz J, Slater G, Smit AF, Stupka E, Szustakowski J, Thierry-Mieg D, Thierry-Mieg J, Wagner L, Wallis J, Wheeler R, Williams A, Wolf YI, Wolfe KH, Yang SP, Yeh RF, Collins F, Guyer MS, Peterson J, Felsenfeld A, Wetterstrand KA, Patrinos A, Morgan MJ, Szustakowki J, de Jong P, Catanese JJ, Osoegawa K, Shizuya H, Choi S, Chen YJ; International Human Genome Sequencing Consortium (2001) Initial sequencing and analysis of the human genome. *Nature* **409**: 860–921. Errata in: *Nature* 2001, **411**: 720; **412**: 565.

Lang FF, Gilbert MR, Puduvalli VK, Weinberg J, Levin VA, Yung WK, Sawaya R, Fuller GN, Conrad CA (2002) Toward better early-phase brain tumor clinical trials: A reappraisal of current methods and proposals for future strategies. *Neuro-oncol* **4**: 268–277.

Lapidot T, Sirard C, Vormoor J, Murdoch B, Hoang T, Caceres-Cortes J, Minden M, Paterson B, Caligiuri MA, Dick JE (1994) A cell initiating human acute myeloid leukaemia after transplantation into SCID mice. *Nature* **367**: 645–648.

Lee Y, McKinnon PJ (2002) DNA ligase IV suppresses medulloblastoma formation. *Cancer Res* **62**: 6395–6399.

Lee Y, Miller HL, Jensen P, Hernan R, Connelly M, Wetmore C, Zindy F, Roussel MF, Curran T, Gilbertson RJ, McKinnon PJ (2003) A molecular fingerprint for medulloblastoma. *Cancer Res* **63**: 5428–5437.

Legler JM, Ries LA, Smith MA, Warren JL, Heineman EF, Kaplan RS, Linet MS (1999) Cancer surveillance series [corrected]: brain and other central nervous system cancers: recent trends in incidence and mortality. *J Natl Cancer Inst* **91**: 1382–1390; erratum: 1693.

Liotta LA, Kohn EC (2001) The microenvironment of the tumour-host interface. *Nature* **411**: 375–379.

Liotta L, Petricoin E (2000) Molecular profiling of human cancer. *Nat Rev Genet* **1**: 48–56.

Liu W, Smith DI, Rechtzigel KJ, Thibodeau SN, James CD (1998) Denaturing high performance liquid chromatography (DHPLC) used in the detection of germline and somatic mutations. *Nucleic Acids Res* **26**: 1396–1400.

Lusher ME, Lindsey JC, Latif F, Pearson AD, Ellison DW, Clifford SC (2002) Biallelic epigenetic inactivation of the RASSF1A tumor suppressor gene in medulloblastoma development. *Cancer Res* **62**: 5906–5911.

MacBeath G (2002) Protein microarrays and proteomics. Nat Genet 32: 526–532.

MacDonald TJ, Brown KM, LaFleur B, Peterson K, Lawlor C, Chen Y, Packer RJ, Cogen P, Stephan DA (2001) Expression profiling of medulloblastoma: PDGFRA and the RAS/MAPK pathway as therapeutic targets for metastatic disease. *Nat Genet* **29**: 143–152. Erratum in *Nat Genet* 2003, **35**: 287.

Maity A, Pore N, Lee J, Solomon D, O'Rourke DM (2000) Epidermal growth factor receptor transcriptionally up-regulates vascular endothelial growth factor expression in human glioblastoma cells via a pathway involving phosphatidylinositol 3'-kinase and distinct from that induced by hypoxia. *Cancer Res* **60**: 5879–5886.

Mantripragada KK, Buckley PG, de Stahl TD, Dumanski JP (2004) Genomic microarrays in the spotlight. *Trends Genet* **20**: 87–94.

Maris JM, Matthay KK (1999) Molecular biology of neuroblastoma. *J Clin Oncol* **17**: 2264–2279.

Nicholson JC, Ross FM, Kohler JA, Ellison DW (1999) Comparative genomic hybridization and histological variation in primitive neuroectodermal tumours. *Br J Cancer* **80**: 1322–1331.

Nishizaki T, Ozaki S, Harada K, Ito H, Arai H, Beppu T, Sasaki K (1998) Investigation of genetic alterations associated with the grade of astrocytic tumor by comparative genomic hybridization. *Genes Chromosomes Cancer* **21**: 340–346.

Pardal R, Clarke MF, Morrison SJ (2003) Applying the principles of stem-cell biology to cancer. *Nat Rev Cancer* **3**: 895–902.

Petricoin EF, Hackett JL, Lesko LJ, Puri RK, Gutman SI, Chumakov K, Woodcock J, Feigal DW, Zoon KC, Sistare FD (2002a) Medical applications of microarray technologies: a regulatory science perspective. *Nat Genet* **32**: 474–479.

Petricoin EF, Zoon KC, Kohn EC, Barrett JC, Liotta LA (2002b) Clinical proteomics: translating benchside promise into bedside reality. *Nat Rev Drug Discov* **1**: 683–695.

Pinkel D, Segraves R, Sudar D, Clark S, Poole I, Kowbel D, Collins C, Kuo WL, Chen C, Zhai Y, Dairkee SH, Ljung BM, Gray JW, Albertson DG (1998) High resolution analysis of DNA copy number variation using comparative genomic hybridization to microarrays. *Nat Genet* **20**: 207–211.

Plass C (2002) Cancer epigenomics. *Hum Mol Genet* **11**: 2479–2488.

Pomeroy SL, Tamayo P, Gaasenbeek M, Sturla LM, Angelo M, McLaughlin ME, Kim JY, Goumnerova LC, Black PM, Lau C, Allen JC, Zagzag D, Olson JM, Curran T, Wetmore C, Biegel JA, Poggio T, Mukherjee S, Rifkin R, Califano A, Stolovitzky G, Louis DN, Mesirov JP, Lander ES, Golub TR (2002) Prediction of central nervous system embryonal tumour outcome based on gene expression. *Nature* **415**: 436–442.

Pui CH, Campana D, Evans WE (2001) Childhood acute lymphoblastic leukaemia—current status and future perspectives. *Lancet Oncol* **2**: 597–607.

Raffel C, Frederick L, O'Fallon JR, Atherton-Skaff P, Perry A, Jenkins RB, James CD (1999) Analysis of oncogene and tumor suppressor gene alterations in pediatric malignant astrocytomas reveals reduced survival for patients with PTEN mutations. *Clin Cancer Res* **5**: 4085–4090.

Reardon DA, Michalkiewicz E, Boyett JM, Sublett JE, Entrekin RE, Ragsdale ST, Valentine MB, Behm FG, Li H, Heideman RL, Kun LE, Shapiro DN, Look AT (1997) Extensive genomic abnormalities in childhood medulloblastoma by comparative genomic hybridization. *Cancer Res* **57**: 4042–4047.

Reardon DA, Entrekin RE, Sublett J, Ragsdale S, Li H, Boyett J, Kepner JL, Look AT (1999) Chromosome arm 6q loss is the most common recurrent autosomal alteration detected in primary pediatric ependymoma. *Genes Chromosomes Cancer* **24**: 230–237.

Romer JT, Kimura H, Magdaleno S, Sasai K, Fuller C, Baines H, Connelly M, Stewart CF, Gould S, Rubin LL, Curran T (2004) Suppression of the Shh pathway using a small molecule inhibitor eliminates medulloblastoma in Ptc1(+/–)p53(–/–) mice. *Cancer Cell* **6**: 229.

Ruiz i Altaba A, Sanchez P, Dahmane N (2002) Gli and hedgehog in cancer: tumours, embryos and stem cells. *Nat Rev Cancer* **2**: 361–372.

Sausville EA, Elsayed Y, Monga M, Kim G (2003) Signal transduction—directed cancer treatments. *Annu Rev Pharmacol Toxicol* **43**: 199–231.

Scheil S, Bruderlein S, Eicker M, Herms J, Herold-Mende C, Steiner HH, Barth TF, Moller P (2001) Low frequency of chromosomal imbalances in anaplastic ependymomas as detected by comparative genomic hybridization. *Brain Pathol* **11**: 133–143.

Singh SK, Hawkins C, Clarke ID, Squire JA, Bayani J, Hide T, Henkelman RM, Cusimano MD, Dirks PB (2004) Identification of human brain tumour initiating cells. *Nature* **432**: 396–401.

Smiraglia DJ, Plass C (2002) The study of aberrant methylation in cancer via restriction landmark genomic scanning. *Oncogene* **21**: 5414–5426.

Sung T, Miller DC, Hayes RL, Alonso M, Yee H, Newcomb EW (2000) Preferential inactivation of the p53 tumor suppressor pathway and lack of EGFR amplification distinguish de novo high-grade pediatric astrocytomas from de novo adult astrocytomas. *Brain Pathol* **10**: 249–259.

Sure U, Ruedi D, Tachibana O, Yonekawa Y, Ohgaki H, Kleihues P, Hegi ME (1997) Determination of p53 mutations, EGFR overexpression, and loss of p16 expression in pediatric glioblastomas. *J Neuropathol Exp Neurol* **56**: 782–789.

Szyf M (2000) The DNA methylation machinery as a therapeutic target. *Curr Drug Targets* **1**: 101–118.

Taipale J, Chen JK, Cooper MK, Wang B, Mann RK, Milenkovic L, Scott MP, Beachy PA (2000) Effects of oncogenic mutations in Smoothened and Patched can be reversed by cyclopamine. *Nature* **406**: 1005–1009.

Takeshima H, Sawamura Y, Gilbert MR, Van Meir EG (2000) Application of advances in molecular biology to the treatment of brain tumors. *Curr Oncol Rep* **2**: 425–433.

Temple S (2001) The development of neural stem cells. *Nature* **414**: 112–117.

Trask BJ (2002) Human cytogenetics: 46 chromosomes, 46 years and counting. *Nat Rev Genet* **3**: 769–778.

Van Dyke T, Jacks T (2002) Cancer modeling in the modern era: progress and challenges. *Cell* **108**: 135–144.

Versteege I, Sevenet N, Lange J, Rousseau-Merck MF, Ambros P, Handgretinger R, Aurias A, Delattre O (1998) Truncating mutations of hSNF5/INI1 in aggressive paediatric cancer. *Nature* **394**: 203–206.

Vogel CL, Cobleigh MA, Tripathy D, Gutheil JC, Harris LN, Fehrenbacher L, Slamon DJ, Murphy M, Novotny WF, Burchmore M, Shak S, Stewart SJ, Press M (2002) Efficacy and safety of trastuzumab as a single agent in first-line treatment of HER2-overexpressing metastatic breast cancer. *J Clin Oncol* **20**: 719–726.

Vogelstein B, Kinzler KW (2004) Cancer genes and the pathways they control. *Nat Med* **10**: 789–799.

Ward S, Harding B, Wilkins P, Harkness W, Hayward R, Darling JL, Thomas DG, Warr T (2001) Gain of 1q and loss of 22 are the most common changes detected by comparative genomic hybridisation in paediatric ependymoma. *Genes Chromosomes Cancer* **32**: 59–66.

Wechsler-Reya R, Scott MP (2001) The developmental biology of brain tumors. *Annu Rev Neurosci* **24**: 385–428.

Weiss WA, Israel M, Cobbs C, Holland E, James CD, Louis DN, Marks C, McClatchey AI, Roberts T, Van Dyke T, Wetmore C, Chiu IM, Giovannini M, Guha A, Higgins RJ, Marino S, Radovanovic I, Reilly K, Aldape K (2002) Neuropathology of genetically engineered mice: consensus report and recommendations from an international forum. *Oncogene* **21**: 7453–7463.

Wong AJ, Bigner SH, Bigner DD, Kinzler KW, Hamilton SR, Vogelstein B (1987) Increased expression of the epidermal growth factor receptor gene in malignant gliomas is invariably associated with gene amplification. *Proc Natl Acad Sci USA* **84**: 6899–6903.

Wong AJ, Ruppert JM, Bigner SH, Grzeschik CH, Humphrey PA, Bigner DS, Vogelstein B (1992) Structural alterations of the epidermal growth factor receptor gene in human gliomas. *Proc Natl Acad Sci USA* **89**: 2965–2969.

Xiao W, Oefner PJ (2001) Denaturing high-performance liquid chromatography: A review. *Hum Mutat* **17**: 439–474.

Yoshida M, Furumai R, Nishiyama M, Komatsu Y, Nishino N, Horinouchi S (2001) Histone deacetylase as a new target for cancer chemotherapy. *Cancer Chemother Pharmacol* **48**: S20–S26.

Yuan X, Curtin J, Xiong Y, Liu G, Waschsmann-Hogiu S, Farkas DL, Black KL, Yu JS (2004) Isolation of cancer stem cells from adult glioblastoma multiforme. *Oncogene* **23**: 9392–9400.

Zardo G, Tiirikainen MI, Hong C, Misra A, Feuerstein BG, Volik S, Collins CC, Lamborn KR, Bollen A, Pinkel D, Albertson DG, Costello JF (2002) Integrated genomic and epigenomic analyses pinpoint biallelic gene inactivation in tumors. *Nat Genet* **32**: 453–458.

Zhu Y, Parada LF (2002) The molecular and genetic basis of neurological tumours. *Nat Rev Cancer* **2**: 616–626.

Zuzak TJ, Steinhoff DF, Sutton LN, Phillips PC, Eggert A, Grotzer MA (2002) Loss of caspase-8 mRNA expression is common in childhood primitive neuroectodermal brain tumour/medulloblastoma. *Eur J Cancer* **38**: 83–91.

6
SURGICAL MANAGEMENT OF CNS TUMOURS IN THE PAEDIATRIC POPULATION

Jerard Ross and John Thorne

Primary tumours of the central nervous system (CNS) are the most frequent solid neoplasms of childhood, occurring in around 2.5–4.0 children per 100,000 per annum (Packer 1999). The management of children with brain tumours is truly a multidisciplinary task and involves a number of medical specialists including general practitioners, radiologists, neurosurgeons, neurologists, oncologists, radiotherapists and endocrinologists. Moreover, the role played by the nursing and paramedical specialists is vital to the holistic management of these children.

Paediatric brain tumours comprise a spectrum of disease superficially similar to, but in many ways quite distinct from, adult neuro-oncological practice. Whereas for adult practice the majority of tumours occur in the supratentorial compartment, a large proportion of paediatric tumours are found infratentorially. As well as age-related differences in location for individual tumour types, age-dependent differences in tumour diagnosis are well recognized (e.g. teratomas are more common in neonates) (Jooma et al. 1984). The vast majority of adult CNS tumours are metastases or malignant tumours of glial cell origin with a very poor prognosis. For children, although tumours of glial cell origin comprise about a half of CNS tumours, they are more variable in their histology and prognosis, with a significant subgroup being curable with surgery, unlike in the adult population (Pollack 1994). Similarly, unlike in adult practice, tumours arising from neuroepithelial cells are common.

Surgery for paediatric brain tumours encompasses a range of aims varying from curative intent, to purely facilitating a biopsy, to the management of tumour or treatment-related complications. In some situations, there is no role for surgery. As with every treatment modality, consideration must be given to the limitation of morbidity associated with treatment, and it is sometimes better to limit resectional surgery to avoid functional, cognitive and endocrinological complications. Rather than listing all possible surgical interventions across the histopathological spectrum, a range of possible interventions in common paediatric tumours will be discussed, as well as general aspects of perioperative care of children with brain tumours.

General care
As tumours grow in a confined space, one of the pathological consequences can be raised

151

intracranial pressure (ICP). This can be secondary to tumour mass, peritumoural oedema and/or obstruction of CSF flow and a resultant hydrocephalus. Steroid therapy (e.g. dexamethasone 0.5 mg/kg/day) is an important adjunct to therapy and vital for preoperative management. Steroids reduce peritumoural oedema and ICP, and can improve the function in peritumoural brain. They are given in high doses initially and tapered postoperatively.

There are occasions when hydrocephalus requires treatment prior to surgery for the causative tumour, e.g. when a child is obtunded and has not responded to high dose steroids or has signs of brainstem compression. However, most surgeons would prefer to perform both a CSF diversionary procedure and resection at the same time, thereby limiting the potential for complications. CSF diversion, with an external ventricular drain, carries a risk of infection, haemorrhage, upward herniation of posterior fossa contents and subsequent brainstem compression, but is sometimes necessary. It is no longer common for ventriculo-peritoneal shunts to be inserted as this exposes patients to the risk of infection or dissemination of disease into the peritoneal cavity. Endoscopic third ventriculostomy allows internal CSF diversion and can reduce ICP safely without the need for external drainage, thus reducing the risk of infection (MacArthur et al. 2001, Sainte-Rose et al. 2001).

Tumours in the supratentorial compartment can result in seizures and it is important that these are controlled medically. Seizures, particularly focal motor or temporal lobe seizures, which are difficult to control with medication, may be the only sign of a low-grade tumour, and as resectional surgery can improve symptomatic control, imaging is always worthwhile. In the context of raised ICP, postictal states predispose to airway obstruction, and for a child with raised ICP, an obstructed or partially obstructed airway – to which children are more prone than adults – can result in retention of CO_2, further raising the ICP. For the same reason preoperative sedation should be avoided. Infratentorial tumours do not predispose to seizures.

Perioperative management
Consideration must be given to a number of different factors during surgery including the positioning of the patient and of their head, cranial stability during the operation, blood loss and ICP.

Children are positioned intraoperatively to allow easy access to the tumour. As indicated, a large proportion of paediatric tumours are in the posterior fossa, and these patients are positioned prone, reducing the risk of air embolism, pneumocephalus and systemic hypotension. Children should have no pressure on their orbits, should have their pressure areas padded to avoid ulceration and nerve damage, and be appropriately insulated to allow use of monopolar diathermy. Children with supratentorial tumours are positioned supine with their head turned or lateral. Infant's heads are generally placed in a jelly head ring or on a well padded horseshoe head rest. Older children can have their heads fixed with the Mayfield pin head rest, although it is important to ensure that the pins are not overtightened as there is a risk of skull fracture and even extradural haemorrhage (Baerts et al. 1984).

It is crucial that all steps are taken to minimize operative blood loss. Scalp bleeding, which can be significant, is reduced by infiltrating with local anaesthetic and adrenaline (e.g. 0.5% lignocaine and 1:200,000 epinephrine), and can be further reduced by elevating the level of the child's head slightly above the heart, reducing venous pressure. Haemostatic clips (e.g. Raney clips) can be applied to the skin edge, and bipolar diathermy should be used liberally. Blood loss should be accurately charted and appropriately replaced.

Elevated ICP can be aggravated by anaesthesia, and if CSF diversion has not already been employed then some neurosurgeons place a drain or perform a ventriculostomy immediately before resection. Similarly, it may be necessary to give a bolus of mannitol (an osmotic diuretic) intraoperatively to reduce this pressure. If ICP is high and the tumour has a large cystic component, then early intraoperative decompression of the cyst may improve the situation. This is of particular importance in infants as, unlike in adults, their less myelinated brain is more likely to herniate through any dural opening.

Access to tumours varies depending on the anatomical site involved. The approach to tumours of the posterior fossa is fairly standard, with a midline incision from just above the inion to the spinous process of C2–3 depending on the inferior extent of the tumour. The muscles are stripped from the occipital bone laterally to the mastoid processes on both sides and down to the foramen magnum and the posterior elements of C1 and C2. Care must be exercised in working laterally around C1 because the vertebral artery is vulnerable as it courses over C1. Generally a craniectomy is performed to open the posterior fossa, limiting the risks of postoperative swelling, allowing identification of the transverse sinus and the dura opened in a Y incision. Tumour is removed piecemeal by a combination of diathermy, suction and aspiration with the ultrasonic aspirator, with meticulous attention to haemostatic detail.

Postoperative brain swelling is always a concern, especially in posterior fossa tumours. Children who have not had CSF diversion who deteriorate should be urgently imaged looking for evidence of obstructive hydrocephalus. There are particular complications of tumour surgery in the posterior fossa that are slightly less obvious in their aetiology to the non-specialist. Dissection around the roof of the fourth ventricle while trying to achieve maximal cytoreduction can result in ocular pareses (particularly of upgaze), but these will generally recover, and when maximal tumour removal is warranted are viewed as an acceptable morbidity. Another is the phenomenon of cerebellar mutism seen postoperatively and probably secondary to dissection around the origin of the cerebellar peduncles and the brainstem, or possibly secondary to splitting the vermis. Again this tends to improve spontaneously, although speech may not return to preoperative levels (Steinbok et al. 2003).

Surgical roles in common tumours
The most common paediatric brain tumours include primitive neuroectodermal tumours, pilocytic astrocytomas, high-grade gliomas, brainstem gliomas, ependymomas and cranio-pharyngiomas.

INFRATENTORIAL TUMOURS
For infratentorial tumours a fundamental management point is the determination of tumour origin. Tumours arising from the cerebellar hemispheres, vermis or fourth ventricular floor are potentially resectable unlike those arising diffusely within the substance of the brainstem. Diffuse brainstem gliomas are best managed non-operatively, and the role of diagnostic

biopsy is questionable with the availability of high quality magnetic resonance imaging (Albright et al. 1993).

Once a decision has been made that the tumour is potentially resectable, intraoperative decisions depend on the nature of the tumour and intraoperative pathological diagnosis. Frequently a frozen section for histology is very helpful in this regard.

Around 20% of all primary CNS neoplasms are primitive neuroectodermal tumours (PNETs), and included in this group is the most common subtype, medulloblastoma, which occurs in the posterior fossa arising most frequently in the cerebellar vermis and on the floor of the fourth ventricle. These tumours have a propensity to spread early within the neuraxis, and at presentation between 11% and 43% of children have metastases (either on imaging or on CSF cytopathology). The presence of solid metastases (i.e. other than purely positive CSF cytology) has been correlated with worse outcome (Zeltzer et al. 1999). The cornerstone of therapy has historically been craniospinal irradiation; however, the long-term neurocognitive effects of irradiation on the developing nervous system are significant and chemotherapy is playing an increasingly important role in the management of these tumours, especially in children under 3 years of age (Mason et al. 1998).

Surgery, although not curative, is important, as children who undergo total or near-total resection have a better outcome (Albright et al. 1996). PNETs arising from the floor of the fourth ventricle can be shaved down to their attachment on the floor of the ventricle and out into the lateral recesses. However, there is little reason to attempt to remove tumour from below the floor, tiny fragments on cranial nerves or tumour encasing important vascular structures, e.g. the posterior inferior cerebellar artery, as to do so can significantly add to morbidity without improving outcome. This, however, is a group of patients in whom early postoperative re-scanning can show tumour foci missed at primary surgery, and if there is no evidence of metastatic disease then re-operative surgery probably has a role. Although important for the treatment of PNETs, surgery is fundamental to the management of two of the next most common posterior fossa tumours in childhood, namely low-grade gliomas (astrocytomas) and ependymomas.

Low-grade cerebellar astrocytomas comprise around 15% of primary tumours and are notable for their generally favourable long-term outcome (Garcia et al. 1989). Pathologically they can be divided into pilocytic tumours that are generally well circumscribed and form the majority of these tumours, and non-pilocytic tumours that can exhibit invasion into surrounding structures. Received wisdom would indicate that there is a difference in outcome between these two groups, although that is questionable. Gross total resection can lead to survival rates in excess of 90% at 10 years, and if early postoperative scanning shows an operable area of tumour residuum then re-operative surgery is indicated (Pollack 1999). Where initial total resection is contraindicated, i.e. where there is brainstem involvement, then follow-up scanning is generally performed and patients showing progression of disease are offered re-operative surgery. Radiotherapy probably has little role in the initial management of these tumours, although some would combine radiotherapy with re-operative surgery after disease progression.

Ependymomas account for around 5% of paediatric brain tumours, and overall 5-year survival is around 60%, with 10-year survival of 45% (Healey et al. 1991, Vanuytsel et al.

1992). Again, the extent of surgical resection is strongly linked to outcome and gross total resection improves the prognosis significantly. For example, the 5-year progression-free and overall survivals were 8.9% and 22%, respectively, among patients who had evidence of residual disease on postoperative imaging studies, compared with 68% and 80% rates among patients with no apparent residual disease (Pollack et al. 1995b). Imaging of the whole of the neuraxis is indicated, as these tumours can metastasize. Evidence of metastasis will change postoperative radiotherapy from local tumour bed radiotherapy, where most recurrences occur, to craniospinal irradiation. Given that more than half of ependymomas arise in children under 5 years of age, there has been increasing interest in chemotherapeutic strategies to limit the application of craniospinal irradiation to the immature brain.

Not all brainstem gliomas are diffuse and inoperable. A significant proportion are indolent, especially tectal plate tumours, and in this situation, CSF diversion and observation is a reasonable strategy. Some brainstem gliomas are more histologically aggressive but can be well demarcated or exophytic, rather than diffuse, and respond well to resection. The diffuse brainstem gliomas have a very poor prognosis, and even with radiotherapy most children do not survive for 1 year. Surgery seldom has a role for these patients, although with improvements in chemotherapy, stereotactic biopsy may be indicated in future support of molecular targeted therapies.

SUPRATENTORIAL TUMOURS

As in adults, the most common supratentorial primary tumours of the CNS in children are of glial origin. Unlike in adults, where such tumours tend to be high grade and incurable, even children with what appear to be malignant tumours can do relatively well after appropriate therapy.

As in the posterior fossa, the most common type of glioma in the supratentorial compartment is of low-grade histology. These can be pilocytic, non-pilocytic, mixed or oligodendrogliomas. As in the posterior fossa, pilocytic tumours often have distinct margins making resection easier, although resection of tumours, of whatever pathological subtype, is limited by the functional constraints of surrounding brain. As in the posterior fossa, total resection is associated with significant survival, up to 93% at 10 years in selected series (Pollack et al 1995a). Radiotherapy is not generally employed unless there is subtotal resection and evidence of progression on serial imaging, and there is a trend to administration of chemotherapy for treatment of unresectable disease (Packer et al. 1997). Early postoperative imaging and second-look surgery may have a role in these tumours. High-grade gliomas are treated with maximal resection, and although numbers are limited it seems to improve outcome, as does the use of adjuvant chemotherapy (Wisoff et al. 1998).

Tumours of the optic pathway or optico-hypothalamic gliomas are tumours of childhood, which are variable in their extent, behaviour and outcome. They are strongly associated with type 1 neurofibromatosis (NF1); 20% of children with NF1 have these tumours, and 50% of children with these tumours have stigmata of NF1. It is while performing MR screening of children with this condition that the full range of appearance of these tumours has become apparent, from mild thickening of the optic nerves to large tumour masses involving the optic chiasm, hypothalamus, third ventricle and even the frontal and temporal

155

lobes. Tumours can be asymptomatic, or present with mild visual symptomatology or with full blown optical impairment, endocrinological dysfunction and hydrocephalus, although this latter presentation is rare (Pollack and Mulvihill 1996).

In children without NF1 and with exophytic tumours causing mass effect (i.e. shifting the surrounding brain), some would argue that there is a role for debulking surgery, although this will not be curative and runs the risk of hypothalamic injury (Wisoff et al. 1990). Others would suggest biopsy and then adjuvant therapy (Pierce et al. 1990). Radiotherapy has long been used in the treatment of these tumours, although the side-effects of irradiating this area are significant and chemotherapy is having an increased role especially for children less than 5 years of age (Petronio et al. 1991). The role of surgery is much more difficult in the minimally symptomatic patient, especially in the context of NF1 where these tumours have been demonstrated to remain stable for years. It is reasonable to suggest that the majority of optic pathway gliomas do not require urgent therapy, and such therapy can be delayed until disease progression is documented. This delay often avoids the harmful long-term sequelae of radiotherapy in the developing brain (Duffner et al. 1985, Radcliffe et al. 1992).

When considering tumours that arise close to the optic tract, one other tumour type that is more frequently found in children is the craniopharyngioma. This is a histologically benign tumour that is cystic and often calcified, which because of its site of occurrence around the pituitary stalk, and adherence to important structures, the optic nerves, the hypothalamus and vessels of the circle of Willis, presents a significant surgical challenge.

Management of these tumours is controversial and discussed in more detail elsewhere in this volume (Chapter 16). Full surgical resection of these tumours can result in cure, but aggressive surgery, particularly around the feeding vessels to the hypothalamus, can give rise to very severe postoperative sequelae. Children in the postoperative period can have severe metabolic disturbance including diabetes insipidus and temperature dysregulation (both of which can be fatal). If children get over these initial complications, then they can develop severe appetite and weight problems, growth failure, behavioural and cognitive difficulties, and predispostition to pan-hypopituitarism secondary to damage to the pituitary stalk. Although there has been a vogue to aggressive resection from both North America and Europe (Yasargil et al 1990, Hoffman et al 1992), there may be a role for less aggressive surgery to debulk the tumour and to decompress the cyst, followed by external beam or intracavitary radiotherapy depending on the age of the patient (Habrand et al. 1999).

Supratentorial PNETs and ependymomas are similar to their infratentorial counterparts but carry a worse prognosis, and their resection is often limited by the eloquence of surrounding tissue. For both tumour types radiotherapy has a role, and for PNETs there is a role for chemotherapy.

Adjuncts to surgical management
FUNCTIONAL MRI
One of the questions that must be asked when planning surgery for paediatric brain tumours is the relationship of the tumour to eloquent areas of the brain. With deep seated tumours such as those of the brainstem or basal ganglia this may be easy to predict, but for more

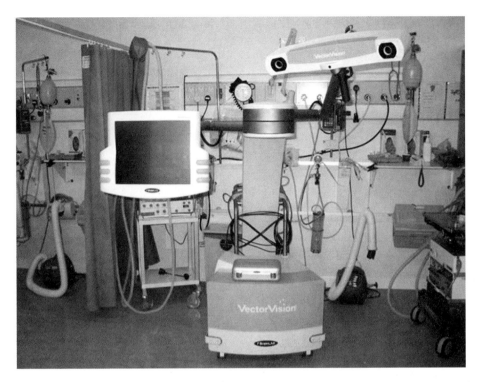

Fig. 6.1. Image guidance system (courtesy of BrainLAB, Cambridge, England).

superficial tumours anatomically close to the motor strip it may be more difficult. The possibility that what appears to be tumour on standard imaging may actually be functioning brain, especially in the case of low-grade gliomas, must also be considered.

Functional MRI is not easy to perform in adults and can be even more complicated in children. To allow accurate mapping of the motor cortex, a patient must be compliant and able to consistently perform a repetitive task. In young children this cannot be achieved, but with older children it can be considered. The ability to plot eloquent areas of the brain in relation to a tumour can make aggressive surgical resection safer. Unfortunately, a guarantee can never be offered that a deficit will not result from resection of a brain tumour, as the vascular supply to the motor cortex may go through the tumour under resection.

IMAGE-GUIDED SURGERY

In the past 10–15 years image guided surgery using frameless stereotaxy has become routine (Fig. 6.1). Frameless stereotaxy depends on computerized systems that allow the correlation of the patient's head position on the operating table with preoperative scan images (CT, MRI or cerebral angiograms). Many different systems are available and they allow the surgeon to know exactly where they are in the brain while operating (Sandeman et al. 1995, Wirtz et al. 1998). The preoperative scans are reconstructed to allow a computer generated three-dimensional image of the head to be produced. This is registered to the patient once they are in the operating theatre, and images of the brain are then displayed on a screen. Using the system allows the surgeon both to plan the safest operative approach (for deep seated tumours) and to use the smallest useful incision and craniotomy (for superficial cortical tumours). When the demarcation between normal brain and tumour is not clear, a more aggressive resection can be achieved as the surgeon can have greater certainty in deciding which tissue is abnormal and which is normal.

AWAKE CRANIOTOMY

Many of the first neurosurgical operations were performed without general anaesthesia. With the introduction of safe anaesthetics, operating under general anaesthesia became the norm. However, for tumours situated in eloquent cortex, another method of reducing the risk of producing a motor deficit and maximizing resection of a tumour is to operate under local anaesthetic, and to stimulate the affected cortex prior to resection. In principle this reduces the risk of producing a deficit (Jaaskelainen and Randell 2003).

However, the technique of neurosurgery under local anaesthesia is extremely complicated. Unless the patient is extremely compliant they will require a general anaesthetic to perform the craniotomy, and then need to be safely woken up before the surgical resection can take place. The process of the operation is extremely frightening and the effect of cortical stimulation often very unpleasant. It is therefore not a technique that is suitable for younger children. Whether better results can be achieved is debatable and it is only considered for a small percentage of tumours.

INTRAOPERATIVE MRI

One of the problems with image-guided surgery is that the brain anatomy changes per-operatively. This happens in two ways: first, on opening the dura CSF leaks out of the skull, which can lead to brain shift; and second the local anatomy of the brain changes during brain resection. As has been emphasized previously, the degree of surgical resection is related to outcome with many different brain tumours, and often the differentiation between normal and abnormal tissue can be difficult during surgery. This has led to the use of intraoperative MRI to allow maximal resection (Vitaz et al. 2003).

However, this poses many logistical problems. MRI scanners are large and bulky, and therefore specific suites have to be built to accommodate them. The strengths of the magnetic fields produced by the magnets mandates that the suites have specially built walls, and all equipment within the suites has to be non-ferrous, which produces difficulties for not just surgical but also anaesthetic equipment.

All these difficulties have been overcome, and brain suites such as the one shown in Figure 6.2 are now commercially available. The patient can undergo surgical resection and then, on the same operating table, be placed in the MRI. Any residual tumour can then be identified and resected. In principal this should lead to complete resection whenever this is anatomically possible. It is as yet unclear as to which tumours will be most suitable for this technique, but the technique may be most useful for those tumours where complete surgical resection makes a significant difference to long-term survival.

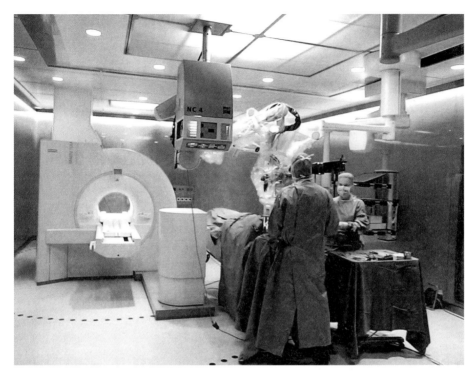

Fig. 6.2. Operative MRI suite (courtesy of BrainLAB, Cambridge, England).

The role of neuroendoscopy in tumour management

Endoscopy is involved in the diagnosis of paediatric brain tumours, the management of obstructive hydrocephalus, and occasionally the surgical resection of, or treatment of, brain tumours.

Hydrocephalus is a common complication of infratentorial tumours. Although surgical removal of the tumour is normally indicated, this does not always lead to cure of the hydrocephalus, and up to 20% of children who undergo surgical resection of an infratentorial tumour will, subsequently, require a CSF diversionary procedure (Gnanalingham et al. 2003). This high rate has led some centres to advocate pre-resection third ventriculostomy for posterior fossa tumours, both to improve the operative conditions and to avoid the possible complications of external ventricular drain and shunt insertion.

At the same time as performing a third ventriculostomy it is also sometimes possible to biopsy fourth ventricular tumours by passing the flexible endoscope through the dilated sylvian aqueduct. The endoscope can also be used to biopsy tumours situated in the lateral or third ventricles. This is particularly relevant to pineal region tumours where there is often hydrocephalus, and again a biopsy can be obtained at the same time as a third ventriculostomy is performed.

Some tumours, such as craniopharyngiomas, are very cystic. The management of craniopharyngiomas has historically been based on very aggressive surgical resection but

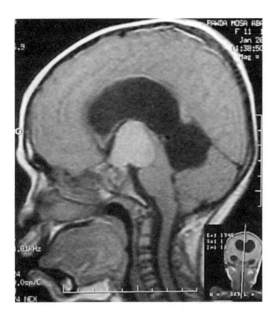

Fig. 6.3. MRI of cystic craniopharyngioma that is suitable for endoscopic drainage and marsupialization.

as many centres now move toward a more conservative approach the endoscope can be used to drain and marsupialize cysts prior to radiotherapy (Fig. 6.3). Some surgeons use the endoscope to remove small intraventricular lesions, although this can be technically difficult and hazardous because of the difficulties in controlling bleeding.

Epilepsy surgery

One of the classical ways in which space-occupying lesions in the brain may present is with seizures. This is particularly common with benign lesions. With improved imaging techniques smaller abnormal foci can be found and this often present difficult surgical decisions.

If there is any doubt about the pathological nature of a brain tumour, then surgery, either to biopsy or remove the lesion, is indicated. Often, however, the histological diagnosis can be predicted from the imaging alone. Good seizure control may be achieved easily using only one antiepileptic drug and then the question of whether or not surgical resection can be justified is raised.

Surgery for epilepsy is an expanding area of paediatric neurosurgery. As surgical resection has become safer with better anaesthesia and improved surgical techniques, the risk/benefit ratio has changed. From published large series the chances of cure or significant improvement of epilepsy for temporal lesions is 90% and for non-temporal lesions is 70%. It must be remembered that the risk of sudden death from epilepsy is at least 1 in 1000 per year. The possibility of surgery in children presenting with epilepsy who have resectable lesions must always be considered.

Many benign lesions, such as dysembryoplastic neuroepithelial tumours (DNETs) and low-grade gliomas, are now being resected for epilepsy management when in the past they would not have been picked up on imaging (with MRI now being routinely available in

160

place of CT) or would have been watched on serial imaging (as the risks of surgery were not felt to be justified).

Conclusion

The surgical approach to paediatric brain tumours differs to that in the adult population. In many of the common paediatric tumours the degree of surgical resection has been shown to make a significant difference to the long-term outcome. A child's brain has a greater degree of plasticity and this allows the surgeon to take a more aggressive approach to resection.

Improvements in imaging and the development of image guided surgery (using frameless stereotaxy) have made surgery safer and are helping to reduce the morbidity associated with removal of brain tumours. Although developments in chemotherapeutic regimens are improving the long-term outcomes of many paediatric tumours, surgery seems likely to remain vital to their initial management.

REFERENCES

Albright AL, Packer RJ, Zimmerman R, Rorke LB, Boyett J, Hammond GD (1993) Magnetic resonance scans should replace biopsies for the diagnosis of diffuse brainstem gliomas: a report from the Children's Cancer Group. *Neurosurgery* **33**: 1026–1030.

Albright AL, Wisoff JH, Zeltzer PM, Boyett JM, Rorke LB, Stanley P (1996) Effects of medulloblastoma resections on outcome in children: a report from the Children's Cancer Group. *Neurosurgery* **38**: 265–271.

Baerts WD, de Lange JJ, Booij LH, Broere G (1984) Complications of the Mayfield skull clamp. *Anesthesiology* **61**: 460–461.

Duffner PK, Cohen ME, Voorhess ML, MacGillivray MH, Brecher ML, Panahon A, Gilani BB (1985) Long-term effects of cranial irradiation on endocrine function in children with brain tumors. A prospective study. *Cancer* **56**: 2189–2193.

Garcia DM, Latifi HR, Simpson JR, Picker S (1989) Astrocytomas of the cerebellum in children. *J Neurosurg* **71**: 661–664.

Gnanalingham KK, Lafuente J, Thompson D, Harkness W, Hayward R (2003) The natural history of ventriculo-megaly and tonsillar herniation in children with posterior fossa tumours—an MRI study. *Pediatr Neurosurg* **39**: 246–253.

Habrand J-L, Ganry O, Couanet D, Rouxel V, Levy-Piedbios C, Pierre-Kahn A, Kalifa C (1999) The role of radiation therapy in the management of craniopharyngioma: a 25 year experience and review of the literature. *Int J Radiat Oncol Biol Phys* **44**: 255–263.

Healey EA, Barnes PD, Kupsky WJ, Scott RM, Sallan SE, Black PM, Tarbell NJ (1991) The prognostic significance of postoperative residual tumor in ependymoma. *Neurosurgery* **28**: 666–671.

Hoffman HJ, De Silva M, Humphreys RP, Drake JM, Smith ML, Blaser SI (1992) Aggressive surgical manage-ment of craniopharyngiomas in children. *J Neurosurg* **76**: 47–52.

Jaaskelainen J, Randell T (2003) Awake craniotomy in glioma surgery. *Acta Neurochir* **88** (Suppl.): 31–35.

Jooma R, Hayward RD, Grant DN (1984) Intracranial neoplasms during the first year of life: analysis of one hundred consecutive cases. *Neurosurgery* **14**: 31–41.

MacArthur DC, Buxton N, Vloeberghs M, Punt J (2001) The effectiveness of neuroendoscopic interventions in children with brain tumours. *Child's Nerv Syst* **17**: 589–594.

Mason WP, Grovas A, Halpern S, Dunkel IJ, Garvin J, Heller G, Rosenblum M, Gardner S, Lyden D, Sands S, Puccetti D, Lindsley K, Merchant TE, O'Malley B, Bayer L, Petriccione MM, Allen J, Finlay JL (1998) Intensive chemotherapy and bone marrow rescue for young children with newly diagnosed malignant brain tumors. *J Clin Oncol* **16**: 210–221.

Packer RJ, Ater J, Allen J, Phillips P, Geyer R, Nicholson HS, Jakacki R, Kurczynski E, Needle M, Finlay J, Reaman G, Boyett JM (1997) Carboplatin and vincristine chemotherapy for children with newly diagnosed progressive low-grade gliomas. *J Neurosurg* **86**: 747–754.

Packer RJ (1999) Brain tumours in children. *Arch Neurol* **56**: 421–425.

Petronio J, Edwards MS, Prados M, Freyberger S, Rabbitt J, Silver P, Levin VA (1991) Management of chiasmal and hypothalamic gliomas of infancy and childhood with chemotherapy. *J Neurosurg* **74**: 701–708.

Pierce SM, Barnes PD, Loeffler JS, McGinn C, Tarbell NJ (1990) Definitive radiation therapy in the management of symptomatic patients with optic glioma. Survival and long-term effects. *Cancer* **65**: 45–52.

Pollack IF (1994) Brain tumours in children. *N Engl J Med* **331**: 1500–1507.

Pollack IF (1999) The role of surgery in paediatric gliomas. *J Neurooncol* **42**: 271–288.

Pollack IF, Mulvihill JJ (1996) Special issues in the management of gliomas in children with neurofibromatosis 1. *J Neurooncol* **28**: 257–268.

Pollack IF, Claassen D, al-Shboul Q, Janosky JE, Deutsch M (1995a) Low-grade gliomas of the cerebral hemispheres in children: an analysis of 71 cases. *J Neurosurg* **82**: 536–547.

Pollack IF, Gerszten PC, Martinez AJ, Lo KH, Shultz B, Albright AL, Janosky J, Deutsch M (1995b) Intracranial ependymomas of childhood: long-term outcome and prognostic factors. *Neurosurgery* **37**: 655–666.

Radcliffe J, Packer RJ, Atkins TE, Bunin GR, Schut L, Goldwein JW, Sutton LN (1992) Three- and four-year cognitive outcome in children with noncortical brain tumors treated with whole-brain radiotherapy. *Ann Neurol* **32**: 551–554.

Sainte-Rose C, Cinalli G, Roux FE, Maixner R, Chumas PD, Mansour M, Carpentier A, Bourgeois M, Zerah M, Pierre-Kahn A, Renier D (2001) Management of hydrocephalus in pediatric patients with posterior fossa tumors: the role of endoscopic third ventriculostomy. *J Neurosurg* **95**: 791–797.

Sandeman DR, Gill SS (1995) The impact of interactive image guided surgery: the Bristol experience with the ISG/Elekta viewing Wand. *Acta Neurochir Suppl* **64**: 54–58.

Steinbok P, Cochrane DD, Perrin R, Price A (2003) Mutism after posterior fossa tumour resection in children: incomplete recovery on long-term follow-up. *Pediatr Neurosurg* **39**: 179–183.

Vanuytsel LJ, Bessell EM, Ashley SE, Bloom HJ, Brada M (1992) Intracranial ependymoma: long-term results of a policy of surgery and radiotherapy. *Int J Radiat Oncol Biol Phys* **23**: 313–319.

Vitaz TW, Hushek S, Shields CB, Moriarty T (2003) Intraoperative MRI for pediatric tumor management. *Acta Neurochir Suppl* **85**: 73–78.

Wirtz CR, Knauth M, Hassfeld S, Tronnier VM, Albert FK, Bonsanto MM, Kunze S (1998) Neuronavigation – first experiences with three different commercially available systems. *Zentralbl Neurochir* **59**: 14–22.

Wisoff JH, Abbott R, Epstein F (1990) Surgical management of exophytic chiasmatic–hypothalamic tumors of childhood. *J Neurosurg* **73**: 661–667.

Wisoff JH, Boyett JM, Berger MS, Brant C, Hao L, Yates AJ, McGuire-Cullen P, Turski PA, Sutton LN, Allen JC, Packer RJ, Finlay JL (1998) Current neurosurgical management and the impact of the extent of resection in the treatment of malignant gliomas of childhood: a report of the Children's Cancer Group Trial No. CCG-945. *J Neurosurg* **89**: 52–59.

Yasargil MG, Curcic M, Kis M, Siegenthaler G, Teddy PJ, Roth P (1990) Total removal of craniopharyngioma. *J Neurosurg* **73**: 3–11.

Zeltzer PM, Boyett JM, Finlay JL, Albright AL, Rorke LB, Milstein JM, Allen JC, Stevens KR, Stanley P, Li H, Wisoff JH, Geyer JR, McGuire-Cullen P, Stehbens JA, Shurin SB, Packer RJ (1999) Metastasis stage, adjuvant treatment, and residual tumor are prognostic factors for medulloblastoma in children: conclusions from the Children's Cancer Group 921 randomized phase III study. *J Clin Oncol* **17**: 832–845.

162

7
GENERAL PRINCIPLES OF RADIOTHERAPY

Eddy Estlin and Stephen Lowis

Radiotherapy has been the mainstay of therapy for childhood CNS tumours for the past 50 years. The recognition that children required craniospinal radiotherapy for the treatment of medulloblastoma led to the first reported cures of children with this cancer (Paterson and Farr 1953), and the advent of supervoltage technology in the 1950s provided better distribution of radiation throughout the tumour while sparing normal tissues. With radiation treatment, the improvements in survival for children with medulloblastoma in the 1950s and 1960s were comparable to those achieved for children with acute lymphoblastic leukaemia and Wilms' tumour over the same period (Vines and Betsch 2001). In more recent years, the development of computerized treatment planning, simulation exercises, customized blocking and more precisely defined margins of radiotherapy delivery have increased both efficacy and tolerability.

The aim of this chapter is to introduce the physical and biological principles of radiotherapy, to describe contemporary techniques for radiotherapy administration, to highlight the role of radiotherapy for the treatment of childhood CNS tumours, and to summarize treatment-related toxicity. Finally, we will discuss the possible future directions for radiotherapy in the treatment of childhood CNS tumours.

Radiotherapy physics and biology

Radiation energy causes ionization of water molecules and free radical generation, which cause damage to cellular macromolecules. Damage to cells is caused by the effect of radiotherapy on DNA, with cell death resulting from DNA strand breaks, apoptosis or necrosis.

The interaction of radiation with matter – in particular, living tissue - is a function of the energy of the radiation, the type of radiation (photon, electron, protons, alpha particles), and the tissue itself. For example, a photon with energy between 50 and 550 keV typically produces Compton scattering: a photon interacts with an outer electron of an atom, and transfers part of its energy to that electron. The photon is scattered, and the electron is ejected from the atom, to impart its energy to another atom. The scattered photon, which has a lower energy than the original, may go on to interact with another electron, and may transfer all of its energy, producing a so-called photo-electron. The interaction of photons with matter is infrequent compared to other forms of radiation, and the beam may penetrate to deep within the exposed tissue.

The interaction of charged particles – electrons, protons and alpha particles – differs significantly. Electrical interactions with matter are frequent, and result in more complete transfer of energy to the tissue within a shorter interval. Interactions lead to excitation of atoms – promotion of an inner orbital electron to an outer orbit – or ionization, with ejection of an electron from the atom. The absorbed dose of energy per unit mass from radiotherapy is measured in Grays (1 Gy = 1 Joule/kg), and the amount of energy transferred to a tissue by a radiation beam per unit distance is referred to as the linear energy transfer (LET). Photons have a low LET, are relatively sparing of superficial structures such as skin, and will penetrate right through the patient. Electrons, protons and alpha particles have a high LET, and deposit their energy within a few centimetres of the skin surface. Photons will therefore have an effect at sites along the radiation plane, and will deliver energy to tissues beyond the target field. Electrons penetrate to superficial regions only, and in theory should cause fewer sequelae in structures beyond the target area.

Improved precision in delivery of radiation therapy has been a significant advance in radiotherapy in the last decade. In order for a treatment field to be targeted to a treatment area selectively, radiation fields are collimated using shields within the machine, between the machine and the patient, and sometimes at the surface of the patient's skin. The distribution of radiation energy within the patient can be modelled, and those regions receiving the same exposure to radiation (so-called iso-dose lines) identified for particular planning fields.

Techniques of radiotherapy administration
Immobilization of the patient, such that precise radiation fields can be targeted repeatedly, is of major importance. Adults and older children are able to cooperate, and immobilization by the use of head fixation with a facemask is commonly used (Kortmann et al. 1995). In younger children, this may mean the need for sedation or even a general anaesthetic. For stereotactic fields, more precise localization is required, and anatomical landmarks will be used. A mouth bite is often used, but in very young children with no teeth, the external auditory meatus and nares may be used.

Effective treatment planning involves delineation of the anatomical extent of tumour, selection of a treatment strategy such as craniospinal radiotherapy, computations of radiotherapy distributions within the volume of interest, and definition of the gross tumour volume and clinical target volume. CT or MRI is used to define the extent of the tumour, or gross target volume (GTV). Depending upon the nature of the tumour, and the known pattern of recurrence, an additional margin will be added to this, defining the clinical target volume (CTV). Finally, the planning target volume (PTV) is determined from the CTV, with added margins for movement, breathing and variations in set-up and positioning. Simulation of treatment, with a specially designed diagnostic X-ray machine, allows the accuracy of the proposed therapy to be determined, and dosimetry and verification procedures throughout treatment are standard clinical practice (Vines and Betsch 2001). Treatment with radiotherapy is usually administered in standard daily fractions of 1.8–2.0 Gy, given on 5 days per week until the target dose of radiotherapy is achieved. This protraction of treatment over several weeks allows acutely reacting tissues to recover during treatment, and allows for the relative preservation of late reacting tissues such as the brain and spinal cord. Tumours with a short cellular doubling time may also proliferate during protracted periods of administration of radiotherapy, and both hyperfractionation and accelerated hyperfractionation of the radiotherapy dose have been proposed in order to overcome this.

For hyperfractionated radiotherapy, smaller fractions of radiotherapy are administered on a twice or three times daily basis (e.g. 1 Gy twice daily), resulting in a moderately increased total dose of radiotherapy administered in a time that is similar to conventional dosing. Accelerated fractionation, delivers a conventional dose of radiotherapy in a shorter time, and accelerated hyperfractionated schedules deliver more than one treatment per day. These regimens are thought to result in a higher proportion of cells being irradiated while they are in the radiosensitive stage of the cell cycle, but with relative sparing of late reacting tissues (Fowler 1984).

Standard practice for radiotherapy in children with CNS tumours is the use of three-dimensional conformal radiotherapy, with the incorporation into computerized treatment planning of three-dimensional information on the anatomy, radiation beams and dosimetry. Conformal therapy seeks to shape the iso-dose volume to closely approximate the contours of any given target volume, and may therefore spare adjacent CNS structures from the late effects of radiotherapy (Fallai and Olmi 1997). Using several (typically four to six) radiation fields along perpendicular axes, it is possible to produce steep gradients of radiation dose, minimizing the radiation dose to normal brain. Stereotactic radiotherapy fields such as these are practical up to perhaps 5 cm; beyond this, the sparing of normal tissue is limited. For very small targets, it may be possible to use numerous fine radiation fields, and to administer a very high radiation dose locally – sufficient to cause cell necrosis – while almost completely sparing adjacent structures. Stereotactic radiosurgery (so-called 'gamma knife' surgery) has proven extremely effective in patients with small inaccessible tumours, for whom conventional surgery is best avoided (Hodgson et al. 2001).

Intensity modulated radiation therapy (IMRT) is a novel technique for conformal treatment planning that optimizes the concept of computer-controlled radiation deposition within a tumour while sparing adjacent structures, and is in the early stages of clinical evaluation for children with CNS tumours (Teh et al. 2002). Another technique that is undergoing evaluation in some North American treatment centres is proton irradiation. Proton irradiation is characterized by a highly constricted dose distribution in tissue, with the potential of enhanced tissue sparing when compared with photon irradiation despite an equivalent potential for tumour cell kill (Wambersie et al. 1992).

Although employed much less frequently than conventional, external beam radiotherapy techniques, brachytherapy has an established place for carefully selected patients with certain low-grade tumours. Brachytherapy involves the placement of a radioactive source directly within the tumour, or a cavity within the tumour. Instillation of colloidal ^{90}yttrium into cystic craniopharyngioma and low-grade astrocytoma has been shown to be an effective way of controlling recurrence while avoiding significant irradiation of surrounding normal brain (Blackburn et al. 1999).

Side-effects of radiotherapy

Acute side-effects have their onset during or immediately following radiotherapy, and are generally a function of age, the volume of tissue irradiated and the quality of the radiation. Acute side-effects commonly found with brain irradiation include fatigue, nausea, anorexia, vomiting, headache, otitis externa, hair loss and radiation dermatitis. Early delayed effects may occur up to 6 months after irradiation and include Lhermitte's sign (a feeling of electric shock brought on by flexion of the neck) and radiation-induced somnolence (Jeremic et al. 1991, Fein et al. 1993). Lhermitte's sign usually appears within 6–8 weeks of completion of craniospinal radiotherapy, and resolves within 9 months of onset (Sheline 1975). Somnolence, with preceding anorexia and irritability, appears between the 4th and 8th weeks after completion of whole brain irradiation, and usually lasts for between 10 and 38 days (Vines and Betsch 2001, Freeman et al. 2002).

The late effects of radiotherapy carry more importance in terms of cognitive function and quality of life than do more immediate side-effects. The late effects of radiotherapy for CNS tumours include neurocognitive deficits, endocrine dysfunction, secondary tumours, alopecia, hearing loss and radiation necrosis. The latter is an increasingly likely consequence of radiotherapy following doses >60 Gy. Radiation necrosis typically presents of a mass lesion with surrounding oedema, and may therefore be confused with a second primary tumour. Surgical excision is necessary for diagnosis and treatment. A similar, but extremely rare consequence to spinal cord sensory and motor function, termed radiation myelopathy, is also described following localized radiotherapy to the spinal cord (Koehler et al. 1996).

The effect of whole brain radiotherapy on full scale IQ is related to the age of the patient and the dose of radiotherapy received. Thus whole brain radiotherapy doses of 24 Gy that have no major impact on intellectual outcome for children over 6 years of age may cause impairment in younger children, and doses >24 Gy cause reductions in full scale IQ even in older children (Fuss et al. 2000). The consideration of late effects is particularly important when considering patients with tumours such as low-grade glioma, where long-term control of disease will be achieved with treatment. Children with hypothalamic and optic chiasm tumours, particularly younger children and those with type 1 neurofibromatosis (NF1), are at increased risk of endocrinopathy with growth and thyroid hormone failures, moya-moya vasculopathy and other cerebrovascular accidents, and an adverse neurocognitive outcome (Kortmann et al. 2003). Children receiving cranial radiotherapy are also at risk of sensorineural deafness, a risk that is amplified by the concomitant use of cisplatin (Schell et al. 1989).

Nonperioperative cerebrovascular accidents are more common in children with a diagnosis of a CNS tumour. One retrospective institutional review found these to occur within a range of 0.3–15.8 years from diagnosis. Treatment with radiotherapy and the finding of an optic pathway glioma were the only associated variables (Bowers et al. 2002).

Radiation-induced tumours are a reported late effect of CNS irradiation, occur in or immediately adjacent to the radiation portals, and are a significant cause of death in long-term survivors of childhood CNS tumour therapy. The occurrence of secondary CNS tumours may be as high as 19% at 30 years follow-up, and patients with an inherited risk of tumour predisposition, such as retinoblastoma or neurofibromatosis, are at an increased risk of sarcoma, leukaemia, lymphoma and secondary CNS tumours (Jenkin 1996). Salvati et al. (2003) described the occurrence of secondary gliomas with an average latency of 9.6 years following radiotherapy, and meningiomas, predominantly malignant forms, in the second decade of life following childhood radiotherapy.

Radiotherapy and the treatment of CNS tumours of childhood

Radiotherapy is the most important treatment modality for many childhood CNS tumours, including medulloblastoma/PNET, glioma and ependymoma. The indications for radiotherapy, the dose administered, and the extent of irradiation of the neuraxis vary with tumour type and age, and strategies to refine and develop the role of radiotherapy for the treatment of childhood CNS tumours are central to national and international studies. In this section the current role of radiotherapy will be discussed for childhood CNS glioma, PNET/medulloblastoma and ependymoma. The role of radiation therapy for intracranial germ cell tumours is discussed in detail in Chapter 14. For other diseases such as craniopharyngioma, the reader is referred to the disease-specific chapters that follow.

LOW- AND HIGH-GRADE ASTROCYTOMA

A dose–response relationship exists for the use of radiotherapy for both low- and high-grade astrocytomas (Mornex et al. 1993). Radiotherapy doses that exceed 60 Gy are more frequently associated with complications such as radionecrosis: for adults with low-grade glioma, equivalent survival has been found for patients who were randomized to receive either 50.4 Gy or 64 Gy by conventional fractionation (Shaw et al. 2002).

For children, the role of radiotherapy in low-grade astrocytoma is less clear than in adults, reflecting the greater risk and more severe sequelae from radiotherapy at a young age. Radiotherapy has been shown to improve progression-free, but not overall, survival in adults with low-grade glioma (Karim et al. 2002), and similar results after radiotherapy in childhood have also been reported. No benefit in overall survival for either supra- or infratentorial tumours was seen in the series reported by Garcia et al. (1989) or by Pollack et al. (1995a). This becomes an important consideration in view of the risk of secondary malignancy or malignant transformation of low-grade tumours following radiotherapy (Vines and Betsch 2001).

The surgical resectability of a tumour is an important determinant of whether radiotherapy should be used. Incompletely resected cerebral cortical lesions may have a good prognosis without further therapy, and subsequent progression may not adversely affect either survival or quality of life. A 'watch and wait' policy is often acceptable for such patients. For children with incomplete resection of a cerebellar astrocytoma involving the floor of the fourth ventricle, recurrence may involve infiltration of the cerebellar peduncle or brainstem and consequent cranial nerve palsies, and for these patients radiotherapy may be indicated at an early stage given the potential serious nature of local recurrence.

Patients with hypothalamic region tumours present particular difficulties given the reported very poor prognosis without radiotherapy, and favourable prognosis for those who do receive radiotherapy (Montgomery et al. 1977, Tenny et al. 1982). The need to avoid irradiation of the diencephalon at an early age means that radiotherapy is not considered as a first line therapy for children below the age of 5–7 years and, as will be discussed in Chapter 10, the role of chemotherapy is being defined for this situation. In addition, a report by Tihan et al. (1999) indicated a particularly poor prognosis for infants with hypothalamic astrocytoma. Whilst these data may reflect a different pathology in infants, the poor overall survival seems, at least in part, to be accounted for by the lack of radiotherapy given to these patients. It has been our experience that such tumours typically respond well to chemotherapy, and radiotherapy can be successfully delayed for up to 4 years.

The age at which radiotherapy can be considered acceptable must be decided for the individual patient, balancing the potential risks of repeated surgical interventions, uncertainty of chemotherapy response and risks to specific areas such as visual pathways, with the overall adverse effects of radiotherapy to intellectual or endocrine function. Chemotherapy is preferred for younger children, and for all children with NF1.

Radiotherapy is indicated for recurrent or progressive tumours where chemotherapy or surgery is not considered appropriate. Response to radiotherapy may be less than that seen in patients who have received no prior therapy (Janss et al. 1995), although this was not seen in the recent SIOP low-grade glioma study (Gnekow et al. 2000).

Given the potential sequelae of radiotherapy, which are numerous and potentially severe, and the lack of evidence for improvement in overall survival in low-grade glioma (LGG), attempts have been made to reduce overall exposure. A dose–response relationship is apparent for LGG, with exposure to doses of less than 40 Gy being associated with higher failure rates. Most regimes adopt a total dose of 45–54 Gy, with fractions of 1.8 Gy or less. Conversely, there seems to be no benefit to increasing radiation dose beyond 50 Gy. A study in adult patients by Shaw et al. (2002) reported no benefit from escalation to 64 Gy by conventional fractionation, but rather an increased risk of radiation necrosis.

The importance of radiation field planning is high in low-grade astrocytoma as for other more aggressive tumours. Local control can be achieved for the majority of patients, but accurately defined fields may reduce long-term sequelae by limiting the amount of normal brain exposed to radiation. Computer assisted treatment planning is necessary to determine the target volume, and conformal treatment techniques should be used wherever possible.

The role of radiotherapy is well established for high-grade glioma, and is summarized in Chapter 10. Studies in adults have demonstrated a clear survival advantage. A dose–effect relationship exists, with radiotherapy doses of 54–60 Gy being more effective than 35–50 Gy (Marchese and Chang 1990). High-grade astrocytoma is typically infiltrative, spreading beyond the resection margin even where surgical clearance appears to be complete. Recurrence occurs most often within 2 cm of the original tumour site, and it is conventional to irradiate these tumours locally, with a 2 cm margin in all directions (Vines and Betsch 2001).

The effectiveness of radiotherapy is also influenced by the extent of tumour resection, with radical resection improving the survival of patients with high-grade glioma who receive subsequent radiotherapy and chemotherapy (Wisoff et al. 1998). In tumours with a very poor prognosis, such as inoperable diffuse intrinsic pontine glioma, both hyperfractionated and accelerated therapy have been evaluated but found to confer no advantage over conventional radiotherapy schedules (Lewis et al. 1997, Mandell et al. 1999).

In summary, radiotherapy may cause varied and severe adverse effects, and is generally recommended only for tumours that are inoperable and progressive or recurrent, where surgery or chemotherapy have failed to achieve control. In locations such as the optic chiasm/hypothalamus, localized radiotherapy (50–55 Gy) results in high progression-free survival rates (65–80% at 10 years – Tao et al. 1997, Cappelli et al. 1998). The role of chemotherapy in young patients is increasing, but it is clear that for some, radiotherapy remains the most effective and rapid treatment available.

There have been no randomized trials to compare radiotherapy and observation alone for residual cerebellar and cerebral LGG (Cokgor et al. 1998), but local field radiotherapy, at a dose of 54 Gy administered over 30 fractions, is generally used for incompletely resected and progressive low-grade tumours. A somewhat higher dose of 54–60 Gy is used for high-grade tumours.

PRIMITIVE NEUROECTODERMAL TUMOURS

Medulloblastoma (PNET-MB) and primitive neuroectodermal tumours (PNETs) at sites within the CNS other than the cerebellum have a high potential for seeding throughout the CSF space, and hence the target volume for radiotherapy must encompass the entire CNS axis. This is extremely challenging in terms of radiotherapy planning, and care must be taken to minimize dose inhomogeneity due to abutment of adjacent radiotherapy fields and variations in anatomical contours and the depth of target tissue. Planning of radiotherapy is of considerable importance in PNETs. Dose inhomogeneity between adjacent radiotherapy fields and variations due to anatomical contours and varying depths of the target tissue may lead to adverse effects, including radiation damage or (more likely) disease recurrence. Deviations from planning protocol have been correlated with relapse risk in medulloblastoma, as in other tumours (Carrie et al. 1992, 1999). Deficiencies in the radiation field covering the cranial meninges, especially in the area of the cribriform plate, have been shown to increase the risk for supratentorial relapse of medulloblastoma (Miralbell et al. 1997, Chojnacka and Skowronska-Gardas 2004). The bottom of the spinal field should provide an adequate margin around the dural sac, and the bottom of S3 is taken as the landmark for this purpose. Conventional treatment involves craniospinal radiation (craniospinal radiotherapy, CSRT) to 36 Gy with a boost to the tumour bed to a total of 50–55 Gy. With this strategy, a progression-free survival of around 55–70% for children with standard-risk medulloblastoma can be anticipated at 5 years (Kun and Constine 1991, Packer et al. 1994).

The importance of radiation therapy in PNET, both posterior fossa and supratentorial, is clear. Attempts to avoid radiation completely, or to avoid supratentorial irradiation, in very young children have in general produced very poor results. For example, the SIOP M4 study used the '8 drugs in 1 day' chemotherapy regime without CSRT, avoiding supratentorial irradiation (Bouffet et al. 1992), but only 1 of 8 children survived. It is clear, however, that radiation, particularly to the whole brain, has significant adverse effects in the long term (Spunberg et al. 1981, Danoff et al. 1982, Duffner et al. 1983, Jannoun and Bloom 1990, Radcliffe et al. 1994).

Recently, the standard of care in terms of radiotherapy for patients with 'average' risk (non-infant, non-metastatic and with minimal postoperative disease) has undergone a re-evaluation. For many years, postoperative radiotherapy to a dose of 35–36 Gy to the craniospinal axis, followed by a boost to the entire posterior fossa to a total dose of 54–55 Gy, was standard (Freeman et al. 2002). When used as the sole adjuvant therapy, reduction in the dose of radiation to the neuraxis has been associated with a significantly greater risk of relapse, and this strategy cannot be considered appropriate in the present day. A joint study

169

by the Paediatric Oncology Group (POG) and the Children's Cancer Group (CCG) (Deutsch et al. 1996) enrolled 126 patients with localized disease who had undergone a complete or subtotal surgical resection of tumour. Patients received conventional radiotherapy (36 Gy with a boost to 54 Gy for the posterior fossa), or reduced-dose RT (23.4 Gy with a boost again to 54 Gy). The study was stopped early, because a clear difference in outcome became apparent. Event-free survival (EFS) at 5 years was later reported to be $52\pm7.7\%$ for the reduced-dose cohort, compared to $67\pm7.4\%$ in the standard radiotherapy cohort (Thomas et al. 2000). It was clear that dose reduction without chemotherapy could not be safely accomplished.

The first report of a significantly improved survival with chemotherapy came from Packer et al. (1994), who used vincristine administered during radiotherapy, and a combination of cisplatin, lomustine (CCNU) and vincristine for 48 weeks after radiotherapy. EFS for patients with no evidence of leptomeningeal spread was reported to be $90\pm6\%$. Only 6 of the 63 patients reported originally by Packer et al. received reduced-dose radiation, but a subsequent pilot study which enrolled 65 patients with localized disease, treating with 23.4 Gy, and a boost to 55.8 Gy to the posterior fossa. EFS was $79\pm7\%$ at 5 years for these patients. Failure of control was principally away from the primary site (Packer et al. 1999).

One further small study reported by Goldwein et al. (1993, 1996) looked at the effect of reducing the dose of CSRT even further. Ten patients aged under 5 years with localized disease received very low dose radiotherapy (18 Gy CSRT and a boost to 50.4–55.8 Gy to the posterior fossa). Seven of these patients remained alive without disease at the time of the second report.

Although reduced-dose CSRT has become the standard therapy for medulloblastoma, the current European study (HIT-SIOP PNET 4) of average-risk medulloblastoma is comparing conventional reduced-dose CSRT and hyperfractionated dosing (36 Gy to the head and spine). For this randomized trial to compare the EFS, overall survival and late sequelae, radiotherapy will be followed by cisplatin, CCNU and vincristine (Packer regimen). Hyperfractionated radiotherapy has shown promising results for children with higher risk PNET (Allen et al. 1996).

The prognosis for children with higher risk disease, principally those with metastatic disease at presentation, is worse than for those with standard-risk disease. Radiotherapy is less effective in achieving a cure, and survival in many series has been less than 40% even in combination with adjuvant chemotherapy, and there is now an effort to improve the efficacy by means of escalation, hyperfractionation and/or acceleration. Early results from the Pediatric Oncology Group's POG#9031 study show initial promise for children with metastatic medulloblastoma receiving a craniospinal dose of 40 Gy in addition to chemotherapy, with boost up to 45 Gy for sites of macroscopic tumour, regardless of site within the CNS axis. However, for the CCG-9931 study, aggressive pre-radiotherapy chemotherapy has not been as successful, although this may be related to the long interval between diagnosis and radiotherapy (Freeman et al. 2002).

Hyperfractionated radiotherapy (HFRT) or hyperfractionated accelerated radiotherapy (HART) schedules, in combination with chemotherapy, are currently being evaluated by European study groups. Results have been reported by several authors using HFRT, but to date the evidence for this approach is equivocal. Allen et al. (1996) reported good results

170

from patients with standard risk medulloblastoma, but only small numbers with high-risk disease. Similarly, Prados et al. (1999) reported no benefit over radiotherapy with chemotherapy. The value of HART is currently under investigation in high-risk patients in the UK.

EPENDYMOMA

Ependymoma accounts for approximately 10% of paediatric brain tumours, and half develop in children under 5 years of age. Radiotherapy has been central to the treatment of ependymoma for many years, and until recently, CSRT was accepted as necessary for all patients. Many of the issues discussed for PNET are therefore relevant to the treatment of ependymoma, although large, multi-institutional studies have only recently been developed. It is clear, however, that the significance of radiotherapy remains limited in comparison to the prognostic significance of the extent of resection or of residual disease (Oya et al. 2002, van Veelen-Vincent et al. 2002). Patients with incomplete surgical resection fare badly, regardless of the radiation modality chosen. Fortunately, technological advances such as the use of the Cavitron ultrasonic aspirator (CUSA), and recognition of the value of second-look surgery mean that the proportion of children with incomplete resection has fallen.

There are no randomized studies of radiotherapy in ependymoma, but the best reported survival data come from those studies with a high rate of surgical complete resection followed by radical radiotherapy. Historical data for patients treated with surgery and local radiotherapy at doses of less than 45 Gy show inferior survival rates compared with doses in the range of 45–55 Gy (Salazar 1983). In addition, a high recurrence rate was reported by Grill et al. (2001) following a protocol aiming to avoid radiotherapy: 40% of children did manage to remain free of radiotherapy, but this corresponded to a high local recurrence rate.

Treatment until the 1990s was directed at the entire neuraxis, given the known capacity of ependymoma to disseminate. It has been shown, however, that the large majority of recurrences occur locally, and this risk is not reduced by whole brain radiotherapy, nor is the risk of dissemination reduced by CSRT (Goldwein et al. 1991, Vanuytsel and Brada 1991, Timmermann et al. 2000, Paulino 2001). The majority of local recurrences occur within 1 cm of the primary tumour bed, and this may be used to define the local radiotherapy field.

Current strategies involve local radiotherapy for all patients, with a dose in the region of 54 Gy for intracranial and intraspinal tumours. The omission of CSRT is not universally accepted, and does not form part of the current SIOP strategy, which requires local radiation for completely resected tumours. Patients with incomplete resection receive four cycles of chemotherapy followed by further surgery if possible, and local radiotherapy.

A possible exception is the myxopapillary ependymoma, which may not require radiotherapy provided complete surgical clearance is achieved. Such tumours typically present in the spine, behave in a more indolent manner than other ependymomas, and have a good overall prognosis. Recurrence is usually local, and radiotherapy is indicated at this time. Late dissemination is reported in some patients (Davis and Barnard 1985, Sonneland et al. 1985, Ross et al. 1993).

DELAY IN OR OMISSION OF RADIOTHERAPY IN YOUNG PATIENTS

There is evidence that chemotherapy may permit radiotherapy to be delayed, and for some children, avoided completely. Whereas progression-free survival for most series with delayed or omitted irradiation has to date been typically less than 40% at 2 years, the current strategy operating in the UK for treatment of children under the age of 3 years shows a PFS at 2 years of 60% (Finlay et al. 1994, Kuhl et al. 1998, White et al. 1998, Timmermann et al. 2000, Grill et al. 2001). This protocol involves surgical resection, immediate second-look surgery if resectable residual tumour is identified, and sequential, intermediate intensity cycles of chemotherapy given every 2 weeks for 1 year. Local field radiotherapy is recommended after this time if there is evidence of progression, but a proportion of these patients remain well without, and only 62% of patients have received radiotherapy to date. Survival after relapse with this strategy is possible in 25% of patients (Richard Grundy, personal communication 2004). Furthermore, the extent of surgical resection was found to have a significant effect on survival in the infant protocols of the Pediatric Oncology Group (POG) and the Société Française d'Oncologie Pédiatrique (SFOP), in which radiotherapy is delayed or avoided (Duffner et al. 1993). The presence of residual disease carries a significant adverse prognosis, even with radiotherapy (Healey et al. 1991, Pollack et al. 1995b).

Stereotactic radiosurgery in recurrent ependymoma

The prognosis for patients who relapse is poor, with reported survival of between 10% and 27%. Surgical resection remains important in these patients, but where there are multiple deposits, or the morbidity of surgery is likely to be great, alternatives have been sought. Encouraging results were reported by Stafford et al. (2000) using radiosurgery in 12 patients with recurrent disease at 17 sites. High rates of local control were achieved (14 of 17 sites), and this approach may be of value in combination with other modalities such as chemotherapy. Stereotactic radiosurgery of multiple sites was feasible and associated with minimal morbidity, and may offer effective palliation in a group of patients unlikely to survive.

Attempts to improve local control with HFRT and stereotactic radiosurgery have not yet been shown to improve outcome (Bouffet et al. 1998, Massimino et al. 2004). International studies are needed to resolve these controversies.

Conclusions and future directions

Radiotherapy is a central part of the treatment regimens for many types of childhood CNS tumour, including PNET, glioma and ependymoma. Future strategies to improve the efficacy and safety of this treatment modality include variations in radiotherapy scheduling, as seen with hyperfractionation, and improvements in the precision of radiotherapy delivery with conformal planning techniques. For example, hyperfractionated CSRT is associated with a lower risk of thyroid dysfunction when compared with conventional scheduling (Ricardi et al. 2001). Similarly, intensity-modulated radiation therapy (IMRT) to the posterior fossa reduces both the dose of radiotherapy to the auditory apparatus and overall ototoxicity scores for children (Huang et al. 2002). Proton radiotherapy appears to be safe and efficacious for children with LGG (Hug et al. 1999), and may confer further advantage when compared with IMRT in terms of sparing normal tissue radiation doses (Miralbell et al. 1997, St Clair et al. 2004). Further studies and ongoing trials will determine the longer-term efficacy of these recent innovations in radiotherapy, and their optimal role for the treatment of children with CNS tumours.

The authors would like to thank Dr Frank Saran for his helpful comments in preparing this chapter.

REFERENCES

Allen JC, Donahue B, DaRosso R, Nirenberg A (1996) Hyperfractionated craniospinal radiotherapy and adjuvant chemotherapy for children with newly diagnosed medulloblastoma and other primitive neuro-ectodermal tumors. *Int J Radiat Oncol Biol Phys* **36**: 1155–1161.

Blackburn TP, Doughty D, Plowman PN (1999) Stereotactic intracavitary therapy of recurrent cystic cranio-pharyngioma by instillation of 90yttrium. *Br J Neurosurg* **13**: 359–365.

Bouffet E, Bernard JL, Frappaz D, Gentet JC, Roche H, Tron P, Carrie C, Raybaud C, Joannard A, Lapras C, et al. (1992) M4 protocol for cerebellar medulloblastoma: supratentorial radiotherapy may not be avoided. *Int J Radiat Oncol Biol Phys* **24**: 79–85.

Bouffet E, Perilongo G, Canete A, Massimino M (1998) Intracranial ependymomas in children: a critical review of prognostic factors and a plea for cooperation. *Med Pediatr Oncol* **30**: 319–329; discussion 329–331.

Bowers DC, Mulne AF, Reisch JS, Elterman RD, Munoz L, Booth T, Shapiro K, Doxey DL (2002) Nonperi-operative strokes in children with central nervous system tumors. *Cancer* **94**: 1094–1101.

Cappelli C, Grill J, Raquin M, Pierre-Kahn A, Lellouch-Tubiana A, Terrier-Lacombe MJ, Habrand JL, Couanet D, Brauner R, Rodriguez D, Hartmann O, Kalifa C (1998) Long-term follow up of 69 patients treated for optic pathway tumours before the chemotherapy era. *Arch Dis Child* **79**: 334–338.

Carrie C, Alapetite C, Mere P, Aimard L, Pons A, Kolodie H, Seng S, Lagrange JL, Pontvert D, Pignon T, et al. (1992) Quality control of radiotherapeutic treatment of medulloblastoma in a multicentric study: the contribution of radiotherapy technique to tumour relapse. The French Medulloblastoma Group. *Radiother Oncol* **24**: 77–81.

Carrie C, Hoffstetter S, Gomez F, Moncho V, Doz F, Alapetite C, Murraciole X, Maire JP, Benhassel M, Chapet S, Quetin P, Kolodie H, Lagrange JL, Cuillere JC, Habrand JL (1999) Impact of targeting deviations on outcome in medulloblastoma: study of the French Society of Pediatric Oncology (SFOP). *Int J Radiat Oncol Biol Phys* **45**: 435–439.

Chojnacka M, Skowronska-Gardas A (2004) Medulloblastoma in childhood: Impact of radiation technique upon the outcome of treatment. *Pediatr Blood Cancer* **42**: 155–160.

Cokgor I, Friedman AH, Friedman HS (1998) Gliomas. Eur J Cancer 34: 1910–1915; discussion 1916–1918.

Danoff BF, Cowchock FS, Marquette C, Mulgrew L, Kramer S (1982) Assessment of the long-term effects of primary radiation therapy for brain tumors in children. *Cancer* **49**: 1580–1586.

Davis C, Barnard RO (1985) Malignant behavior of myxopapillary ependymoma. Report of three cases. *J Neurosurg* **62**: 925–929.

Deutsch M, Thomas PR, Krischer J, Boyett JM, Albright L, Aronin P, Langston J, Allen JC, Packer RJ, Linggood R, Mulhern R, Stanley P, Stehbens JA, Duffner P, Kun L, Rorke L, Cherlow J, Freidman H, Finlay JL, Vietti T (1996) Results of a prospective randomized trial comparing standard dose neuraxis irradiation (3,600 cGy/20) with reduced neuraxis irradiation (2,340 cGy/13) in patients with low-stage medulloblastoma. A combined Children's Cancer Group–Pediatric Oncology Group Study. *Pediatr Neurosurg* **24**: 167–176; discussion 176–177.

Duffner PK, Cohen ME, Anderson SW, Voorhess ML, MacGillivray MH, Panahon A, Brecher M L (1983) Long-term effects of treatment on endocrine function in children with brain tumors. *Ann Neurol* **14**: 528–532.

Duffner PK, Horowitz ME, Krischer JP, Friedman HS, Burger PC, Cohen ME, Sanford RA, Mulhern RK, James HE, Freeman CR, et al. (1993) Postoperative chemotherapy and delayed radiation in children less than three years of age with malignant brain tumors. *N Engl J Med* **328**: 1725–1731.

Fallai C, Olmi P (1997) Hyperfractionated and accelerated radiation therapy in central nervous system tumors (malignant gliomas, pediatric tumors, and brain metastases). *Radiother Oncol* **43**: 235–246.

Fein DA, Marcus RB, Parsons JT, Mendenhall WM, Million RR (1993) Lhermitte's sign: incidence and treatment variables influencing risk after irradiation of the cervical spinal cord. *Int J Radiat Oncol Biol Phys* **27**: 1029–1033.

Finlay JL, Geyer JR, Turski PA, Yates AJ, Boyett JM, Allen JC, Packer RJ (1994) Pre-irradiation chemotherapy in children with high-grade astrocytoma: tumor response to two cycles of the '8-drugs-in-1-day' regimen. A Children's Cancer Group study, CCG-945. *J Neurooncol* **21**: 255–265.

Fowler JF (1984) Review: total doses in fractionated radiotherapy — implications of new radiobiological data. *Int J Radiat Biol Relat Stud Phys Chem Med* **46**: 103–120.

Freeman CR, Taylor RE, Kortmann RD, Carrie C (2002) Radiotherapy for medulloblastoma in children: a perspective on current international clinical research efforts. *Med Pediatr Oncol* **39**: 99–108.

Fuss M, Poljanc K, Hug EB (2000) Full Scale IQ (FSIQ) changes in children treated with whole brain and partial brain irradiation. A review and analysis. *Strahlenther Onkol* **176**: 573–581.

Garcia DM, Latifi HR, Simpson JR, Picker S (1989) Astrocytomas of the cerebellum in children. *J Neurosurg* **71**: 661–664.

Gnekow AK, Kaatsch P, Kortmann R, Wiestler OD (2000) [HIT-LGG: effectiveness of carboplatin–vincristine in progressive low-grade gliomas of childhood — an interim report.] *Klin Pädiatr* **212**: 177–184 (German).

Goldwein JW, Corn BW, Finlay JL, Packer RJ, Rorke LB, Schut L (1991) Is craniospinal irradiation required to cure children with malignant (anaplastic) intracranial ependymomas? *Cancer* **67**: 2766–2771.

Goldwein JW, Radcliffe J, Packer RJ, Sutton LN, Lange B, Rorke LB, D'Angio GJ (1993) Results of a pilot study of low-dose craniospinal radiation therapy plus chemotherapy for children younger than 5 years with primitive neuroectodermal tumors. *Cancer* **71**: 2647–2652.

Goldwein JW, Radcliffe J, Johnson J, Moshang T, Packer RJ, Sutton LN, Rorke LB, D'Angio GJ (1996) Updated results of a pilot study of low dose craniospinal irradiation plus chemotherapy for children under five with cerebellar primitive neuroectodermal tumors (medulloblastoma). *Int J Radiat Oncol Biol Phys* **34**: 899–904.

Grill J, Le Deley MC, Gambarelli D, Raquin MA, Couanet D, Pierre-Kahn A, Habrand JL, Doz F, Frappaz D, Gentet JC, Edan C, Chastagner P, Kalifa C (2001) Postoperative chemotherapy without irradiation for ependymoma in children under 5 years of age: a multicenter trial of the French Society of Pediatric Oncology. *J Clin Oncol* **19**: 1288–1296.

Healey EA, Barnes PD, Kupsky WJ, Scott RM, Sallan SE, Black PM, Tarbell NJ (1991) The prognostic significance of postoperative residual tumor in ependymoma. *Neurosurgery* **28**: 666–671; discussion 671–672.

Hodgson DC, Goumnerova LC, Loeffler JS, Dutton S, Black PM, Alexander E, Xu R, Kooy H, Silver B, Tarbell NJ (2001) Radiosurgery in the management of pediatric brain tumors. *Int J Radiat Oncol Biol Phys* **50**: 929–935.

Huang E, Teh BS, Strother DR, Davis QG, Chiu JK, Lu HH, Carpenter LS, Mai WY, Chintagumpala MM, South M, Grant WH, Butler EB, Woo SY (2002) Intensity-modulated radiation therapy for pediatric medulloblastoma: early report on the reduction of ototoxicity. *Int J Radiat Oncol Biol Phys* **52**: 599–605.

Hug EB, Loredo LN, Slater JD, DeVries A, Grove RI, Schaefer RA, Rosenberg AE, Slater JM (1999) Proton radiation therapy for chordomas and chondrosarcomas of the skull base. *J Neurosurg* **91**: 432–439.

Jannoun L, Bloom HJ (1990) Long-term psychological effects in children treated for intracranial tumors. *Int J Radiat Oncol Biol Phys* **18**: 747–753.

Janss AJ, Grundy R, Cnaan A, Savino PJ, Packer RJ, Zackai EH, Goldwein JW, Sutton LN, Radcliffe J, Molloy PT, et al. (1995) Optic pathway and hypothalamic/chiasmatic gliomas in children younger than age 5 years with a 6-year follow-up. *Cancer* **75**: 1051–1059.

Jenkin D (1996) Long-term survival of children with brain tumors. *Oncology (Huntingt)* **10**: 715–719; discussion 720, 722, 728.

Jeremic B, Djuric L, Mijatovic L (1991) Incidence of radiation myelitis of the cervical spinal cord at doses of 5500 cGy or greater. *Cancer* **68**: 2138–2141.

Karim AB, Afra D, Cornu P, Bleehan N, Schraub S, De Witte O, Darcel F, Stenning S, Pierart M, Van Glabbeke M (2002) Randomized trial on the efficacy of radiotherapy for cerebral low-grade glioma in the adult: European Organization for Research and Treatment of Cancer Study 22845 with the Medical Research Council study BRO4: an interim analysis. *Int J Radiat Oncol Biol Phys* **52**: 316–324.

Koehler PJ, Verbiest H, Jager J, Vecht CJ (1996) Delayed radiation myelopathy: serial MR-imaging and pathology. *Clin Neurol Neurosurg* **98**: 197–201.

Kortmann RD, Hess CF, Hoffmann W, Jany R, Bamberg M (1995) Is the standardized helmet technique adequate for irradiation of the brain and the cranial meninges? *Int J Radiat Oncol Biol Phys* **32**: 241–244.

Kortmann RD, Timmermann B, Taylor RE, Scarzello G, Plasswilm L, Paulsen F, Jeremic B, Gnekow AK, Dieckmann K, Kay S, Bamberg M (2003) Current and future strategies in radiotherapy of childhood low-grade glioma of the brain. Part I: Treatment modalities of radiation therapy. *Strahlenther Onkol* **179**: 509–520.

Kuhl J, Muller HL, Berthold F, Kortmann RD, Deinlein F, Maass E, Graf N, Gnekow A, Scheurlen W, Gobel U, Wolff JE, Bamberg M, Kaatsch P, Kleihues P, Rating D, Sorensen N, Wiestler OD (1998) Preradiation chemotherapy of children and young adults with malignant brain tumors: results of the German pilot trial HIT'88/'89. *Klin Pädiatr* 210: 227–233.

Kun LE, Constine LS (1991) Medulloblastoma—caution regarding new treatment approaches. *Int J Radiat Oncol Biol Phys* **20**: 897–899.

Lewis J, Lucraft H, Gholkar A (1997) UKCCSG study of accelerated radiotherapy for pediatric brain stem gliomas. United Kingdom Childhood Cancer Study Group. *Int J Radiat Oncol Biol Phys* **38**: 925–929.

Mandell LR, Kadota R, Freeman C, Douglass EC, Fontanesi J, Cohen ME, Kovnar E, Burger P, Sanford RA, Kepner J, Friedman H, Kun LE (1999) There is no role for hyperfractionated radiotherapy in the management of children with newly diagnosed diffuse intrinsic brainstem tumors: results of a Pediatric Oncology Group phase III trial comparing conventional vs. hyperfractionated radiotherapy. *Int J Radiat Oncol Biol Phys* **43**: 959–964.

Marchese MJ, Chang CH (1990) Malignant astrocytic gliomas in children. *Cancer* **65**: 2771–2778.

Massimino M, Gandola L, Giangaspero F, Sandri A, Valagussa P, Perilongo G, Garre ML, Ricardi U, Forni M, Genitori L, Scarzello G, Spreafico F, Barra S, Mascarin M, Pollo B, Gardiman M, Cama A, Navarria P, Brisigotti M, Collini P, Balter R, Fidani P, Stefanelli M, Burnelli R, Potepan P, Podda M, Sotti G, Madon E (2004) Hyperfractionated radiotherapy and chemotherapy for childhood ependymoma: final results of the first prospective AIEOP (Associazione Italiana di Ematologia–Oncologia Pediatrica) study. *Int J Radiat Oncol Biol Phys* **58**: 1336–1345.

Miralbell R, Bleher A, Huguenin P, Ries G, Kann R, Mirimanoff RO, Notter M, Nouet P, Bieri S, Thum P, Toussi H (1997) Pediatric medulloblastoma: radiation treatment technique and patterns of failure. *Int J Radiat Oncol Biol Phys* **37**: 523–529.

Montgomery AB, Griffin T, Parker RG, Gerdes AJ (1977) Optic nerve glioma: the role of radiation therapy. *Cancer* **40**: 2079–2080.

Mornex F, Nayel H, Taillandier L (1993) Radiation therapy for malignant astrocytomas in adults. *Radiother Oncol* **27**: 181–192.

Oya N, Shibamoto Y, Nagata Y, Negoro Y, Hiraoka M (2002) Postoperative radiotherapy for intracranial ependymoma: analysis of prognostic factors and patterns of failure. *J Neurooncol* **56**: 87–94.

Packer RJ, Sutton LN, Elterman R, Lange B, Goldwein J, Nicholson HS, Mulne L, Boyett J, D'Angio G, Wechsler-Jentzsch K, et al. (1994) Outcome for children with medulloblastoma treated with radiation and cisplatin, CCNU, and vincristine chemotherapy. *J Neurosurg* **81**: 690–698.

Packer RJ, Goldwein J, Nicholson HS, Vezina LG, Allen JC, Ris MD, Muraszko K, Rorke LB, Wara WM, Cohen BH, Boyett JM (1999) Treatment of children with medulloblastomas with reduced-dose craniospinal radiation therapy and adjuvant chemotherapy: A Children's Cancer Group Study. *J Clin Oncol* **17**: 2127–2136.

Paterson E, Farr RF (1953) Cerebellar medulloblastoma: treatment by irradiation of the whole central nervous system. *Acta Radiol* **39**: 323–336.

Paulino AC (2001) The local field in infratentorial ependymoma: does the entire posterior fossa need to be treated? *Int J Radiat Oncol Biol Phys* **49**: 757–761.

Pollack IF, Claassen D, al-Shboul Q, Janosky JE, Deutsch M (1995a) Low-grade gliomas of the cerebral hemispheres in children: an analysis of 71 cases. *J Neurosurg* **82**: 536–547.

Pollack IF, Gerszten PC, Martinez AJ, Lo KH, Shultz B, Albright AL, Janosky J, Deutsch M (1995b) Intracranial ependymomas of childhood: long–term outcome and prognostic factors. *Neurosurgery* **37**: 655–666; discussion 666–667.

Prados MD, Edwards MS, Chang SM, Russo C, Davis R, Rabbitt J, Page M, Lamborn K, Wara WM (1999) Hyperfractionated craniospinal radiation therapy for primitive neuroectodermal tumors: results of a Phase II study. *Int J Radiat Oncol Biol Phys* **43**: 279–285.

Radcliffe J, Bunin GR, Sutton LN, Goldwein JW, Phillips PC (1994) Cognitive deficits in long-term survivors of childhood medulloblastoma and other noncortical tumors: age-dependent effects of whole brain radiation. *Int J Dev Neurosci* **12**: 327–334.

Ricardi U, Corrias A, Einaudi S, Genitori L, Sandri A, di Montezemolo LC, Besenzon L, Madon E, Urgesi A

175

(2001) Thyroid dysfunction as a late effect in childhood medulloblastoma: a comparison of hyperfractionated versus conventionally fractionated craniospinal radiotherapy. *Int J Radiat Oncol Biol Phys* **50**: 1287–1294.

Ross DA, McKeever PE, Sandler HM, Muraszko KM (1993) Myxopapillary ependymoma. Results of nucleolar organizing region staining. *Cancer* **71**: 3114–3118.

Salazar OM (1983) A better understanding of CNS seeding and a brighter outlook for postoperatively irradiated patients with ependymomas. *Int J Radiat Oncol Biol Phys* **9**: 1231–1234.

Salvati M, Frati A, Russo N, Caroli E, Polli FM, Minniti G, Delfini R (2003) Radiation-induced gliomas: report of 10 cases and review of the literature. *Surg Neurol* **60**: 60–67; discussion 67.

Schell MJ, McHaney VA, Green AA, Kun LE, Hayes FA, Horowitz M, Meyer W H (1989) Hearing loss in children and young adults receiving cisplatin with or without prior cranial irradiation. *J Clin Oncol* **7**: 754–760.

Shaw E, Arusell R, Scheithauer B, O'Fallon J, O'Neill B, Dinapoli R, Nelson D, Earle J, Jones C, Cascino T, Nichols D, Ivnik R, Hellman R, Curran W, Abrams R (2002) Prospective randomized trial of low- versus high-dose radiation therapy in adults with supratentorial low-grade glioma: initial report of a North Central Cancer Treatment Group/Radiation Therapy Oncology Group/Eastern Cooperative Oncology Group study. *J Clin Oncol* **20**: 2267–2276.

Sheline GE (1975) Radiation therapy of tumors of the central nervous system in childhood. *Cancer* **35** (Suppl.): 957–964.

Sonneland PR, Scheithauer BW, Onofrio BM (1985) Myxopapillary ependymoma. A clinicopathologic and immunocytochemical study of 77 cases. *Cancer* **56**: 883–893.

Spunberg JJ, Chang CH, Goldman M, Auricchio E, Bell JJ (1981) Quality of long-term survival following irradiation for intracranial tumors in children under the age of two. *Int J Radiat Oncol Biol Phys* **7**: 727–736.

St Clair WH, Adams JA, Bues M, Fullerton BC, La Shell S, Kooy HM, Loeffler JS, Tarbell NJ (2004) Advantage of protons compared to conventional X-ray or IMRT in the treatment of a pediatric patient with medulloblastoma. *Int J Radiat Oncol Biol Phys* **58**: 727–734.

Stafford SL, Pollock BE, Foote RL, Gorman DA, Nelson DF, Schomberg PJ (2000) Stereotactic radiosurgery for recurrent ependymoma. *Cancer* **88**: 870–875.

Tao ML, Barnes PD, Billett AL, Leong T, Shrieve DC, Scott RM, Tarbell NJ (1997) Childhood optic chiasm gliomas: radiographic response following radiotherapy and long-term clinical outcome. *Int J Radiat Oncol Biol Phys* **39**: 579–587.

Teh BS, Mai WY, Grant WH, Chiu JK, Lu HH, Carpenter LS, Woo SY, Butler EB (2002) Intensity modulated radiotherapy (IMRT) decreases treatment-related morbidity and potentially enhances tumor control. *Cancer Invest* **20**: 437–451.

Tenny RT, Laws ER, Younge BR, Rush JA (1982) The neurosurgical management of optic glioma. Results in 104 patients. *J Neurosurg* **57**: 452–458.

Thomas PR, Deutsch M, Kepner JL, Boyett JM, Krischer J, Aronin P, Albright L, Allen JC, Packer RJ, Linggood R, Mulhern R, Stehbens JA, Langston J, Stanley P, Duffner P, Rorke L, Cherlow J, Friedman HS, Finlay JL, Vietti TJ, Kun LE (2000) Low-stage medulloblastoma: final analysis of trial comparing standard-dose with reduced-dose neuraxis irradiation. *J Clin Oncol* **18**: 3004–3011.

Tihan T, Fisher PG, Kepner JL, Godfraind C, McComb RD, Goldthwaite PT, Burger PC (1999) Pediatric astrocytomas with monomorphous pilomyxoid features and a less favorable outcome. *J Neuropathol Exp Neurol* **58**: 1061–1068.

Timmermann B, Kortmann RD, Kuhl J, Meisner C, Slavc I, Pietsch T, Bamberg M (2000) Combined postoperative irradiation and chemotherapy for anaplastic ependymomas in childhood: results of the German prospective trials HIT 88/89 and HIT 91. *Int J Radiat Oncol Biol Phys* **46**: 287–295.

van Veelen-Vincent ML, Pierre-Kahn A, Kalifa C, Sainte-Rose C, Zerah M, Thorne J, Renier D (2002) Ependymoma in childhood: prognostic factors, extent of surgery, and adjuvant therapy. *J Neurosurg* **97**: 827–835.

Vanuytsel L, Brada M (1991) The role of prophylactic spinal irradiation in localized intracranial ependymoma. *Int J Radiat Oncol Biol Phys* **21**: 825–830.

Vines E, Betsch HF (2001) Radiotherapy. In: Keating RF, Goodrich JT, Packer RJ, eds. *Tumors of the Pediatric Central Nervous System*. New York: Thieme, pp. 135–156.

Wambersie A, Gregroire V, Brucher JM (1992) Potential clinical gain of proton (and heavy ion) beams for brain tumors in children. *Int J Radiat Oncol Biol Phys* **22**: 275–286.

White L, Kellie S, Gray E, Toogood I, Waters K, Lockwood L, Macfarlane S, Johnston H (1998) Postoperative chemotherapy in children less than 4 years of age with malignant brain tumors: promising initial response to a VETOPEC-based regimen. A Study of the Australian and New Zealand Children's Cancer Study Group (ANZCCSG). *J Pediatr Hematol Oncol* **20**: 125–130.

Wisoff JH, Boyett JM, Berger MS, Brant C, Li H, Yates AJ, McGuire-Cullen P, Turski PA, Sutton LN, Allen JC, Packer RJ, Finlay JL (1998) Current neurosurgical management and the impact of the extent of resection in the treatment of malignant gliomas of childhood: a report of the Children's Cancer Group trial no. CCG-945. *J Neurosurg* **89**: 52–59.

8
GENERAL PRINCIPLES OF CHEMOTHERAPY

Eddy Estlin

In comparison to other solid tumours of childhood such as Wilms' tumour and rhabdo-myosarcoma, the role of chemotherapy in the treatment of many childhood CNS cancers such as glioma and ependymoma is less well established. This may reflect a previous un-willingness to employ treatment regimens that are associated with significant toxicity, given the barriers to the effectiveness of chemotherapy such as the blood–brain barrier and a perception that CNS tumours lack chemosensitivity. However, increasing cooperation at national and international level over recent years is allowing the evaluation of contemporary chemotherapy drugs in the therapy of childhood CNS tumours.

Modern anticancer drugs are expected to progress through an evaluation process that includes pre-clinical pharmacology and toxicology, followed by phase I trial to determine the maximum tolerated dose and pharmacokinetics. Phase II trials to determine efficacy in a given tumour type then follow, usually in the setting of relapsed disease, and then phase III evaluation as part of a treatment comparison with standard or previous best treatment is undertaken. The preclinical and early clinical evaluation of contemporary anticancer agents usually includes studies of the pharmacology and cellular determinants of chemo-sensitivity in the cancers to be targeted by the drug (Estlin and Veal 2003). However, for several of the drugs employed against paediatric CNS tumours, this knowledge is lacking. The aim of this chapter is to highlight the current knowledge of pharmacology and the cellular determinants of chemosensitivity in relation to CNS tumours, and in this context the example of the clinical and cellular pharmacological determinants of sensitivity to the methylating agents temozolomide and CCNU will be discussed.

Pharmacology and tumours of the CNS

The delivery of effective concentrations of drug to tumour cells in the CNS is determined in the first instance by the dose and schedule of administration of the drug, which may determine the effective systemic exposure in the clinical setting. However, a wide variation in pharmacokinetic variability exists for the majority of anticancer drugs in children (Rodman et al. 1993). Furthermore, where this phenomenon has been studied, it has been found to be important in relation to response for solid tumours (Rodman et al. 1987) and outcome for childhood acute lymphoblastic leukaemia (Evans et al. 1998).

In addition to the pharmacokinetic variability inherent in the delivery of anticancer drugs to their targets, drug penetration into CNS tumours is modulated by the blood–brain barrier (BBB) and blood–tumour barrier (BTB). The BBB consists of capillary endothelial cells

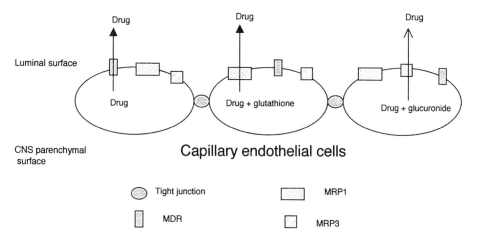

Fig. 8.1. Schematic representation of the blood–brain barrier.
MDR = multidrug resistance protein; MRP-1 = multidrug resistance associated protein-1; MRP-3 = multidrug resistance associated protein-3.

that lack fenestrations, and that are connected together with continuous tight junctions with a high electrical resistance (Bart et al. 2000). The BBB helps to maintain CNS homeostasis, and acts as a barrier to most hydrophilic substances and to large hydrophilic substances. Therefore, passive transport across the BBB is highly dependent on the physicochemical features of the drugs in question, and unless actively transported into the brain, only lipophilic drugs can enter the CNS, albeit to varying degrees (Bart et al. 2000).

Since the majority of anticancer drugs, such as vincristine, carboplatin, cisplatin and methotrexate, are hydrophilic, the BBB forms a substantial barrier for entry of the drug into the CNS. For drugs such as etoposide, CCNU and BCNU, the more lipophilic nature of the drug should facilitate a higher CNS penetration (Blasberg and Groothius 1986). However, drugs such as etoposide and vincristine show a lower CNS penetration than expected on the basis of their lipophilicity. This may be explained by the presence of transmembrane efflux pump mechanisms that span the luminal surface of capillary endothelial cells in the CNS (Fig. 8.1). These energy dependent transport mechanisms include P-glycoprotein (MDR-1), and the multidrug resistance associated proteins MRP1 and MRP3 (Bart et al. 2000). Therefore the CNS penetration of drugs such as doxorubicin, vincristine and etoposide are further limited by MDR-1 and MRP1 activity, and methotrexate is a substrate for MRP3 (Bart et al. 2000).

In contrast to the normal BBB, a number of alterations in the capillary ultrastructure have been described within primary and metastatic CNS tumours. These vary from subtle alterations in tight junction structure to a very irregular appearance of the capillary endothelium, with many fenestrations and an increase in the number and size of pinocytic vacuoles or a totally irregular basal lamina (Bart et al. 2000). These changes in tumour-related capillary ultrastructure, or tumour–brain barrier, result in increased permeability to drugs such that

179

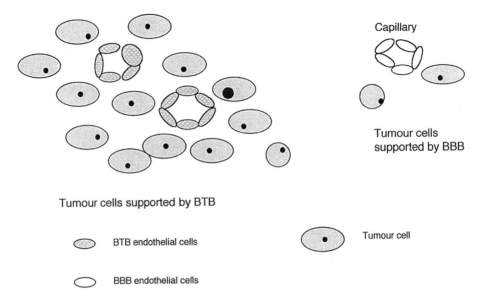

Capillary

Tumour cells
supported by BBB

Tumour cells supported by BTB

BTB endothelial cells

Tumour cell

BBB endothelial cells

Fig. 8.2. Schematic representation of cancer cells supported by blood–tumour barrier (BTB) and blood–brain barrier (BBB).

the concentrations of drugs such as etoposide, cisplatin and BCNU reach cytotoxic levels within human CNS tumours (Donelli et al. 1992). However, parenchymal concentrations of these drugs decrease as a function of distance from the tumour, such that drug levels are markedly reduced at a distance of 5cm from the tumour (Donelli et al. 1992). This reflects the increasing functionality of the BBB as distance increases from the tumour, and has implications for the treatment of locally invasive or metastatic disease, where tumour cells may be supported by capillary endothelial cells with intact BBB function (Fig. 8.2).

Chemosensitivity and CNS tumours

One popular understanding of paediatric CNS tumours such as glioma is that these tumours are primarily relatively resistant to chemotherapy. However, a meta-analysis of the chemosensitivity of glioma cell lines in vitro showed that these cell lines were sensitive to a wide range of anticancer agents. These ranged from actinomycin-D (most active agent) and CCNU (least active agent), with sensitivity also found for drugs such as vincristine, cisplatin and methotrexate (Wolff et al. 1999). Moreover, the inter-individual differences for in vitro sensitivity of tumours derived from paediatric medulloblastoma, ependymoma and glioma cases are large, and differ between tumour type (Lewandowicz et al. 2000). For example, a 2- to 4-fold range in sensitivity to CCNU was found, with glioma found to be less sensitive than medulloblastoma and ependymoma. For vincristine, a larger range of sensitivity was found between different patients (7- to 15-fold), and cultures derived from ependymomas were markedly less sensitive than cultures derived from medulloblastoma or high-grade glioma.

Thus, there is considerable inter-patient variation in the sensitivity of paediatric CNS tumours to CCNU, at least in the in vitro setting. The recent pre-clinical and clinical development of the methylating agent temozolomide may help to explain this potentially important clinical phenomenon. Temozolomide is active by virtue of the formation of O^6-methylguanine DNA adduct that results in a futile round of mismatch repair that is cytotoxic if large numbers of adducts are formed and repair attempted. O^6-alkylguanine DNA alkyltransferase (AGT) acts as a suicide acceptor protein for the alkyl group of temzolomide, thereby restoring DNA to normal. Thus, sensitivity to temozolomide is reduced with increasing levels of intracellular AGT, and this phenomenon also applies to the sensitivity to the chloroethylating agent CCNU, which also forms DNA adducts at the O^6-guanine position (Gerson 2002). For human glial tumour xenografts, thresholds of AGT activity have been characterized to confer significant resistance to BCNU or temozolomide, indicating the potential importance of this repair protein as a mechanism of intrinsic resistance to these agents in vivo (Kokkinakis et al. 2001). AGT may also modulate the activity of cyclophosphamide against human medulloblastoma cells in vitro (Friedman et al. 1999).

However, the resistance of CNS tumours to temozolomide or nitrosoureas is multifaceted. For both human medulloblastoma and glioma cell lines, AGT levels are not the only determinant of cytotoxicity for these drugs (Silber et al. 1992, Bobola et al. 1996). For example, differences in the p53 response and p21-related cell cycle arrest in relation to temozolomide also relate to the sensitivity to the drug (Bocangel et al. 2002). Resistance to temozolomide and CCNU may also occur in the face of deficiency in the repair of the DNA mismatches that result from methylation and chloroethylation, respectively (Fink et al. 1998). The relative importance of AGT levels and mismatch repair status as a determinant of sensitivity to temozolomide has been investigated for a panel of 17 paediatric cancer xenografts. Although AGT levels were found to be the primary mechanism for temozolomide resistance, mismatch repair proficiency determined the sensitivity to temzolomide when AGT levels were low (Middlemass et al. 2000).

In the pre-clinical setting, the depletion of AGT with agents such as O^6-benzylguanine has been shown to improve the efficacy of BCNU or temozolomide against human high-grade glioma xenografts (Kokkinakis et al. 2001), and of BCNU against human medullo-blastoma xenografts (Kokkinakis et al. 1999). For the medulloblastoma xenografts in particular, optimization of the doses of O^6-benzylguanine and BCNU to avoid host toxicity allowed the development of treatment schedules that eradicated established xenografts in the majority of cases (Kokkinakis et al. 1999).

Other potential mechanisms of drug resistance that may be relevant to paediatric CNS tumours include the modulation of chemosensitivity by glutathione (GSH) and glutathione-S-transferase (GST), and MDR/MRP mediated drug efflux. Intracellular GSH is known to confer resistance to cyclophosphamide in medulloblastoma cell lines (Friedman et al. 1992) and to cisplatin in human glioblastoma cell lines in vitro (Iida et al. 1999). For human glioblastoma cell lines, expression of GST, the enzyme that conjugates GSH to the target drug or substrate with subsequent inactivation, also relates to sensitivity to chloroethylating agents (Ali-Osman et al. 1990). MRP_3 shares the properties of MRP_1 in that it transports organic anions such as methotrexate. However, drugs are transported as conjugates with glucuronide rather than glutathione (Bart et al. 2000). Although MDR-1 expression has not been found for tumour samples derived from children with high-grade glioma, the majority of tumours express this protein in the endothelium of their blood vessels (Billson et al. 1994). This indicates that the capillary endothelial cells themselves may play a role in conferring resistance to drugs such as vincristine and etoposide. Moreover, MRP_1 and MRP_3 expression has been found for human glioblastoma cell lines (Decleves et al. 2002), indicating the possible importance of multidrug resistance associated proteins as a potential mechanism of resistance to methotrexate, and also to drugs that are MDR-1 substrates.

The usage of dexamethasone in clinical practice may, at least in theory, add to the limitation of drug efficacy conferred by the BBB and the cellular determinants of chemosensitivity described above. Dexamethasone, a corticosteroid commonly employed for the therapy of peritumoural oedema, also decreases the sensitivity of human glioma cell lines to a wide variety of anticancer agents (Weller et al. 1997). Therefore, although several mechanisms exist that may potentially limit the effectiveness of the drugs currently employed in the therapy of childhood CNS tumours, their clinical importance is not yet known.

Clinical trials involving paediatric CNS tumours

Novel anticancer drugs brought into clinical practice today are subject to very rigorous preclinical and clinical evaluation, particularly in the area of early clinical trials. However, this approach has been used very patchily in relation to paediatric neuro-oncology. For example, in a phase I trial, dose limiting toxicities and pharmacokinetics are defined during a cohort escalation study, and the maximum tolerated dose (MTD) of the new drug is taken forward into phase II or efficacy evaluation (Estlin et al. 1996). Although modern phase I trials have determined the MTD for drugs such as carboplatin (Gaynon et al. 1987) and temozolomide (Estlin et al. 1998) in children, more established drugs such as vincristine and CCNU have not been evaluated in this way.

However, one of the largest deficiencies in this process relates to the area of phase II trials. Phase II studies are required to determine whether or not a new agent or treatment strategy appears sufficiently active to warrant further study, as determined by objective response rates of 20–30%, but may also further define the toxicity profile and pharmacokinetics of new agents. As with phase I studies, phase II studies in paediatric oncology are now conducted on a multi-institutional or group collaborative basis, and usually follow a two-stage design that allows early termination of studies if the activity level is too low or is adequately high (Estlin and Ablett 2001). However, a review of phase II trials published in the area of paediatric neuro-oncology over the past 20 years indicated several areas of deficiency (Chastagner et al. 2001). For example, methodological problems such as a lack of central histopathological and radiological review, mixed-tumour trials resulting in few patients per given tumour type and arbitrary response definitions are frequent occurrences. Nevertheless, the review of Chastagner et al. (2001) indicates the difficulty in selecting agents for rational phase III evaluation in paediatric neuro-oncology. For example, the calculated overall phase II response rate was 2.8% for high-grade glioma, 37% for medulloblastoma and 10% for ependymoma. However, from this analysis the response rates for medulloblastoma were highest when platinum agents were included, the most active agent in ependymoma therapy was cisplatin, and the response rates were much higher for phase II studies performed at initial diagnosis than at the time of relapse. Thus, there is less evidence, based on the findings of early clinical trials, with which to define the appropriate drugs and combinations of agents to take forward to phase III study.

In addition, the few phase II trials that have been performed in the context of chemotherapy or radiotherapy naïve disease have related the response rates observed to the clinical or cellular pharmacological determinants of chemosensitivity. For example, for children with high-grade glioma, response to pre-radiotherapy chemotherapy with the 8-drugs-in-1-day regimen was only 18% (Finlay et al. 1994). However, a significantly higher response rate was observed for children less than 36 months of age (33%) when compared with older children (11%), although the latter were less likely to progress in the pre-radiotherapy treatment period. Whether these differences were the result of age-specific differences in drug disposition or chemosensitivity is not known. Similarly, a 62% response rate was reported for 16 children with high risk medulloblastoma receiving two courses of carboplatin as a single agent prior to conventional therapy. Although inter-patient pharmacokinetic variability was not felt to be important, cellular determinants of chemosensitivity were not measured in the tumour samples (Mastrangelo et al. 1995).

In comparison with other areas of paediatric cancer therapy, there has been a relative paucity of randomized phase III studies in paediatric neuro-oncology to date. Moreover, the design of the trials, and the treatment regimens compared, have usually not been progressed from knowledge of phase I or phase II clinical trials. For example, for medullo-blastoma, a randomized comparison of the 8-drugs-in-1-day regimen (which included two courses of chemotherapy prior to radiotherapy) with immediate radiotherapy followed by chemotherapy with CCNU, vincristine and prednisone showed a clear superiority for the latter regimen (Zeltzer et al. 1999). This finding has cast doubt over the rationale for pre-radiotherapy chemotherapy for the treatment of medulloblastoma, but may have been ex-pected if the activity for the regimen for this disease was as poor as that for high-grade glioma.

In contrast, the experience of the German Society of Paediatric Haematology and Oncology with respect to pre-radiotherapy chemotherapy was more encouraging. Children randomized to receive two courses of chemotherapy with ifosfamide, etoposide, high-dose methotrexate, cisplatin and cytosine arabinoside (HIT) prior to radiotherapy, followed by further treatment with HIT, experienced a statistically poorer event-free survival than those treated with early radiotherapy and maintenance chemotherapy with cisplatin, CCNU and vincristine. However, this effect was mainly found in children aged between 6 and 18 years, where post-radiotherapy treatment with CCNU, vincristine and cisplatin was associated with an improved outcome (Kortmann et al. 2000). Again, age-related differences in pharmaco-logical variables may at least partly explain this effect. For patients with high-grade glioma, HIT therapy with pre- and post-irradiation chemotherapy has been found to produce a superior event-free survival when compared with post-irradiation maintenance chemo-therapy with cisplatin, CCNU and vincristine (Wolff et al. 2002). Therefore, although chemotherapy appears to be beneficial for the therapy of CNS tumours such as high-grade glioma and medulloblastoma, the drugs that are the most active components of multi-agent regimens have not been identified by prior early clinical studies.

In an attempt to overcome the physical barrier to chemotherapy imposed by the BBB, several studies have employed high doses of chemotherapy, with bone marrow or peripheral haematological stem cell rescue. The treatment regimens most frequently contained agents or combinations of agents such as carboplatin, etoposide, busulphan, thiotepa and BCNU (Kalifa et al. 1999). High response rates have been described for medulloblastoma and CNS germ cell tumours, and durable survival has been described for selected patients with medulloblastoma, germ cell tumour and high-grade glioma. This is especially true in the context of minimal residual disease at the time of high dose therapy (Kalifa et al. 1999, Chastagner et al. 2001). However, for diffuse intrinsic pontine glioma and ependymoma, high dose chemotherapy has not been found to be effective (Kalifa et al. 1999).

Relationship between pharmacology, chemosensitivity and clinical effect
There have been few studies that relate the intrinsic sensitivity of tumour cells derived from patients with CNS tumours to measures of clinical outcome such as response, time to progression or survival. For adults with high-grade glioma, in vitro BCNU sensitivity has been related to outcome, with a longer relapse-free interval found for patients whose disease was more sensitive to the drug, with an average 15 months versus 6 months time to progression for patients with BCNU-resistant disease, respectively (Bogdahn 1983).

In relation to the pharmacokinetics of the nitrosoureas, and their potential influence for disease response or survival, these have only been reported for CCNU in adults. For patients receiving the standard dose of $130 \, mg/m^2$, a narrow range of inter-patient pharmacokinetic variability was found, and the systemic exposures observed were at the low end for those required for cytotoxicity in a panel of human and rodent cancer cells (Lee et al. 1985). Furthermore, Lewandowicz et al. (2000) related the plasma CCNU concentrations reported for adults to the drug sensitivity of the paediatric tumours in their series. Only 50% of medulloblastoma, 17% of ependymoma and none of the glioblastoma tumours tested in their series had CCNU IC50 (the concentration of drug required to kill 50% of cells in comparison to control) values below the lower range of plasma CCNU concentrations achieved in adult patients. Therefore, the cellular determinants of chemosensitivity for CCNU in paediatric CNS tumours are likely to be relevant at clinically achievable concentrations for this drug in children.

In relation to the cellular determinants of chemosensitivity and clinical effect, the relationship between AGT and mismatch repair status and response to therapy with temzolomide has been studied extensively in relation to adult high-grade glioma. AGT levels in tumour samples are generally 5-fold higher than histologically normal brain, are lower for oligo-dengroglial than astroglial tumours, and in glial tumours are inversely related to age (Silber et al. 1998). The characterization of AGT in adult high-grade glioma has revealed a large (>300-fold) inter-patient range in AGT expression, with 24% of cases lacking detectable AGT activity (Silber et al. 1999). This inter-individual difference in tumoural AGT expression may be significant in the setting of therapy with methylating and chloroethylating agents. For patients with newly diagnosed high-grade glioma, response to therapy with temzolomide was more likely to occur in the face of tumours where <20% of cells stained for AGT, and where >60% of cells stained for the mismatch repair proteins MSH2 and MLH1 (Friedman et al. 1998). However, whereas the frequency of tumours lacking AGT activity (Mer−) is unchanged in relapse following surgery and radiotherapy alone, prior therapy with an alkylating reduces the incidence of the Mer− phenotype to 4%. Although this finding suggests that alkylating agent-containing therapy can kill Mer− cell in vivo, no difference in the median time to progression was found for the Mer− and Mer+ cases in one study (Silber et al. 1999).

However, other studies have indicated the potential importance of Mer+ status for high-grade glioma. In a retrospective study of AGT levels from patients with primary brain tumours receiving BCNU-containing therapy, a significantly shorter time to treatment failure and death was found for those cases with high tumoural AGT levels, when compared to those with those with low AGT levels. In particular, for glioblastoma multiforme, AGT levels were more strongly related to survival than age (Belanich et al. 1996). Similarly, for patients receiving BCNU and radiotherapy for treatment of high-grade glioma in a separate study, significant reductions in median times to treatment failure and survival were found to relate to AGT levels. For the 60% of patients with high AGT levels, the hazard ratios for high AGT expression were higher for patients under 60 years than for those aged 60 years or over (Jaeckle et al. 1998). A more recent analysis has also related methylation of the AGT gene promoter in high-grade glioma samples, which occurs in 40% of samples, with consequent reduction in tumoural AGT levels, with improved response to BCNU and prolonged overall and disease-free survival. Moreover, AGT gene methylation status was found to be an independent and stronger prognostic factor than age, stage, histological grade or performance status (Esteller et al. 2000).

Therefore, AGT levels may be an important determinant of response and prognosis with methylating and chloroethylating agents in adult high-grade glioma. In relation to paediatric CNS tumours, a very large (>100-fold) inter-patient range for cellular AGT levels has been found for high-grade glioma, medulloblastoma, ependymoma and low-grade tumours. Moreover, for high-grade glioma and medulloblastoma/primitive neuroectodermal tumour, the variability in AGT levels was very large, with a range of 550- and 1200-fold, respectively. In contrast to adult tumours, only 5% of paediatric high-grade glioma tumours carried a Mer− phenotype. In general, tumour AGT levels were 9-fold higher than that for adjacent normal brain, and a 4-fold higher AGT level is found for high-grade versus low-grade tumours. AGT levels are also found to relate to age, with tumour AGT content being 5-fold higher for children aged 3–12 years than for infants and adolescents (Bobola et al. 2001). The impact of tumour AGT levels on the efficacy of temozolomide in the therapy of paediatric high-grade glioma is unknown, but the finding that only a small minority of tumours are Mer− may be important. Moreover, the finding that temozolomide had only moderate activity in the phase II setting for children with high-grade glioma and brainstem glioma (Lashford et al. 2002) may serve to highlight this point.

Summary and conclusions
Paediatric CNS tumours remain a major challenge for the effective delivery of treatment with conventional chemotherapy. Although the main body of a tumour mass may be supplied by capillaries that are relatively permeable to chemotherapy agents, the presumed supply

185

of locally invasive or metastatic tumour with capillaries that have an intact BBB remains a major limitation for drug access and effectiveness. This difficulty would apply to many of the drugs employed in first line chemotherapeutic regimens.

Strategies to increase local drug delivery to CNS tumours have included intra-arterial delivery of chemotherapy, osmotic opening of the BBB, and the use of the bradykinin agonist RMP-7. Although intra-arterial delivery of drugs such as methotrexate and cisplatin has been achieved in adults, this technique is invasive and associated with neurological toxicity on the ipsilateral side of the infusion (Shapiro and Shapiro 1986). Similarly, although osmotic disruption of the BBB with mannitol increases the penetration of drug into the brain parenchyma, this technique also requires carotid arterial cannulation and has yet to find widespread clinical practice (Kroll and Neuwelt 1998). The bradykinin agonist RMP-7 has been developed as a means to promote short-lived opening of the BBB with a systemically administered drug. Although RMP-7 has associated toxicities including hypotension, flushing and gastrointestinal complaints, the compound is tolerated in combination with carboplatin in children, and phase II studies of this combination are planned (Warren et al. 2001).

Therefore, for the time being at least, conventional cytotoxic agents will form part of the mainstay of front line chemotherapy regimens for the treatment of childhood CNS tumours. However, as discussed above, there is a paucity of early clinical trials on which to base treatment regimens on the basis of the properly documented efficacy for each drug. Perhaps more importantly, the cellular determinants of chemosensitivity for the drugs employed in combination therapy for individual tumours need to be understood so that treatment can be optimized. The adult experience with temozolomide/nitrosoureas may serve as a paradigm in this regard. Not only does this information at least partly inform the prognosis of high-grade glioma in relation to chemotherapy, but it may also explain the greater success of nitrosourea-based chemotherapy for oligoastrocytomas in adults (Kim et al. 1996). Early clinical trials of AGT inhibitors in combination with temozolomide and nitrosoureas are ongoing in adults (Gerson 2002), and the lessons learned from these may have important applications in paediatric practice.

REFERENCES

Ali-Osman F, Stein DE, Renwick A (1990) Glutathione content and glutathione-S-transferase expression in 1,3 bis(2-choroethyl)-1-nitrosourea-resistant human malignant astrocytoma cell lines. *Cancer Res* **50**: 6976–6980.

Bart J, Groen HJM, Hendrkse NH, van der Graaf WTA, Vaalburg W, de Vries EGE (2000) The blood–brain barrier and oncology: new insights into function and modulation. *Cancer Treat Rev* **26**: 449–462.

Belanich M, Pastor M, Randall T, Guerra D, Kibitel J, Alas L, Li B, Citron M, Wasserman P, White A, Eyre H, Jaeckle K, Schulman S, Rector D, Prados M, Coons S, Shapiro W, Yarosh D (1996) Retrospective study of the correlation between the DNA repair protein alkyltransferase and survival of brain tumor patients treated with carmustine. *Cancer Res* **56**: 783–788.

Billson AL, Palmer JB, Walker DA, Lowe J (1994) Multidrug resistance gene (MDR 1) expression in neuroaxial tumours of children and young adults. *Br J Neurosurg* **8**: 585–591.

Blasberg RG, Groothius DR (1986) Chemotherapy of brain tumours: physiological and pharmacokinetic considerations. *Semin Oncol* **13**: 70–82.

Bobola MS, Tseng SH, Blank A, Berger MS, Silber JR (1996) Role of O^6-methylguanine–DNA methyltransferase in resistance of human brain tumour cell lines to the clinically relevant methylating agents temozolomide and streptozotocin. *Clin Cancer Res* **2**: 735–741.

Bobola MS, Berger MS, Ellenbogen, Roberts TS, Geyer JR, Silber JR (2001) O^6-methylguanine-DNA-methyl-transferase in paediatric primary brain tumours: relation to patient and tumour characteristics. *Clin Cancer Res* **7**: 613–619.

Bocangel DB, Finkelstein S, Schold SC, Bhakat KK, Mitra S, Kokkinakis DM (2002) Multifaceted resistance of gliomas to temozolomide. *Clin Cancer Res* **8**: 2725–2734.

Bogdahn U (1983) Chemosensitivity of malignant human brain tumours. Preliminary results. *J Neurooncol* **1**: 149–166.

Chastagner P, Bouffet E, Grill J, Kalifa C (2001) What have we learnt from previous phase II trials to help in the management of childhood brain tumours? *Eur J Cancer* **37**: 1981–1993.

Decleves X, Fajac A, Lehmann-Che J, Tardy M, Mercier C, Hurbain I, Laplanche JL, Bernaudin JF, Schermann JM (2002) Molecular and functional MDR1-Pgp and MRP's expression in human glioblastoma multiforme cell lines. *Int J Cancer* **10**: 173–180.

Donelli MG, Zucchetti M, D'Incalci M (1992) Do anticancer agents reach the tumour target within the human brain? *Cancer Chemother Pharmacol* **30**: 251–260.

Esteller M, Garcia-Foncillas J, Andion E, Goodman SN, Hidalgo OF, Vanaclocha V, Baylin SB, Herman JG (2000) Inactivation of the DNA-repair gene MGMT and the clinical response of gliomas to alkylating agents. *N Engl J Med* **343**: 1350–1354.

Estlin EJ (2001) Novel targets for therapy in paediatric oncology. *Curr Drug Targets Immune Endocr Metabol Disord* **2**: 141–150.

Estlin EJ, Ablett S (2001) Practicalities and ethics of running clinical trials in paediatric oncology – the UK experience. *Eur J Cancer* **37**: 1394–1398.

Estlin EJ, Veal GJ (2003) Clinical and cellular pharmacology in relation to solid tumours of childhood. *Cancer Treat Rev* **29**: 253–273.

Estlin EJ, Ablett S, Newell DR, Lewis IJ, Lashford L, Pearson ADJ (1996) Phase I trials in paediatric oncology – the European perspective. *Invest New Drugs* **14**: 23–32.

Estlin EJ, Lashford L, Ablett S, Price L, Gowing R, Gholkar A, Kohler J, Lewis IJ, Morland B, Pinkerton CR, Stevens MCG, Mott M, Stevens R, Newell DR, Walker D, Dicks-Mireaux C, McDowell H, Reidenberg P, Statkevich P, Marco A, Batra V, Dugan M, Pearson ADJ (1998) Phase I study of temozolomide in paediatric patients with advanced cancer. *Br J Cancer* **78**: 652–661.

Evans WE, Relling M, Rodman JH, Crom WR, Boyett JM, Pui C-H (1998) Conventional compared with individualized chemotherapy for childhood acute lymphoblastic leukaemia. *New Engl J Med* **338**: 499–505.

Fink D, Aebi S, Howell SB (1998) The role of DNA mismatch repair in drug resistance. *Clin Cancer Res* **4**: 1–6.

Finlay JL, Geyer JR, Turski PA, Yates AJ, Boyett JM, Allen JC, Packer RJ (1994) Pre-irradiation chemotherapy in children with high grade astrocytoma: tumour response to two cycles of the '8-drugs-in-1-day' regimen. A Children's Cancer Group study, CCG-945. *J Neurooncol* **21**: 255–265.

Friedman HS, Colvin OM, Kaufman SM, Bullock N, Bigner DD, Griffith OW (1992) Cyclophosphamide resistance in medulloblastoma. *Cancer Res* **52**: 5373–5378.

Friedman HS, McLendon RE, Kerby T, Dugan M, Bigner SH, Henry AJ, Ashley DM, Krisher J, Lovell S, Rasheed K, Marchev F, Seman AJ, Cokgor I, Rich J, Stewart E, Colvin OM, Provencale JM, Bigner DD, Haglund MM, Friedman AH, Modrich PL (1998) DNA mismatch repair and O^6-alkylguanine-DNA alkyltransferase analysis and response to Temodal in newly diagnosed malignant glioma. *J Clin Oncol* **16**: 3851–3857.

Friedman HS, Pegg AE, Johnson SP, Loktionova NA, Dolan ME, Modrich P, Moschel RC, Struck R, Brent TP, Ludeman S, Bullock N, Kilborn C, Keir S, Dong Q, Bigner DD, Colvin OM (1999) Modulation of cyclophosphamide activity by O^6-alkylgunaine-DNA alkyltransferase. *Cancer Chemother Pharmacol* **43**: 80–85.

Gaynon PS, Ettinger LJ, Moel D, Siegel SE, Baum ES, Krivit W, Hammond GD (1987) Pediatric phase I trial of carboplatin: a Children's Cancer Group report. *Cancer Treat Rep* **71**: 1039–1042.

Gerson SL (2002) Clinical relevance of MGMT in the treatment of cancer. *J Clin Oncol* **20**: 2388–2399.

Iida M, Doi H, Asamoto S, Sugiyama H, Kuribayashi N, Takeda M, Okamura Y, Matsumoto K (1999) Effect of glutathione-modulating compounds on platinum compounds-induced cytotoxicity in human glioma cell lines. *Anticancer Res* **19**: 5383–5384.

Jaeckle KA, Eyre HJ, Townsend JJ, Schulman S, Knudson HM, Belanich M, Yarosh DB, Bearman SI, Giroux DJ, Schold SC (1998) Correlation of tumor O^6 methylguanine-DNA methyltransferase levels with survival of malignant astrocytoma patients treated with bis-chloroethnylnitrosourea: a Southwest Oncology Group study. *J Clin Oncol* **16**: 3310–3315.

Kalifa C, Valteau D, Pizer B, Vassal G, Grill J, Hartmann O (1999) High-dose chemotherapy in childhood brain tumours. Child's Nerv Syst 15: 498–505.

Kim L, Hochberg FH, Thornton AF, Harsh GR, Patel H, Finklestein D, Louis DN (1996) Procarbazine, lomustine and vincristine (PCV) chemotherapy for grade III and grade IV oligoastrocytomas. *J Neurosurg* **85**: 602–607.

Kokkinakis DM, Moschel RC, Pegg AE, Schold SC (1999) Eradication of human medulloblastoma tumour xenografts with a combination of O^6-benzyl-$2'$-deoxyguanosine and 1,3-Bis(2-chlroethyl)-1-nitrosourea. *Clin Cancer Res* **5**: 3676–3681.

Kokkinakis DM, Bocangel DB, Schold SC, Moschel RC, Pegg AE (2001) Thresholds of O^6-alkylguaine-DNA alkyltransferase which confer significant resistance of human glial tumour xenografts to treatment with 1,3-bis(2-chloroethyl)-1-nitrosourea or temozolomide. *Clin Cancer Res* **7**: 421–428.

Kortmann RD, Kuhl J, Timmerann B, Mittler U, Urban C, Budach V, Richter E, Willich N, Flentje M, Brthold F, Slavc I, Wolff J, Meisner C, Wiestler O, Sorensen N, Warmuth-Metz M, Bamberg M (2000) Postoperative neoadjuvant chemotherapy before radiotherapy as compared to immediate radiotherapy followed by maintenance chemotherapy in the treatment of medulloblastoma in childhood: results of the German prospective randomized trial HIT '91. *Int J Radiat Oncol Biol Phys* **46**: 261–263.

Kroll RA, Neuwelt EA (1998) Outwitting the blood–brain barrier for therapeutic purposes: osmotic opening and other means. *Neurosurgery* **42**: 1083–1100.

Lashford LS, Thiesse P, Jouvet A, Jaspan T, Couanet D, Griffiths PD, Doz F, Ironside J, Robson K, Hobson R, Dugan M, Pearson ADJ, Vassal G, Frappaz D (2002) Temozolomide in malignant gliomas of childhood. A United Kingdom Children's Cancer Study Group and French Society for Pediatric Oncology Intergroup study. *J Clin Oncol* **20**: 4684–4691.

Lee FYF, Workman P, Roberts JT, Bleehen NM (1985) Clinical pharmacokinetics of oral CCNU (lomustine). *Cancer Chemother Pharmacol* **14**: 125–131.

Lewandowicz GM, Harding B, Harkness W, Hayward R, Thomas DGT, Darling JL (2000) Chemosensitivity in childhood brain tumours in vitro: evidence of differential sensitivity to lomustine (CCNU) and vincristine. *Eur J Cancer* **36**: 1955–1964.

Mastrangelo R, Lasorella A, Riccardi R, Colosimo C, Iavarone A, Tornesello A, Mastrangelo S, Ausili-Cefaro G, Di Rocco C (1995) Carboplatin in childhood medulloblastoma/PNET: feasibility of an in vivo test in an "up-front" study. *Med Pediatr Oncol* **24**: 188–196.

Middelmass DS, Stewart CF, Kirstein MN, Poquette C, Friedman HS, Houghton PJ, Brent TP (2000) Biochemical correlates of temozolomide sensitivity in pediatric solid tumour xenograft models. *Clin Cancer Res* **6**: 998–1007.

Rodman JH, Abromowitch M, Sinkule JA, Hayes FA, Rivera GK, Evans WE (1987) Clinical pharmacodynamics of continuous infusion teniposide: systemic exposure as a determinant of response in a phase I trial. *J Clin Oncol* **5**: 1007–1014.

Rodman JH, Relling MV, Stewart CF, Synold TW, McLeod H, Kearns C, Stute N, Crom WR, Evans WE (1993) Clinical pharmacokinetics and pharmacodynamics of anticancer drugs in children. *Semin Oncol* **20**: 18–29.

Shapiro WR, Shapiro JR (1986) Principles of brain tumour chemotherapy. *Semin Oncol* **13**: 56–69.

Silber JR, Bobola MS, Ewers TG, Muramoto M, Berger MS (1992) O^6-alkylguanine DNA-alkyltransferase is not a major determinant of sensitivity to 1,3-bis(2-chloroethyl)-1-nitrosourea in four medulloblastoma cell lines. *Oncol Res* **4**: 241–248.

Silber JR, Bobola MS, Ghatan S, Blank A, Kolstoe DD, Berger MS (1998) O^6-methylguanine-DNA methyltransferase activity in adult gliomas: relation to patient and tumour characteristics. *Cancer Res* **58**: 1068–1073.

Silber JR, Blank A, Bobola MS, Ghatan S, Kolstoe DD, Berger MS (1999) O^6-methylguainine-DNA methyltransferase-deficient phenotype in human gliomas: frequency and time to tumour progression after alkylating agent-based chemotherapy. *Clin Cancer Res* **5**: 807–814.

Warren KE, Patel MC, Aikin AA, Widemann B, Libucha M, Adamson PC, Neuwirth R, Benziger D, O'Toole D, Ford K, Patronas N, Packer RJ, Balis FM (2001) Phase I trial of lobradimil (RMP-7) and carboplatin in children with brain tumours. *Cancer Chemother Pharmacol* **48**: 275–282.

Weller M, Schmidt C, Roth W, Dichgans J (1997) Chemotherapy of human malignant glioma: prevention of efficacy by dexamethasone? *Neurology* **48**: 1704–1709.

Wolff JEA, Trilling T, Molenkamp G, Egeler RM, Jurgens H (1999) Chemosensitivity of glioma cells in vitro: a meta analysis. *J Cancer Res Clin Oncol* **125**: 481–486.

Wolff JE, Gneko AK, Kortmann RD, Pietsch T, Urban C, Graf N, Kuhl J (2002) Preradiation chemotherapy for paediatric patients with high grade glioma. *Cancer* **94**: 264–271.

Zeltzer PM, Boyett JM, Finaly JL, Albright AL, Rorke LB, Milstein JM, Allen JC, Stevens KR, Stanley P, Hao Li, Wisoff JH, Geyer JR, McGuire-Cullen P, Stehbens JA, Shurin SB, Packer RJ (1999) Metastases stage, adjuvant treatment, and residual tumour are prognostic factors for medulloblastoma in children: conclusions from the Children's Cancer Group 921 randomized Phase III study. *J Clin Oncol* **17**: 832–845.

9
MANAGEMENT OF COMPLICATIONS AT PRESENTATION FOR CHILDREN WITH CNS TUMOURS

Stephen Lowis

Patients with brain tumours are similar to, but different from other neurosurgical and oncological patients.

The presentation of intracranial tumours is often associated with severe neurological impairment, the result of acute hydrocephalus, haemorrhage or tumour-related infiltration or oedema. The supportive care of such patients should be directed by experienced teams, but at presentation the majority of children will be seen in an accident and emergency department. Initial management must be rapid in order to minimize secondary disability not directly produced by the tumour, and it is important that appropriate management protocols for specific situations are available.

At a later stage of therapy, patients undergoing chemotherapy or radiotherapy may suffer similar complications to other oncology patients, and once again, management protocols are necessary for optimal recovery. In this chapter, some of the more important hazards for neuro-oncology patients are reviewed.

Impaired consciousness, encephalopathy

Alterations in the level of consciousness of a patient, confusion, disorientation and convulsions must always be regarded as serious events. The spectrum of illness leading to reduced consciousness is wide, but consideration of intracranial space tumour should be made particularly in the child presenting with profound impairment or focal signs, or who is afebrile.

Changes in neurological states are more common in patients with brain tumours, but may occur in any patient undergoing treatment for malignant disease. The process involved in managing such events is similar to that for any other patient, but important additional considerations exist, reflecting a different spectrum of potential causes of such problems. In the immediate postoperative period, delayed recovery from general anaesthetic is likely to be related to the immediate surgical and anaesthetic procedure. Important causes that must be rapidly excluded include postoperative raised intracranial pressure (ICP) (including brain oedema), electrolyte imbalance, hypoglycaemia, vascular complications (haemorrhage, infarction or iscahaemia), high or low blood CO_2, and a post-ictal state. Patients with delayed recovery are at risk of further complications, particularly if their airway is inadequately protected, and early postoperative imaging should be performed.

TABLE 9.1
Modified Glasgow Coma Scale: modified James scale*

Eye opening	4	Spontaneous		
	3	To voice		
	2	To pain		
	1	None		
Verbal	5	*>5 years* Orientated	*<5 years*	Alert, babbles, coos, words or sentences: normal
	4	*>5 years* Confused	*<5 years*	Less than usual ability, irritable cry
	3	*>5 years* Inappropriate words	*<5 years*	Cries to pain
	2	*>5 years* Incomprehensible sounds	*<5 years*	Moans to pain
	1	*>5 years* No response to pain	*<5 years*	No response to pain
Motor	6	*>5 years* Obeys commands	*<5 years*	Normal spontaneous movements
	5	Localizes to supra-ocular pain (>9 months)		
	4	Withdraws from nailbed pressure		
	3	Flexion to supraocular pain		
	2	Extension to supraocular pain		
	1	No response to supraocular pain		

*Tatman et al. (1997).

Beyond the initial postoperative period, the approach to investigation of an acute change in neurological state should be the same as for any acutely unwell child, although the relative likelihood of particular causes differs. The initial management for all patients must be to ensure adequate ventilation, and to maintain the systemic circulation. If there is evidence of metabolic disturbance, this should be corrected. Blood pressure may be elevated, but this is an appropriate response in a patient with raised ICP and should not be reduced precipitously. Patients with hypothalamic or pituitary tumours may have established endocrine deficits and may show electrolyte disturbances or hypoglycaemia, or have inadequate perfusion, which should be corrected immediately.

If a child is suffering generalized seizures, these must be controlled, and initial investigations undertaken while this is begun. Diazepam should be used initially, but if more than one bolus dose is required in an unconscious patient, ventilation will be necessary. Rectal paraldehyde may be effective, and has less effect on respiratory drive than either benzodiazepines or barbiturates. If seizures continue, intravenous phenytoin may be given (slowly, with ECG monitoring). Phenytoin is less likely to cause respiratory depression than phenobarbitone, although when given intravenously carries a risk of inducing extrapyramidal movement disorders.

It is important to document the level of consciousness of any neurologically ill child. The Glasgow Coma scale is appropriate for all children, and is familiar to most medical and nursing staff. An adaptation of this, suitable for use with children below the age of 5 years, has been reported to be reproducible between observers (Tatman et al. 1997) and is given in Table 9.1. A low score in a child of any age indicates a high risk of further deterioration, and urgent need for investigation and treatment. A change in GCS of two points is

TABLE 9.2
Causes of impaired level of consciousness in oncology patients, additional to those affecting all children

Metabolic	Drug-related
Hypoglycaemia	Steroid psychosis/depression
Hyperglycaemia (diabetic ketoacidosis)	Ifosfamide-related encephalopathy
Hyponatraemia	Melphalan, busulphan neurotoxicity
Hypernatraemia	Cyclosporin neurotoxicity
Uraemia	L-asparaginase induced thromboembolic disease
	Cytarabine encephalopathy
Infection: meningitis, encephalitis	Methotrexate leukoencephalopathy
Bacterial	Sedative analgesia
Viral	Opiates, benzodiazepines, phenothiazines,
Opportunistic, include fungal	cannabinoids
Neurosurgery-related (ventriculitis, shunt infection)	
	Tumour-related
Haemorrhage, thrombosis	Primary CNS tumour
Thrombocytopenia	Metastatic tumour
Diffuse intravascular coagulation	Paraneoplastic
Thrombotic thrombocytopenic purpura	Post-neurosurgery complication
Coagulation factor hypoproduction (malnutrition,	Subdural/extradural collection, haematoma
malabsorption, L-asparaginase-related)	Infarction, haemorrhage
Dehydration	Posterior fossa syndrome
Sepsis	Shunt dysfunction

significant and is an indication for ventilation. Severe neurological impairment requires intensive care support, and involvement of a paediatric neurologist and a neurosurgeon.

Further assessment of the patient should assess the possibility of raised ICP and cerebral herniation. Given that cerebral perfusion pressure is the difference between mean arterial pressure and ICP, raised ICP will lead to reduced cerebral perfusion, and this affects particularly the watershed areas between vascular territories. In addition, differences in pressure between parts of the brain may lead to herniation of one or both temporal lobes through the tentorium, or of the medulla or pons through the foramen magnum, causing more severe ischaemia and haemorrhage. Uncal herniation may be compatible with intact recovery, but herniation of the pons or medulla through the foramen magnum is not. It is therefore important to be able to identify these events. These have been summarized by Kirkham (2001). Repeated examination of the patient to assess pupillary response, somatic response to pain, limb tone, posture, reflexes and respiratory pattern is essential for appropriate assessment of the unconscious patient.

Table 9.2 summarizes causes of impaired consciousness that are particularly relevant to the child with malignant disease. An approach to the investigation of non-traumatic coma in children with known malignant disease is given in Table 9.3, which is an adaptation of that published by Kirkham (2001) for children without known malignant disease.

Where a transient change is seen, clearly associated with administration of a chemotherapeutic or other drug, the drug must be stopped immediately. Ifosfamide is well reported to be associated with such an encephalopathy (Cantwell et al. 1988, Lewis et al. 1993). Risk factors for its development include oral administration, renal impairment, bulky abdominal disease and poor nutritional status, although recent brain surgery is likely also to be associated with a greater risk. Discontinuation of the infusion is usually, but not always, associated with rapid recovery (Bruggers et al. 1994, Shuper et al. 2000). Methylene blue has been found to reverse the acute neurotoxic effects rapidly (Pelgrims et al. 2000), and should be routinely available on the oncology ward. Busulphan similarly is associated with a risk of inducing fits, and prophylactic anticonvulsant medications are typically given in high dose conditioning regimes (requiring stem cell rescue) containing this drug.

Table 9.3 lists some suggested investigations that may be of value for patients with impaired consciousness.

Spinal cord compression

Spinal cord compression is a severe and often irreversible complication of intraspinal pathology, which greatly increases the morbidity for any patient regardless of their underlying illness. A patient presenting with symptoms and signs of spinal cord compression must be investigated and treated without delay: whatever the underlying pathology, oedema and obstruction of vascular drainage causes further deterioration and will lead to irreversible infarction if prompt action is not taken.

Symptoms suggestive of cord compression include back pain, a sensory level, bladder or bowel dysfunction (Lewis et al. 1986). Back pain in a young patient must always be investigated fully, unless minor, transient and with a clear history of injury. Signs that may be seen include sensory change at the level of disease, sensory loss, loss of deep tendon and abdominal reflexes, and motor loss. There may be local tenderness at the level of the compression, particularly if this arises as a result of vertebral destruction. There may be an associated scoliosis, particularly with low-grade intrinsic spinal cord tumours. The presence of other features suggestive of systemic malignant disease should prompt a full search for metastatic deposits including bone scan, bone marrow examination, and CT and/or MRI of chest, abdomen and affected regions. Lumbar puncture is contra-indicated in the presence of cord compressive signs until adequate spinal imaging is complete. The urgency for investigation is increased if any neurological deficit is identified: irreversible paraplegia may develop rapidly unless decompression is achieved.

Spinal cord compression may arise from primary, intrinsic spinal cord disease, from intradural or extradural intraspinal tumours, both primary and metastatic. Although spinal cord tumours represent the majority of intrinsic spinal lesions, acute disseminated encephalomyelitis (ADEM) may present in the spine (Hung et al. 2001), and in patients who have previously undergone spinal surgery or radiotherapy, infarction or radiation myelopathy (radiation necrosis) may be indistinguishable clinically or radiologically from tumour. The management of intrinsic spinal cord tumours is discussed in Chapter 18, and of spinal metastatic disease in Chapter 19.

Spinal cord compression is uncommon in childhood, although up to 5% of children with solid malignant tumours have been reported to develop spinal epidural compression, usually in the final stages of their disease (Lewis et al. 1986, Klein et al. 1991). Tumours arising outside the CNS that may present with spinal cord compression include neuroblastoma, peripheral primitive neuroectodermal tumour (pPNET), other sarcomas and non-Hodgkin

TABLE 9.3
Investigations of non-traumatic coma in children with malignant disease

Investigation	Indication	Risk factors	Possible abnormality	Further investigation if abnormal	Possible diagnosis	Immediate action
Blood glucose	All	Nutrition	Hypoglycaemia	Insulin, blood ammonia, lactate, blood and urine amino acids, urine organic acids	Hypoglycaemia secondary to poor intake	Intravenous glucose
		L-asparaginase			Pancreatitis, diabetic ketoacidosis	Supportive
Sodium	All	Poor intake, vomiting, ifosfamide, cisplatin	Hypernatraemia	Urinary sodium, osmolality, tubular resorption of phosphate	Dehydration, possible renal tubular leak	Appropriate fluids
		Pituitary region tumour, hyperhydration	Hyponatraemia	See specific protocol	Fluid overload, SIADH	Fluid restriction
Urea	All	Poor intake, vomiting, ifosfamide, cisplatin	Dehydration	Serum creatinine	Dehydration	Intravenous fluids
		BMT, cyclosporin	Raised		TTP	Correction of coagulopathy. ?IVIG, plasmapheresis
LDH	All	BMT, cyclosporin	Raised		TTP	Correction of coagulopathy. ?IVIG, plasmapheresis
AST/ALT	All	Actinomycin D, 6-thioguanine, busulphan	Hepatic impairment		Veno-occlusive disease	Supportive
		High-dose therapy	Hepatic impairment		Direct organ toxicity	Supportive
FBC and film	All	Recent chemotherapy	Anaemia	CT/MRI brain	Intracranial haemorrhage	Neurosurgical referral
			Thrombocytopenia	CT/MRI brain	Intracranial haemorrhage	Neurosurgical referral
			Leukocytosis	Infection screen	Meningitis	Lumbar puncture if CT, clotting normal. Antibiotic therapy
		Infection, shocked, BMT	DIC/TTP	CT/MRI brain	Intracranial haemorrhage	Neurosurgical referral
PT, APTT, fibrinogen, D-dimers	All	Poor nutrition, malabsorption	Reduced vitamin K dependent factor production	CT/MRI brain	Intracranial haemorrhage	Neurosurgical referral
		Infection, active disease	DIC (TTP)	CT/MRI brain	Intracranial haemorrhage	Neurosurgical referral

Investigation	Indication	Predisposing factors	Finding	Further investigation	Interpretation	Action
Blood culture	All		Bacteraemia			Antibiotic therapy
Stool culture	If clinically indicated		Shigella, enteroviruses			
CT/MRI brain	All	Prior radiotherapy, Leukaemia, L-asparaginase, dehydration, hyperleukocytosis, recent neurosurgery, (intracranial germ cell tumour)	Primary tumour, metastasis	FBC, BM aspiration MRI/angiography	Recurrent or progressive disease	Consider neurosurgical referral
			Mass lesion ± cavitation		Radionecrosis	Neurosurgical referral
			Infiltration		Leukaemic relapse	
			Infarct		Infarct	Appropriate fluids. Consider anticoagulation, defibrotide(?)
			Blood			
			Hydrocephalus		Tumour progression, shunt dysfunction	Neurosurgical referral
			Focal low density			
			Abscess		Abscess, herpes, tumour	
			Diffuse oedema			Mannitol, dexamethasone
			Fronto-temporal abnormality	CSF virology, PCR	Herpes virus encephalopathy	Aciclovir
Lumbar puncture* Cytospin MC+S	All	Leukaemia, lymphoma	Blasts		Relapse	Discussion of chemotherapy
			High non-malignant WCC		Meningitis (bacterial, viral, opportunistic)	Appropriate antibiotics
PCR for TB						Antituberculous therapy
PCR for viruses						Antivirals if available
EEG	All		Epileptiform discharges		Status epilepticus	Control seizure activity

* After CT/MRI, FBC, clotting.

Abbreviations: ALT = alanine transaminase; AST = aspartate transaminase; APTT = activated partial thromboplastin time; BMT = bone marrow transplantation; DIC = diffuse intravascular coagulation; FBC = full blood count; IVIG = intravenous immunoglubulin; MC+S = microscopy, culture and sensitivity; PCR = polymerase chain reaction; PT = prothrombin time; TTP = thrombotic thrombocytopenic purpura; WCC = white cell count.

195

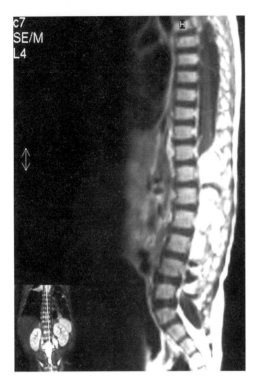

Fig. 9.1. Extensive intraspinal primitive neuro-ectodermal tumour (Ewing sarcoma) presenting in a 6-month-old infant. A macroscopically complete resection was obtained involving multiple hemi-laminotomies.

lymphoma (Lewis et al. 1986). Rarely, germ cell tumour, Wilms tumour or Hodgkin's disease may present in this way. Often, compression may arise as a result of extension through intervertebral foramina, and extensive intraspinal extension may be associated with even a small extraspinal mass (Fig. 9.1).

INITIAL TREATMENT

As is required for all patients with acute neurological symptoms, initial emergency treatment includes provision of adequate airway, breathing and circulation. It must be established that the patient is able to self-ventilate normally, and this may require an arterial blood gas measurement. High flow oxygen should be given unless a specific contraindication exists. Maintenance of normal blood pressure is essential, and rapid reduction of raised blood pressure may lead to irreversible cord damage. The spine should be stabilized before any procedure involving movement. Intravenous dexamethasone should be given either before or immediately after urgent imaging. Very high intravenous doses, up to 1 mg/kg/day, may be used initially, although smaller oral doses may be used in the absence of neurological deficit. If there is a likelihood of cord compression being due to non-Hodgkin's lymphoma, there is a theoretical risk that dexamethasone may induce tumour lysis. The risks of this, and consequent medical problems, must be balanced against the likelihood of permanent neurological deficit if compression is not relieved promptly.

IMAGING

Spinal imaging must be obtained urgently. Plain spine radiographs are often performed, and may indicate a destructive lesion affecting one or more vertebrae, but the diagnostic value of this investigation is significantly lower than in adult patients (Lewis et al. 1986). MRI is the initial investigation of choice, and should be performed unless a specific contra-indication exists (Carmody et al. 1989, Shuper et al. 2000). In very young children, general anaesthesia or sedation may be necessary to perform MRI, and this may not be felt appropriate. For such patients, and for those in whom extraspinal tumour is suspected, CT may allow an assessment of the cord that is sufficient to decide on further therapy. Complete contrast enhanced neuraxis MRI should be obtained at the first safe opportunity.

Myelography has no role in the diagnosis of acute spinal cord compression in childhood, being difficult, invasive, and having a lower sensitivity and specificity than MRI (Godersky et al. 1987, Smoker et al. 1987, Carmody et al. 1989).

THERAPY

Surgery

Surgery, chemotherapy and radiotherapy may have a role in relieving acute compression. For the majority, surgical decompression will be the most appropriate, and for all patients, discussion with the neurosurgical team is essential at the time of presentation. Decompressive laminotomy or laminectomy over multiple segments, preserving normal anatomy where possible, is usually performed. Where there is bony destruction or vertebral collapse, stabilization of the affected vertebrae will be necessary.

For two, normally extraspinal tumours, chemotherapy is the treatment of choice. In non-Hodgkin's lymphoma, the initial response to even single agent corticosteroid may be dramatic, allowing full recovery of neurological deficit. In neuroblastoma, intervertebral foramina may be infiltrated by tumour, leading to a 'dumbbell' tumour that may have ex-tensive intraspinal involvement. There is good evidence that chemotherapy is as effective as surgery or radiotherapy in relieving cord compression in neuroblastoma (Hayes et al. 1984, Sanderson et al. 1989, Plantaz et al. 1996, Hoover et al. 1999), and given the anticipated morbidity of extensive laminectomy or laminotomy, this should be the modality of choice unless neurological impairment is rapidly preogressive or of less than 72 hours duration.

The diagnosis of neuroblastoma can be made on the basis of elevated urinary catechol-amines together with evidence of malignant cells from either a biopsy or (if involved) bone marrow. Most paraspinal dumbbell tumours will be localized at presentation, and will have good prognostic features (histological evidence of ganglion cell differentiation, lack of MycN amplification, lack of chromosome 1p deletion or 17q gain), but this is not always so. Given that therapy of neuroblastoma is now stratified according to stage and MycN status, it is essential that an appropriate diagnostic sample is obtained whenever possible.

Radiotherapy

Radiotherapy is an essential component of therapy for the majority of tumours that may affect the spine, but its use in the emergency relief of compression is limited. Typically this will be in patients with metastatic disease, often in the context of palliative care. For

197

patients in such situations, radiotherapy may offer rapid stabilization of progressive disease, and prevent further bony collapse.

Radiotherapy has been used as initial therapy for intraspinal neuroblastoma, but a high incidence of late kyphosis and scoliosis was seen, particularly with doses of more than 20 Gy and with asymmetrical irradiation fields (Mayfield et al. 1981).

Electrolyte and endocrine disturbance

Patients presenting with a brain tumour will often have a history of vomiting or impaired oral intake. Where a tumour arises in the hypothalamus, suprasellar region, pituitary gland or occasionally the anterior optic pathway, there is risk of endocrine dysfunction, and the patient may already have developed hypopituitarism or diabetes insipidus. Initial management of a patient presenting with raised ICP may include forced diuresis, and patients are therefore at risk of significant dehydration.

Intraoperatively, highly vascular tumours may make large transfusion and fluid resuscitation necessary. It is not uncommon for patients to require whole blood volume, or even two or three times blood volume transfusion. Patients returning from theatre may therefore have significant disturbance of water and electrolyte homeostasis.

Postoperatively, inappropriate ADH secretion is common, and inappropriate fluid management will lead to hyponatraemia and significant fluid shifts. In patients undergoing pituitary surgery, but also in the hypothalamic region, postoperative diabetes insipidus (DI) may be seen. This may be temporary, presumably due to local oedema disrupting normal AVP release, or permanent due to destruction of the posterior pituitary by tumour or surgery. The problem of fluid management is made more difficult by the so-called 'triple' response. An early diuretic phase due to DI is followed after several days by anti-diuresis associated with inappropriate secretion of preformed ADH. Later, after a further interval of several days, DI will return if endogenous secretion was damaged. The rapid changes in fluid output over this time may lead to large fluid shifts, and it is essential that nurses and doctors respond promptly. Rapid dehydration–overhydration cycles are associated with central pontine myelinolysis, with catastrophic results.

A further cause of hyponatraemia in the postoperative patient is cerebral salt wasting (CSW). This is independent of the syndrome of inappropriate ADH secretion (SIADH), and is probably due to production of atrial naturetic peptide. A clinical assessment of the patient is necessary to distinguish CSW from SIADH, and the principal difference seen will be fluid overload in SIADH, and fluid loss in CSW. The management of these conditions is clearly different, and fluid restriction is hazardous in the presence of CSW.

The involvement of a paediatric endocrinologist is essential preoperatively for all patients with pituitary region surgery, both in the management of fluids and for replacement of specific hormones if necessary. Loss of production of any pituitary hormone will be important to the patient's normal development, but the greatest immediate concern is to replace ACTH and vasopressin. Most patients will receive high dose dexamethasone at the time of presentation, and the perioperative period may therefore not lead to potentially dangerous hypoadrenalism. In the postoperative period, however, early discontinuance of steroid may precipitate an Addisonian episode. Patients 'at risk' of hypopituitarism must

receive replacement corticosteroid. The replacement hydrocortisone dose is 12–15 mg/m²
(dose to be doubled if the child is febrile or unwell) until full hypothalamic–pituitary axis
function testing is complete.

REFERENCES

Bruggers CS, Friedman HS, Tien R, Delong R (1994) Cerebral atrophy in an infant following treatment with ifosfamide. *Med Pediatr Oncol* **23**: 380–383.

Cantwell BM, Carmichael J, Ghani S, Harris AL (1988) A phase II study of ifosfamide/mesna with doxorubicin for adult soft tissue sarcoma. *Cancer Chemother Pharmacol* **21**: 49–52.

Carmody RF, Yang PJ, Seeley GW, Seeger JF, Unger EC, Johnson JE (1989) Spinal cord compression due to metastatic disease: diagnosis with MR imaging versus myelography. *Radiology* **173**: 225–229.

Godersky JC, Smoker WR, Knutzon R (1987) Use of magnetic resonance imaging in the evaluation of metastatic spinal disease. *Neurosurgery* **21**: 676–680.

Hayes FA, Thompson EI, Hvizdala E, O'Connor D, Green AA (1984) Chemotherapy as an alternative to laminectomy and radiation in the management of epidural tumor. *J Pediatr* **104**: 221–224.

Hoover M, Bowman LC, Crawford SE, Stack C, Donaldson JS, Grayhack JJ, Tomita T, Cohn SL (1999) Long-term outcome of patients with intraspinal neuroblastoma. *Med Pediatr Oncol* **32**: 353–359.

Hung KL, Liao HT, Tsai ML (2001) The spectrum of postinfectious encephalomyelitis. *Brain Dev* **23**: 42–45.

Kirkham FJ (2001) Non-traumatic coma in children. *Arch Dis Child* **85**: 303–312.

Klein SL, Sanford RA, Muhlbauer MS (1991) Pediatric spinal epidural metastases. *J Neurosurg* **74**: 70–75.

Lewis DW, Packer RJ, Raney B, Rak IW, Belasco J, Lange B (1986) Incidence, presentation, and outcome of spinal cord disease in children with systemic cancer. *Pediatrics* **78**: 438–443.

Lowis SP, Pearson AD, Reid MM, Craft AW (1993) Prohibitive toxicity of a dose-intense regime for metastatic neuroblastoma containing ifosfamide, doxorubicin and cisplatin. *Cancer Chemother Pharmacol* **31**: 415–418.

Mayfield JK, Riseborough EJ, Jaffe N, Nehme ME (1981) Spinal deformity in children treated for neuroblastoma. *J Bone Joint Surg Am* **63**: 183–193.

Pelgrims J, De Vos F, Van den Brande J, Schrijvers D, Prove A, Vermorken JB (2000) Methylene blue in the treatment and prevention of ifosfamide-induced encephalopathy: report of 12 cases and a review of the literature. *Br J Cancer* **82**: 291–294.

Plantaz D, Rubie H, Michon J, Mechinaud F, Coze C, Chastagner P, Frappaz D, Gigaud M, Passagia JG (1996) The treatment of neuroblastoma with intraspinal extension with chemotherapy followed by surgical removal of residual disease. A prospective study of 42 patients—results of the NBL 90 Study of the French Society of Pediatric Oncology. *Cancer* **78**: 311–319.

Sanderson IR, Pritchard J, Marsh HT (1989) Chemotherapy as the initial treatment of spinal cord compression due to disseminated neuroblastoma. *J Neurosurg* **70**: 688–690.

Shuper A, Stein J, Goshen J, Kornreich L, Yaniv I, Cohen IJ (2000) Subacute central nervous system degeneration in a child: an unusual manifestation of ifosfamide intoxication. *J Child Neurol* **15**: 481–483.

Smoker WR, Godersky JC, Knutzon RK, Keyes WD, Norman D, Bergman W (1987) The role of MR imaging in evaluating metastatic spinal disease. *AJR* **149**: 1241–1248.

Tatman A, Warren A, Williams A, Powell JE, Whitehouse W (1997) Development of a modified paediatric coma scale in intensive care clinical practice. *Arch Dis Child* **77**: 519–521.

SECTION TWO

CNS TUMOURS
OF CHILDHOOD

10
LOW-GRADE AND HIGH-GRADE ASTROCYTOMA

Eddy Estlin and Stephen Lowis

Glial cells provide the supportive architecture of the central nervous system. They include astrocytes, oligodendrocytes and ependymal cells, and the corresponding tumours arising from these cells (astrocytomas, oligodendrogliomas and ependymomas) can strictly be referred to as 'gliomas'. More commonly, 'glioma' is used interchangeably with 'astrocytoma' to denote the more common subgroup of tumours. The behaviour and management of ependymomas are sufficiently distinct for these to be discussed separately in Chapter 11.

Astrocytomas account for the majority of CNS tumours in children. Low-grade gliomas are the most common type of paediatric CNS tumour, and account for approximately one-third of cases (Reddy and Packer 1999). High-grade gliomas occur less frequently, and account for 7–11% of cases of CNS malignancy in childhood (Heideman et al. 1997).

As will be discussed below, low- and high-grade gliomas differ markedly in terms of their histological grading, predominant site of disease within the CNS, treatment strategies and prognosis. For each tumour type, the discussion will focus on the epidemiology, clinical presentation, investigation, treatment and prognosis. Current controversies in terms of therapy will be highlighted.

Low-grade glioma
EPIDEMIOLOGY AND PATHOLOGY
The different tumour types within the group of low-grade gliomas (LGGs), which derive from astrocytes and oligodendrocytes, are classified as WHO grade I and grade II (Reddy and Packer 1999). The commonest histological subtype is the juvenile pilocytic astrocytoma, a WHO grade I tumour that is usually well circumscribed and has only a narrow margin of infiltration into the surrounding tissues. The next most common form is the fibrillary astrocytoma (WHO grade II), which has a tendency to be more infiltrative. The pathology of LGGs can be more complex and they may contain mixed glial (oligoastrocytoma) or ganglionic elements (ganglioglioma, see Chapter 13). A monomorphous pilomyxoid variant of LGG has been recently described in infants and young children and is reported to be associated with a poorer outcome (Tihan et al. 1999).

The commonest cytogenetic abnormality for juvenile pilocytic astrocytomas is a high frequency of gains in chromosomes 7 and 8 (Cokgor et al. 1998). Cytogenetic abnormalities do not, however, seem to impact upon progression-free survival (PFS) or overall survival in the context of LGG (Orr et al. 2002). Expression of the nuclear proliferation marker

Ki-67 may relate to a poorer outcome for children with LGG, with average Ki-67 indices >10% relating to a poorer overall survival (Fisher et al. 2002).

The aetiology of the majority of cases of childhood LGG remains unknown, but the phakomatoses are known to predispose to formation of LGGs. Neurofibromatosis type 1 (NF1) is associated with optic pathway tumours in particular, and tuberous sclerosis is associated with subependymal giant cell astrocytomas within the ventricular system (Cokgor et al. 1998).

CLINICAL PRESENTATION AND RADIOLOGY
In their review of a decade of experience at St Jude Children's Research Hospital, Memphis, Gajjar et al. (1997) found LGGs to arise from the cerebral hemispheres (20%), cerebellar hemispheres (35%), hypothalamus (12%), thalamus (12%), brain stem (12%), spinal cord (4%) and optic nerve/chiasm (3%). The median age at diagnosis was 7 years, and 32% of children were younger than 5 years at diagnosis.

The presenting features of the disease depend largely on the site involved in the CNS. For example, children with posterior fossa disease may present with the signs and symptoms of raised intracranial pressure secondary to obstructive hydrocephalus: papilloedema, headache, morning vomiting and ataxia would be expected.

Children with tumours affecting the optic chiasm or hypothalamus may present with visual loss – both visual field and acuity loss – with endocrinopathy and disturbance of hypothalamic function such as the diencephalic syndrome (Cokgor et al. 1998). Approximately half of all children with optic chiasm or hypothalamus tumours present before the age of 5 years (Medlock and Scott 1997), and in such young children these symptoms and signs may be less specific and more difficult to detect. This is especially true with regard to visual field loss, which may prove impossible to assess until after the age of 5 years. Although approximately 33% of these children have NF1 and a more indolent course, the majority of cases progress within 6 years of diagnosis (Janss et al. 1995).

On MRI examination, LGG is typically hypodense or isodense to the surrounding brain on T_1-weighted imaging, and hyperdense on T_2-weighting (Fig. 10.1; see also Fig. 3.3, p. 25, and Fig. 3.34, p. 54). LGG may present as homogenously enhancing mass lesions with gadolinium, a ring enhancing cyst, or a cystic cavity with an enhancing mural nodule (Medlock et al. 1997).

LGGs rarely metastasize within the CNS, and the overall frequency of this phenomenon, which is more likely to occur with tumours affecting the hypothalamic and periventricular areas, has been estimated at approximately 4% (Prados and Mamelak 1994). Furthermore, the risk of transformation to a higher-grade glioma is very small in children (Reddy and Packer 1999), and for these reasons, treatment strategies for LGG are aimed at achieving durable local control, with minimal morbidity. As will be discussed below, this involves site- and age-specific emphasis on surgery, radiotherapy and chemotherapy.

SURGERY AND RADIOTHERAPY
Surgery is the mainstay of therapy for LGG of the cerebral hemispheres (Pollack et al. 1995) or cerebellum (Gajjar et al. 1997), with radiotherapy or chemotherapy being reserved for

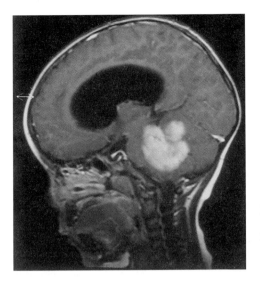

Fig. 10.1. T_1-weighted sagittal MRI post-gadolinium showing a cerebellar tumour. The large
homogeneously enhancing mass compresses
the brainstem anteriorly and there is associated
hydrocephalus.

recurrent or progressive inoperable disease. In the St Jude series, gross total resection of
tumour was achieved for 84% of children with cerebellar disease, and for 68% of children
with cerebral hemisphere tumours (Gajjar et al. 1997).The long-term survival for children
with cerebellar LGG where gross total resection is achieved is excellent, with individual
series reporting survival rates of 90–100%. However, PFS is poorer (40–50% at 10 years)
for children with residual disease post-surgery, although in some cases spontaneous involution
of residual tumour has been reported (Medlock et al. 1997). Similarly, the extent of resection
has been found to be of prognostic significance for children with either pilocytic astrocytomas
or other LGGs of the cerebral hemispheres (Pollack et al. 1995). For tumours of the optic
chiasm/hypothalamus, curative surgery is not usually possible or indicated. Surgery is
usually only indicated to debulk symptomatic tumours, relieve obstruction at the foramen
of Monro, and obtain a diagnostic biopsy (Medlock and Scott 1997).

Although there have been no randomized trials to compare radiotherapy and observation
alone for residual cerebellar and cerebral LGG (Cokgor et al. 1998), local field radiotherapy,
at a dose of 54 Gy administered over 30 fractions, is generally used for incompletely resected
and progressive LGG. Despite this, the use of radiotherapy has not been shown to improve
overall survival for eithersupratentorial (Pollack et al. 1995) or cerebellar astrocytomas (Garcia
et al. 1989). Furthermore, although the development of anaplastic changes in LGG is uncommon in childhood, this occurrence is generally associated with previous radiotherapy
(Dirks et al. 1994, Pollack et al. 1995).

Although the benefit of adjuvant radiotherapy for tumours affecting the cerebellar and
cerebral hemispheres is uncertain, for children with LGG involving the optic chiasm/hypo-
thalamus, local radiotherapy results in long-term disease control and visual preservation
for the majority of patients (Tao et al. 1997). Moreover, vision has been reported to improve
for up to 25% of children with visual impairment following radiotherapy (Cappelli et al.

205

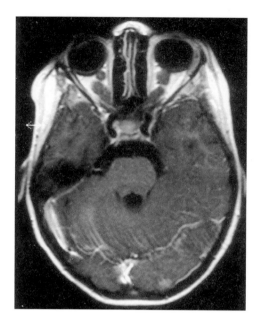

Fig. 10.2. T$_1$-weighted axial MRI post-gadolinium demonstrating grossly enlarged optic nerves and optic chiasm.

1998). When assessed radiologically, the percentage of children achieving a partial response to treatment with radiotherapy increases with time. For example, whereas 18% of children have been shown to demonstrate a partial response at 2 years post-radiotherapy, this rises to 46% by 5 years and is associated with a 10 year PFS rate of approximately 90% (Tao et al. 1997).

CHEMOTHERAPY

The late effects of radiation, such as endocrinopathy, vasculopathy, optic nerve damage and effects upon intellect, have generated interest in the use of chemotherapy in the treatment of LGG. This is especially true for children with hypothalamic or optic chiasm tumours, and for children under the age of 5 years who are at higher risk from radiation-induced long-term sequelae (Cokgor et al. 1998). Visual improvement that is not associated with radiological response has been described for children following chemotherapy (Mitchell et al. 2001). Moreover, much of the international experience in the chemotherapy of LGG derives from the treatment of LGG involving the hypothalamus/optic chiasm (Fig. 10.2).

Considerable variation exists worldwide for the treatment of LGG, both for the agents used and for the duration of therapy. Most institutional, national and international protocols employ a combination of agents, although single agent studies have been performed that may give important clues to the relative effectiveness of each drug in the treatment of LGG. For example, carboplatin given as a monthly dose of 560 mg/m^2 is associated with an objective response (OR) rate of 28% and stabilization rate (OR + stable disease) rate of 85% (Gururangan et al. 2002). When given as a single agent, carboplatin was found to be less effective for children with diencephalic tumours than for tumours at other sites, but the overall

TABLE 10.1

Selected combination chemotherapy for the treatment of childhood low-grade glioma

Regimen	Duration (months)	Objective response	Stable disease	PFS*	Reference
Vincristine, carboplatin	12	42%	37%	49% at 3 years	Walker et al. (2000)
Vincristine, actinomycin-D	28	37%	58%	62% at 4.3 years	Packer et al. (1988)
Cisplatin, etoposide	10	70%	30%	78% at 3 years	Massimino et al. (2002)
Procarbazine, CCNU, dibromodulcitol, 6-thioguanine	12	35%	60%	50% at 2.25 years	Prados et al. (1997)
Vincristine, carboplatin	22	56%	38%	68% at 3 years	Packer et al. (1997)

*PFS = progression-free survival.

PFS rate of 64% supports the role of this drug in the treatment of LGG. In contrast, single agent studies of cyclophosphamide (Kadota et al. 1999) and etoposide (Chamberlain 1997) have demonstrated that these agents have unacceptably high on-treatment progression rates.

The major findings of recently published institutional, national and international LGG treatment protocols based on combination therapy are presented in Table 10.1. Treatment with vincristine and carboplatin has been accepted as the gold standard for therapy in many European and North American centres. However, differences in philosophy exist for the scheduling of vincristine and carboplatin during both the induction and maintenance phases of therapy. For example, Packer et al. (1997) recommended carboplatin according to a fractionated schedule of $175 \, mg/m^2$ weekly ×4 and vincristine $1.5 \, mg/m^2$ weekly ×3 in repeating cycles of 7 weeks duration, following a 10 week induction period where vincristine is given weekly. In contrast, the International Consortium on Low Grade Glioma (ICLGG) recommended a single carboplatin dose of $560 \, mg/m^2$ 3 weekly during induction (with weekly vincristine) and at 4 weekly intervals with vincristine during maintenance therapy (Walker et al. 2000).

The various institutional and national/collaborative protocols have highlighted difficulties in relation to their protocols. For example, the administration of carboplatin according to the recommendations of the ICLGG is associated with the development of hypersensitivity reactions that limit further therapy in 30% of cases (Gnekow et al. 2000). In contrast, a carboplatin hypersensitivity rate of 6% was reported by Packer et al. (1997) in relation to their use of fractionated carboplatin dosing. Massimino et al. (2002) reported a 28% incidence high frequency hearing loss in relation to therapy with cisplatin. Despite these toxicities, chemotherapy is successful in delaying the need for radiotherapy for approximately 50–60% of children over a 3-year period. Individual studies, however, have highlighted clinical groups that are at particular risk of early or on-treatment progression, as well as those children who should do well. Packer and co-workers, for example, described the outcome for 78 children with a newly diagnosed progressive LGG who received chemotherapy with vincristine and carboplatin. The NF1 status of the patient, histological subtype, location and maximum response to chemotherapy did not have an impact on the duration of disease control, but children aged less than 5 years at the time of treatment had a 3-year PFS rate of 74%, which was significantly better than the PFS for older children (39%).

In contrast to the relatively good prognosis found for younger children by Packer and co-workers, where the mean age of the study population was 3 years, other groups have reported a relatively poor outcome for infants and younger children with LGG. For example, the ICLGG has reported that infants diagnosed with LGG under the age of 1 year tend to progress during periods of observation, and approximately one-quarter will progress during or soon after chemotherapy. The medium term efficacy of chemotherapy in this population is yet to be reported (Gnekow et al. 2000). Similarly, the French Society of Paediatric Oncology (SFOP) reported their experience for 84 children commencing chemotherapy according to the BB-SFOP protocol (carboplatin, procarbazine, etoposide, cisplatin, cyclophosphamide and vincristine over a duration of 16 months) at a median age of 25 months. Children commencing chemotherapy in the first year of life experienced a two-year PFS of 51% compared to 82% for older children.In this study, the degree of best partial response and a positive NF1 status were found to confer a positive effect on PFS (Laithier et al. 2000). Accordingly, forthcoming studies of LGG by the International Society of Paediatric Oncology (SIOP) will attempt to answer questions such as the value of intensifying the induction phase of therapy and prolonging the duration of maintenance therapy in improving PFS.

PROGNOSIS AND LATE EFFECTS OF THERAPY
Although overall survival rates for children with LGG are very good, the control of disease at certain sites of the CNS presents particular challenges in terms of prognosis and the late sequelae of therapy. For example, although the overall 4-year survival rate was 90% at 4 years in the St Jude series, the PFS rate was significantly better for children with cerebellar or cerebral hemisphere tumours (85%) than for those with tumours at other sites such as the hypothalamus (40%) and thalamus (55%). In addition, children below the age of 5 years had a poorer PFS than those diagnosed after the age of 5 years, and this difference was most pronounced in children with hypothalamic or thalamic tumours (Gajjar et al. 1997). If radiotherapy is required for disease control in these circumstances, then important neuropsychological and other sequelae may ensue. For 61 children receiving radiotherapy for LGG involving the optic chiasm, 53% were found to have some degree of cognitive impairment on long-term follow-up. This was rated as severe for 50% of children treated under the age of 5 years, although hydrocephalus at presentation may also have contributed to this outcome (Medlock et al. 1997), and has been implicated as an adverse prognostic factor in other series (Yule et al. 2001). Severe intellectual deficiencies were also reported for 18 children of a series of 69 who received radiotherapy for optic pathway gliomas, and again, these were those children who underwent irradiation when very young (median age of 4 years). Despite the lack of certain evidence regarding the role of radiotherapy in the eventual neuropsychological outcome of children treated at a young age, the international

practice of employing chemotherapy as a means to avoid or delay radiotherapy is likely to be preventing significant morbidity.

In addition to potential effects on neuropsychological outcome, the treatment of hypothalamic or optic chiasm tumours is known to be associated with long-term damage to the vessels of the circle of Willis, and an increased risk of cerebrovascular accident. This complication, which has been reported to occur in 20% of cases, is five times more likely to occur with patients who have NF1 (Cappelli et al. 1998). Furthermore, endocrine dysfunction has been reported for 42% of children who received radiotherapy for treatment of a hypothalamus/optic chiasm LGG, with growth hormone deficiency being the most prevalent deficiency (Collet-Solberg et al. 1997).

In summary, LGG, in the face of inoperable disease continues to pose a challenge for the multidisciplinary team. Clinical studies of chemotherapy that are designed to avoid or delay the need for radiotherapy in younger children have identified patients who are at risk for early disease progression or death. International cooperative studies will be essential for the continued improvement in prognosis for these children.

High-grade astrocytoma

High-grade astrocytomas (HGAs) are those graded III (anaplastic astrocytoma) or IV (glioblastoma multiforme) and comprise approximately 7–11% of paediatric tumours (Heideman et al. 1997). A greater proportion of grade III (rather than grade IV) tumours is seen in the paediatric population than in adults, and paediatric HGAs have a slightly better prognosis than in adults, but the outcome, particularly for unresected tumours, remains dismal.

There is evidence that some, but not all HGAs develop from lower grade (II) diffuse astrocytic tumours, and it is therefore important to investigate any intrinsic brain lesion fully at presentation. A previously diagnosed low-grade astrocytic tumour is therefore a predisposing factor leading to the development of HGA: others include prior radiotherapy to the CNS (possibly affected also by chemotherapy) (McLeod et al. 2000), and genetic predisposition syndromes. These latter include those associated with abnormalities of the retinoblastoma gene, NF1, Li–Fraumeni syndrome, tuberous sclerosis, Turcot syndrome and multiple enchondromatosis.

PATHOLOGY
High-grade glial tumours include astrocytomas, oligodendrogliomas, and mixed tumours or oligo-astrocytomas (WHO classification) (Kleihues et al. 2002).

Gross appearance of anaplastic tumours typically shows diffusely infiltrating margins, with or without haemorrhage. Histologically, these tumours are more cellular, pleomorphic and less differentiated than lower grade tumours, but lack necrosis. The presence of gemistocytes (Latin: "stuffed") – rounded cells with abundant cytoplasm and an eccentric nucleus – indicates more aggressive behaviour even without other typical appearances of anaplasia.

Glioblastomas may show macroscopic evidence of necrosis, and haemorrhage is typical. Histologically, tumours have variable features and may appear well differentiated in parts. Necrosis, vascular proliferation and a high mitotic rate are characteristic.

209

Grading of astrocytic tumours is important for prognosis, but remains one of the most difficult areas in pathology. This is made more difficult by the heterogeneous nature of high-grade tumours, and small biopsies that may not be representative of the whole. For a significant number of patients, grade, and therefore prognosis, continues to be uncertain. In the CCG-945 paediatric study, 18% of tumours originally graded as 'high grade' were regarded to low grade after central review. For this reason, multiple biopsies should be taken wherever possible, and central pathological review should be obtained for all patients.

GENETICS AND MOLECULAR BIOLOGY AS PROGNOSTIC FACTORS

In adults, progression of low-grade astrocytomas to high grade is associated with loss of heterozygosity (LOH) of chromosome 17p. Forty per cent of anaplastic astrocytomas and 30% of glioblastomas had this abnormality in the series of Fults et al. (1992), whereas this is most uncommon in pilocytic tumours. In children, the incidence of LOH 17p in high-grade tumours is low – 16% in the report of Raffel (1996) – suggesting a biological difference in at least some paediatric tumours. Expression of mutant p53 is common in adult tumours, particularly those which are believed to have arisen from pre-existent low-grade lesions, but not those which arise de novo. Interestingly, the gene encoding TP53 is found on 17p13.1.

Expression of TP53 in children varies with age at presentation: in a series of 77 patients enrolled in the CCG 945 study, with anaplastic astrocytoma or glioblastoma, a mutation of TP53 occurred in 2/17 below 3 years and in 24/60 older than 3 years. A poorer prognosis was seen in patients with TP53 expression, and particularly in those who also demonstrated a mutation of TP53 (Pollack et al. 2001, 2002a). Infants under the age of 3 years rarely show TP53 overexpression.

Amplification of the epidermal growth factor receptor is common in adult tumours, often with an associated gene rearrangement, and indeed is being pursued as a potential target for novel therapies. It is seen in a few anaplastic astrocytomas, and in about 60% of primary glioblastomas, and is associated closely with loss of chromosome 10. It was not seen at all in two series of paediatric non-brainstem HGAs (Cheng et al. 1999, Raffel et al. 1999).

Many studies have examined the relationship of specific signal transduction pathways in high-grade glioma, including the p53/MDM2/p21 pathway, p16/p15/Rb pathway, PTEN and others. In addition, proliferative activity of tumours is likely to have predictive value. In the B975 study, using patients enrolled in CCG 945 (randomized chemotherapy with PCV or "8 drugs in 1 day"), it was possible to stratify patients into prognostic groups according to labelling index (Pollack et al. 2002b). This study of 179 patients with centrally reviewed biopsies was performed in a rigorous manner, with reporters blinded to pathology, treatment and outcomes, using the MIB-1 monoclonal antibody to determine proliferative activity. Patients with anaplastic astrocytoma had a median MIB-1 labelling index of 11.5%, and those with glioblastoma had an index of 23%, as might be expected given the more aggressive nature of glioblastoma. Thirty-five patients had low MIB-1 labelling, and these were patients who were subsequently regraded as having low-grade tumours. MIB-1 labelling indices of <18%, 18–36% and >36% were associated with a progressively worse outcome, and MIB-1 labelling was a prognostic factor independent of pathological grade.

Paediatric tumours do seem to have a more favourable outcome compared to adults (Duffner et al. 1996), and separate pathways for development seems likely, one requiring overexpression of EGFR, and one associated with mutation of TP53.

PRESENTATION

The majority of HGAs arise within the cerebral hemispheres, or within the thalamus. Tumours arising in the posterior fossa are uncommon. Whilst the majority of astrocytic spinal tumours will also be low grade, high-grade tumours do occur (Lowis et al. 1998).

Clinical features of HGA depend upon the site of presentation, and may include loss of function (if impinging on the motor strip or involving thalamic tracts), new symptoms (such as focal seizures), or raised intracranial pressure. Patients with a long-standing history of epilepsy presenting with deterioration may have developed a high-grade tumour (anaplastic change) within a pre-existent low-grade diffuse astrocytoma or oligoastrocytoma. Spinal cord tumours may present with scoliosis, back pain, and sensory or motor deficits.

ASSESSMENT AND STAGING

Initial assessment involves a history that should include some measure of the duration of symptoms or signs, asking specifically about epilepsy. Examination should first ensure the neurological stability of the patient, and then seek to identify areas of motor or sensory deficit. Imaging may be first by CT. CT appearances of anaplastic tumours are typically mixed density, irregularly enhancing lesions, often with rim enhancement and mass effect. Tumours are usually in the cerebral cortex, and significant mass effect is seen. Calcification is uncommon, as these are rapidly growing tumours, although may be present in a pre-existent low-grade tumour, and does not exclude the diagnosis of a high-grade tumour.

MRI typically shows a poorly demarcated lesion with heterogeneous signal and variable enhancement. High signal seen on T_2-weighted images indicates oedema, and is expected to contain tumour cells. The significance of the area of vasogenic oedema is two-fold. Firstly, it represents the area of abnormal vascular supply, and potentially ischaemic normal brain tissue. Secondly, given the nature of HGAs, it represents the area most likely to contain microscopic residual disease after tumour resection. Spread of tumour may be seen through cortical pathways including the corpus callosum and corticospinal tracts.

Imaging appearances of glioblastomas are more variable. Radiological distinction of tumour grade is not possible, and especially in very young children, no conclusive diagnosis other than a likely malignant tumour can be made. Metastatic disease, which may be truly metastatic or in some cases represent extensive contiguous spread, is seen in a small proportion of cases.

THERAPY

Surgery

Standard therapy of HGAs involves surgical resection (or biopsy) and radiotherapy. There has been a somewhat nihilistic approach to management in some centres, with a very non-aggressive surgical policy, but there is good evidence that aggressive surgical resection is associated with prolonged progression-free and overall survival (Wisoff et al. 1998). Five year PFS rates in the CCG-945 study were 44% vs 22% for anaplastic astrocytoma with or without radical resection, and 26% vs 4% for patients with glioblastoma with or without radical resection.

Radiotherapy

The role of radiotherapy is also certain, and at least six randomized studies in adults have indicated a clear benefit (Shapiro and Young 1976; Andersen 1978; Walker et al. 1978, 1980; Kristiansen et al. 1981; Sandberg-Wollheim et al. 1991). The volume to be irradiated has been debated extensively. Given the known infiltrating nature of HGAs, and the known pattern of recurrence – most often within 2 cm of the original tumour site – it is conventional to irradiate locally, with a 2 cm margin in all directions (Sneed et al. 1994). Radiation dose is also important prognostically, with evidence for improved outcomes in doses up to 55–60 Gy (Walker et al. 1979, Garden et al. 1991). In adults, a randomized study of 45 Gy vs 60 Gy demonstrated a slight survival advantage after 60 Gy (Bleehen and Stenning 1991). Further intensification of dose to 72 Gy with hyperfractionation has been examined but evidence of survival benefit is limited (Fulton et al. 1992, Nelson et al. 1993, Liu et al. 1998).

Chemotherapy

An extensive body of literature has been published on the use of adjuvant chemotherapy in HGAs. Many of the agents used in HGG are old, and no clear phase I or II data exist for their use in this tumour, but for more recently developed agents, these data do exist. Evidence for activity of the nitrosoureas, BCNU and CCNU as single agents was reported by Walker et al. (1978), and these drugs were included in therapy at a very early stage. BCNU is associated with significant pulmonary toxicity, particularly in young patients, and therefore CCNU is more commonly used in therapy in most adult and paediatric units.

Most chemotherapy agents have shown only limited response rates when used as single agents, although some have been reported to have good response rates in small series. Procarbazine, which has been studied in phase II, had a response rate of 9/35 patients, all of whom had previously failed radiotherapy and BCNU, and this led to its early inclusion in paediatric studies (Newton et al. 1990). Cyclophosphamide, which is extensively used in many brain tumour regimes, has only limited single agent data to support its use: in a series of seven children with glioma, Allen and Helson (1981) reported responses in five. In contrast, Abrahamson et al. (1995) reported no responders in a series of 15 children who received high dose cyclophosphamide (1.8–2.25 g/m^2/d for 2 days). Despite encouraging pre-clinical activity, other agents, including cisplatin, carboplatin, etoposide and ifosfamide, have shown only limited single agent activity in HGA.

Temozolomide has received considerable attention following early reports of activity in adult HGG, and improved overall survival compared to procarbazine alone in adults (Bower et al. 1997, Yung et al. 2000). A phase I study run by the UKCCSG demonstrated responses in 3 of 15 patients with HGAs (Estlin et al. 1998), and a phase I study run by the CCG reported response in 1 of 9 patients (Nicholson et al. 1998). Recently, an extended phase I study of temozolomide in patients with HGAs performed by the UKCCSG did not confirm the high response rates seen in adult patients (Lashford et al. 2002).

Topotecan, an inhibitor of topoisomerase I, has been studied in phase II and responses seen in 4 of 9 patients with HGAs. These included two patients with relapsed glioblastoma who had complete responses.

Anthracyclines are not commonly used in brain tumour therapy, although in vitro activity is seen. Recently, liposomal preparations of daunorubicin and doxorubicin have been developed, and greater activity in brain tumours has been proposed on the grounds of greater penetration into brain tissue, and reduced removal from tumour tissue than native anthracycline. There is some evidence for both accumulation (Zucchetti et al. 1999) and activity in malignant brain tumours in children (Lippens 1999), but significant concerns relating to cardiac toxicity are likely to limit the usefulness of these drugs (Lowis et al. 2002).

Combination chemotherapy

Evidence for a beneficial effect of chemotherapy has been seen in a number of studies. Sposto et al. (1989) reported the results of a CCG study for patients with HGG treated with radiotherapy with or without CCNU, vincristine and prednisone, with a significant increase in event-free survival for those receiving chemotherapy (46% vs 18%, p=0.026). This combination has dominated prescribing practice in the USA for many years. A later study in children of "8-drugs-in-one-day" therapy, compared with vincristine, CCNU and prednisone, demonstrated equivalent activity of these regimes (Finlay et al. 1995).

The most common combination regime in the United Kingdom utilizes three agents, CCNU, procarbazine (not prednisone) and vincristine. This combination has a high response rate in anaplastic oligodendrogliomas, particularly those with deletions of chromosomes 1p or 19q (Cairncross et al. 1998, Smith et al. 2000, Fortin et al. 2001), but there is doubt about the efficacy of PCV in HGAs. A recent retrospective study suggested no survival benefit for this regime over use of BCNU alone (Prados et al. 1999, Medical Research Council Brain Tumor Working Party 2001). Furthermore, the Medical Research Council Brain Tumour Working Party has reported a prospective randomized study of PCV and radiotherapy vs radiotherapy alone in newly diagnosed adult patients with grade III and IV astrocytomas. A total of 674 patients were enrolled, and no difference in survival for either arm with grade III or IV tumours was seen (Medical Research Council Brain Tumor Working Party 2001).

More encouraging reports of activity of chemotherapy have been published by the German Paediatric Oncology Group. A significant survival benefit was seen after surgical complete remission if intensive multiagent chemotherapy (ifosfamide, etoposide, methotrexate, cisplatin, cytarabine) followed by radiotherapy was given rather than radiotherapy first followed by a standard regime of PCV (median survival 5.2 years vs 1.3 years, p<0.0005) (Wolff et al. 2002). Patient numbers were small (15 vs 16 patients).

A study by Lopez-Aguilar et al. (2000) of 11 children with HGAs treated with intensive ifosfamide, carboplatin and etoposide ('ICE') reported a complete response in seven, with no relapses in these at the time of publication. An earlier report in 36 adult patients had reported significant activity, with 5 showing a complete response, 5 a partial response, and 9 having stable disease (Sanson et al. 1996). Although clearly limited numbers of patients are reported, this study suggests significant activity and may be worth further consideration.

Another potentially beneficial combination that is under investigation is cisplatin plus alkylating agents such as temozolomide. Resistance to temozolomide seems to involve at least two independent mechanisms: the overexpression of the enzyme O^6-alkyl-guanine-transferase (AGT), and a functional defect of the systems for mismatch repair of DNA. The cellular concentration of AGT is a major determinant of the in vitro cytotoxicity of temozolomide (Wedge and Newlands 1996) and of nitrosoureas (Kokkinakis et al. 2001), and inhibitors of AGT increase the activity of temozolomide, albeit with greater haematological toxicity (Liu et al. 2002). It is expected that cisplatin may deplete AGT and thereby increase the therapeuic efficacy of temozolomide (Britten et al. 1999). The combination of cisplatin and temozolomide is being investigated by the French and UK children's cancer study groups (Geoerger et al. 2002).

High-dose chemotherapy
The role of high-dose therapy and autologous stem cell reconstitution remains uncertain. Patients with unresected glioblastoma have an appalling prognosis, and arguably any survivor in the long term may represent evidence for success. Most published regimes to date have included ThioTEPA, with BCNU, etoposide, carboplatin or cyclophosphamide. These regimes are all extremely toxic, and high toxic death rates have led to early closure of some studies. Nevertheless, long-term survivors have been reported after high-dose therapy with BCNU, thiotepa and etoposide (Grovas et al. 1999), and with thiotepa and etoposide (Finlay et al. 1996). In the CCG-9922 study, 11 patients with glioblastoma were treated with BCNU, thiotepa and etoposide. Five developed severe organ-specific toxicity including grade III and IV pulmonary toxicity. Three patients were alive at the time of the report, all of whom had undergone surgical gross total resection (Grovas et al. 1999). In a series of 9 patients with HGAs, treated with induction chemotherapy of vincristine, cisplatin, cyclophosphamide and etoposide, 7 developed progressive disease and died. Two others proceeded to high-dose therapy with carboplatin, thiotepa and etoposide, and both of these were alive at the time of reporting (Mason et al. 1998).

The role of high-dose therapy appears to be limited in HGA, although occasional patients may be cured with regimens including intensive therapies. For both newly diagnosed and relapsed tumours, there seems to be no benefit where previous response to chemotherapy has not been demonstrated, or where bulky residual disease remains. The dismal prognosis for such patients means that new therapeutic modalities are needed.

RELAPSED ASTROCYTOMA
The prognosis for patients with recurrent HGAs is very poor, and therapies such as the aggressive high-dose regimens described above may be adopted in an attempt to eliminate residual disease. Although it is possible that conventional chemotherapy and radiotherapy based treatments may lead to effective treatment of HGAs, there remain many patients for whom no such cure can be offered. Many preclinical and clinical research programmes exist, aiming to identify alternative tumour targets.

Improvement in the efficacy of conventional agents may come from improved delivery to the site of the tumour. Implantation of a solid preparation of alkylating chemotherapy agent (such as 'Gliadel' wafers) has not been associated with any improvement in local control, but has been associated with a greater complication rate (Subach et al. 1999, Engelhard 2000, McGovern et al. 2003).

Intra-arterial administration of chemotherapy with acceptable rates of CNS toxicity has been reported to show improved PFS in adult patients (Tfayli et al. 1999, Madajewicz et al. 2000). Infusion of agents such as RMP-7, which is designed to disrupt the blood–brain barrier and theoretically improve penetration of chemotherapy to brain tissue, is still being evaluated (Thomas et al. 2000).

Overcoming common resistance mechanisms may improve the efficacy of chemotherapeutic agents. The enzyme O_6-alkyl guanine alkyl transferase is important in tumour resistance to alkylating agents, and its inhibition leads to greater therapeutic efficacy in vitro and in vivo (Kurpad et al. 1997). Inhibitors of AGT, such as O^6-benzyl guanine and 'Patrin' are currently being investigated.

One approach that may offer significant benefit in the future involves the use of viruses such as the herpes simplex virus (HSV) mutant 1716. The normal infective cycle of HSV involves expression of the gene g134.5, which encodes the protein ICP34.5, which then promotes infection of non-dividing cells and inhibits apoptosis by infected cells. HSV mutant 1716 is a null mutant of the g134.5 gene, and does not replicate within healthy adult neurons or cause encephalitis. It can, however, grow in permissive, actively cycling cells, such as malignant tumour cells, and selectively cause tumour cell death. Activity has been seen in relapsed malignant gliomas, with no evidence of adverse clinical symptoms (Rampling et al. 2000).

Finally, there has been considerable interest in recent years in the UK in particular in the drug chlorimipramine. Chlorimipramine is a tricyclic antidepressant drug, noted to have in vitro activity against glial cells in vitro. Anecdotal reports of activity in patients with recurrent tumours, and a low perceived risk of significant adverse effects, led to it being prescribed for patients in an ad hoc manner for several years without formal monitoring. A phase I study is now underway in adult patients, although published data remain sparse.

Conclusions

Surgery remains the most important factor in the management of HGA, and an attempt at complete surgical resection should be made for all patients, unless the anticipated morbidity is considered severe. Adjuvant radiotherapy is clearly beneficial, whilst the role of chemotherapy is not yet proven. A coordinated approach aiming to achieve a complete response of tumour should be taken in all patients, and this may mean repeated surgical procedures for some patients.

Increasingly, it is possible to quantify the risk of recurrence using pre-treatment, biological factors, and these factors need to be incorporated into any future study. At present, treatment reduction is not indicated for any group, but intensification of therapy may be appropriate for some.

The outcome for patients with resistant or relapsed tumours remains extremely poor, and there is a need for novel approaches to the management of these patients. International cooperation will be essential to achieve improvement for these very high-risk patients.

REFERENCES

Abrahamsen TG, Lange BJ, Packer RJ, Venzon DJ, Allen JC, Craig CE, Patronas NJ, Katz DA, Goldwein JW, DeLaney TF, et al. (1995) A phase I and II trial of dose-intensified cyclophosphamide and GM-CSF in pediatric malignant brain tumors. *J Pediatr Hematol Oncol* **17**: 134–139.

Allen JC, Helson L (1981) High-dose cyclophosphamide chemotherapy for recurrent CNS tumors in children. *J Neurosurg* **55**: 749–756.

Andersen AP (1978) Postoperative irradiation of glioblastomas. Results in a randomized series. *Acta Radiol Oncol Radiat Phys Biol* **17**: 475–484.

Bleehen NM, Stenning SP (1991) A Medical Research Council trial of two radiotherapy doses in the treatment of grades 3 and 4 astrocytoma. The Medical Research Council Brain Tumour Working Party. *Br J Cancer* **64**: 769–774.

Bower M, Newlands ES, Bleehen NM, Brada M, Begent RJ, Calvert H, Colquhoun I, Lewis P, Brampton MH (1997) Multicentre CRC phase II trial of temozolomide in recurrent or progressive high-grade glioma. *Cancer Chemother Pharmacol* **40**: 484–488.

Britten CD, Rowinsky EK, Baker SD, Agarwala SS, Eckardt JR, Barrington R, Diab SG, Hammond LA, Johnson T, Villalona-Calero M, Fraass U, Statkevich P, Von Hoff DD, Eckhardt SG (1999) A Phase I and pharmacokinetic study of temozolomide and cisplatin in patients with advanced solid malignancies. *Clin Cancer Res* **5**: 1629–1637.

Cairncross JG, Ueki K, Zlatescu MC, Lisle DK, Finkelstein DM, Hammond RR, Silver JS, Stark PC, Macdonald DR, Ino Y, Ramsay DA, Louis DN (1998) Specific genetic predictors of chemotherapeutic response and survival in patients with anaplastic oligodendrogliomas. *J Natl Cancer Inst* **90**: 1473–1479.

Cappelli C, Grill J, Raquin M, Pierre-Kahn A, Lellouch-Tubiana A, Terrier-Lacombe MJ, Habrand JL, Couanet D, Brauner R, Rodriguez D, Hartmann O, Kalifa C (1998) Long-term follow up of 69 patients treated for optic pathway tumours before the chemotherapy era. *Arch Dis Child* **79**: 334–338.

Chamberlain MC (1997) Recurrent cerebellar gliomas: salvage therapy with oral etoposide. *J Child Neurol* **12**: 200–204.

Cheng Y, Ng HK, Zhang SF, Ding M, Pang JC, Zheng J, Poon WS (1999) Genetic alterations in pediatric high-grade astrocytomas. *Hum Pathol* **30**: 1284–1290.

Cokgor I, Friedman AH, Friedman HS (1998) Gliomas. *Eur J Cancer* **34**: 1910–1915; discussion 1916–1918.

Collet-Solberg PF, Sernyak H, Satin-Smith M, Katz LL, Sutton L, Molloy P, Moshang T (1997) Endocrine outcome in long-term survivors of low-grade hypothalamic/chiasmatic glioma. *Clin Endocrinol* **47**: 79–85.

Dirks PB, Jay V, Becker LE, Drake JM, Humphreys RP, Hoffman HJ, Rutka JT (1994) Development of anaplastic changes in low-grade astrocytomas of childhood. *Neurosurgery* **34**: 68–78.

Duffner PK, Krischer JP, Burger PC, Cohen ME, Backstrom JW, Horowitz ME, Sanford RA, Friedman HS, Kun LE (1996) Treatment of infants with malignant gliomas: the Pediatric Oncology Group experience. *J Neurooncol* **28**: 245–256.

Engelhard HH (2000) Tumor bed cyst formation after BCNU wafer implantation: report of two cases. *Surg Neurol* **53**: 220–224.

Estlin EJ, Lashford L, Ablett S, Price L, Gowing R, Gholkar A, Kohler J, Lewis IJ, Morland B, Pinkerton CR, Stevens MC, Mott M, Stevens R, Newell DR, Walker D, Dicks-Mireaux C, McDowell H, Reidenberg P, Statkevich P, Marco A, Batra V, Dugan M, Pearson AD (1998) Phase I study of temozolomide in paediatric patients with advanced cancer. United Kingdom Children's Cancer Study Group. *Br J Cancer* **78**: 652–661.

Finlay JL, Boyett JM, Yates AJ, Wisoff JH, Milstein JM, Geyer JR, Bertolone SJ, McGuire P, Cherlow JM, Tefft M, et al. (1995) Randomized phase III trial in childhood high-grade astrocytoma comparing vincristine, lomustine, and prednisone with the eight-drugs-in-1-day regimen. Children's Cancer Group. *J Clin Oncol* **13**: 112–123.

Finlay JL, Goldman S, Wong MC, Cairo M, Garvin J, August C, Cohen BH, Stanley P, Zimmerman RA, Bostrom B, Geyer JR, Harris RE, Sanders J, Yates AJ, Boyett JM, Packer RJ (1996) Pilot study of high-dose thiotepa and etoposide with autologous bone marrow rescue in children and young adults with recurrent CNS tumors. The Children's Cancer Group. *J Clin Oncol* **14**: 2495–2503.

Fisher BJ, Naumova E, Leighton CC, Naumov GN, Kerklviet N, Fortin D, Macdonald DR, Cairncross JG, Bauman GS, Stitt L (2002) Ki-67: a prognostic factor for low-grade glioma? *Int J Radiat Oncol Biol Phys* **52**: 996–1001.

Fortin D, Macdonald DR, Stitt L, Cairncross JG (2001) PCV for oligodendroglial tumors: in search of prognostic factors for response and survival. *Can J Neurol Sci* **28**: 215–223.

216

Fulton DS, Urtasun RC, Scott-Brown I, Johnson ES, Mielke B, Curry B, Huyser-Wierenga D, Hanson J, Feldstein M (1992) Increasing radiation dose intensity using hyperfractionation in patients with malignant glioma. Final report of a prospective phase I-II dose response study. *J Neurooncol* **14**: 63–72.

Fults D, Brockmeyer D, Tullous MW, Pedone CA, Cawthon RM (1992) p53 mutation and loss of heterozygosity on chromosomes 17 and 10 during human astrocytoma progression. *Cancer Res* **52**: 674–679.

Gajjar A, Sanford RA, Heideman R, Jenkins JJ, Walter A, Li Y, Langston JW, Muhlbauer M, Boyett JM, Kun LE (1997) Low-grade astrocytoma: a decade of experience at St. Jude Children's Research Hospital. *J Clin Oncol* 15: 2792–2799.

Garcia DM, Latifi HR, Simpson JR, Picker S (1989) Astrocytomas of the cerebellum in children. *J Neurosurg* **71**: 661–664.

Garden AS, Maor MH, Yung WK, Bruner JM, Woo SY, Moser RP, Lee YY (1991) Outcome and patterns of failure following limited-volume irradiation for malignant astrocytomas. *Radiother Oncol* **20**: 99–110.

Geoerger B, Vassal G, Doz F, Raquin MA, Frappaz D, Chastagner P, Rubie H, Gentet J-C, O'Quigley J, Djazouli K, Margison G, Pein F (2002) Dose-finding study and O_6-alkyltransferase depletion of cisplatin combined with temozolomide in pediatric solid malignancies. In: Proceedings of the American Society of Clinical Oncology, Florida, p. 424.

Gnekow AK, Perilongo G, Walker DA (2000) SIOP Low Grade Glioma Study: Low grade glioma diagnosed in children under one year of age: Clinical presentation and treatment outcome. Paper presented at the 9th International Symposium on Paediatric Neuro-Oncology (ISPNO), San Francisco.

Grovas AC, Boyett JM, Lindsley K, Rosenblum M, Yates AJ, Finlay JL (1999) Regimen-related toxicity of myeloablative chemotherapy with BCNU, thiotepa, and etoposide followed by autologous stem cell rescue for children with newly diagnosed glioblastoma multiforme: report from the Children's Cancer Group. *Med Pediatr Oncol* **33**: 83–87.

Gururangan S, Cavazos CM, Ashley D, Herndon JE, Bruggers CS, Moghrabi A, Scarcella DL, Watral M, Tourt-Uhlig S, Reardon D, Friedman HS (2002) Phase II study of carboplatin in children with progressive low-grade gliomas. *J Clin Oncol* **20**: 2951–2958.

Heideman R, Packer RJ, Albright LA, Freeman CR, Rorke LB (1997) Tumors of the central nervous system. In: Pizzo PA, Poplack DG (eds) *Principles and Practice of Pediatric Oncology*. Philadelphia: Lippincott-Raven, pp 633–697.

Janss AJ, Grundy R, Cnaan A, Savino PJ, Packer RJ, Zackai EH, Goldwein JW, Sutton LN, Radcliffe J, Molloy PT, et al. (1995) Optic pathway and hypothalamic/chiasmatic gliomas in children younger than age 5 years with a 6-year follow-up. *Cancer* **75**: 1051–1059.

Kadota RP, Kun LE, Langston JW, Burger PC, Cohen ME, Mahoney DH, Walter AW, Rodman JH, Parent A, Buckley E, Kepner JL, Friedman HS (1999) Cyclophosphamide for the treatment of progressive low-grade astrocytoma: a Pediatric Oncology Group phase II Study. *J Pediatr Hematol Oncol* **21**: 198–202.

Kleihues P, Louis DN, Scheithauer BW, Rorke LB, Reifenberger G, Burger PC, Cavenee WK (2002) The WHO classification of tumors of the nervous system. *J Neuropathol Exp Neurol* **61**: 215–225; discussion 226–229.

Kokkinakis DM, Bocangel DB, Schold SC, Moschel RC, Pegg AE (2001) Thresholds of O_6-alkylguanine-DNA alkyltransferase which confer significant resistance of human glial tumor xenografts to treatment with 1,3-bis(2-chloroethyl)-1-nitrosourea or temozolomide. *Clin Cancer Res* **7**: 421–428.

Kristiansen K, Hagen S, Kollevold T, Torvik A, Holme I, Nesbakken R, Hatlevoll R, Lindgren M, Brun A, Lindgren S, Notter G, Andersen AP, Elgen K (1981) Combined modality therapy of operated astrocytomas grade III and IV. Confirmation of the value of postoperative irradiation and lack of potentiation of bleomycin on survival time: a prospective multicenter trial of the Scandinavian Glioblastoma Study Group. *Cancer* **47**: 649–652.

Kurpad SN, Dolan ME, McLendon RE, Archer GE, Moschel RC, Pegg AE, Bigner DD, Friedman HS (1997) Intraarterial O_6-benzylguanine enables the specific therapy of nitrosourea-resistant intracranial human glioma xenografts in athymic rats with 1,3-bis(2-chloroethyl)-1-nitrosourea. *Cancer Chemother Pharmacol* **39**: 307–316.

Laithier V, Racquin MA, Doz F, Gentet JC, Frappaz D, Chastagner P, Couanet D, Lellouch-Tubiana A, Kalifa C (2000) Chemotherapy for children with hypothalamic and optic pathway glioma: Results of a prospective study by the French Society for Paediatric Oncology (SFOP). Paper presented at the 9th International Symposium on Paediatric Neuro-Oncology (ISPNO), San Francisco.

Lashford LS, Thiesse P, Jouvet A, Jaspan T, Couanet D, Griffiths PD, Doz F, Ironside J, Robson K, Hobson R, Dugan M, Pearson AD, Vassal G, Frappaz D (2000) Chemotherapy for children with hypothalaic and optic pathway glioma: Results of a prospective study by the French Society of Paediatric Oncology (SFOP). 9th International Symposium on Paediatric Neuro-Oncology (ISPNO), San Francisco.

Lashford LS, Thiesse P, Jouvet A, Jaspan T, Couanet D, Griffiths PD, Doz F, Ironside J, Robson K, Hobson R, Dugan M, Pearson AD, Vassal G, Frappaz D (2002) Temozolomide in malignant gliomas of childhood: a United Kingdom Children's Cancer Study Group and French Society for Pediatric Oncology Intergroup Study. *J Clin Oncol* **20**: 4684–4691.

Lippens RJ (1999) Liposomal daunorubicin (DaunoXome) in children with recurrent or progressive brain tumors. *Pediatr Hematol Oncol* **16**: 131–139.

Liu L, Nakatsuru Y, Gerson SL (2002) Base excision repair as a therapeutic target in colon cancer. *Clin Cancer Res* **8**: 2985–2991.

Liu YM, Shiau CY, Wong TT, Wang LW, Wu LJ, Chi KH, Chen KY, Yen SH (1998) Prognostic factors and therapeutic options of radiotherapy in pediatric brain stem gliomas. *Jpn J Clin Oncol* **28**: 474–479.

Lopez-Aguilar E, Sepulveda-Vildosola AC, Rivera-Marquez H, Cerecedo-Diaz F, Hernandez-Contreras I, Ramon-Garcia G, Diegoperez-Ramirez J, Santacruz-Castillo E (2000) Preirradiation ifosfamide, carboplatin, and etoposide for the treatment of anaplastic astrocytomas and glioblastoma multiforme: a phase II study. *Arch Med Res* **31**: 186–190.

Lowis SP, Pizer BL, Coakham H, Nelson RJ, Bouffet E (1998) Chemotherapy for spinal cord astrocytoma: can natural history be modified? *Child's Nerv Syst* **14**: 317–321.

Lowis SP, Lewis I, Elsworth A, Ablett S, Robert J, Frappaz D (2002) Cardiac toxicity may limit the usefulness of Daunoxome. Results of a phase I study in children with relapsed or resistant tumours – a UKCCSG/SFOP study. Paper presented at the 34th meeting of the International Society of Paediatric Oncology (SIOP), Oporto.

Madajewicz S, Chowhan N, Tfayli A, Roque C, Meek A, Davis R, Wolf W, Cabahug C, Roche P, Manzione J, Iliya A, Shady M, Hentschel P, Atkins H, Braun A (2000) Therapy for patients with high grade astrocytoma using intraarterial chemotherapy and radiation therapy. *Cancer* **88**: 2350–2356.

Mason WP, Grovas A, Halpern S, Dunkel IJ, Garvin J, Heller G, Rosenblum M, Gardner S, Lyden D, Sands S, Puccetti D, Lindsley K, Merchant TE, O'Malley B, Bayer L, Petriccione MM, Allen J, Finlay JL (1998) Intensive chemotherapy and bone marrow rescue for young children with newly diagnosed malignant brain tumors. *J Clin Oncol* **16**: 210–221.

Massimino M, Spreafico F, Cefalo G, Riccardi R, Tesoro-Tess JD, Gandola L, Riva D, Ruggiero A, Valentini L, Mazza E, Genitori L, Di Rocco C, Navarria P, Casanova M, Ferrari A, Luksch R, Terenziani M, Balestrini MR, Colosimo C, Fossati-Bellani F (2002) High response rate to cisplatin/etoposide regimen in childhood low-grade glioma. *J Clin Oncol* **20**: 4209–4216.

McGovern, PC, Lautenbach, E, Brennan, PJ, Lustig, RA and Fishman, NO (2003) Risk factors for postcraniotomy surgical site infection after 1,3-bis (2-chloroethyl)-1-nitrosourea (Gliadel) wafer placement. *Clin Infect Dis* **36**: 759–765.

McLeod HL, Krynetski EY, Relling MV, Evans WE (2000) Genetic polymorphism of thiopurine methyl-transferase and its clinical relevance for childhood acute lymphoblastic leukemia. *Leukemia* **14**: 567–572.

Medical Research Council Brain Tumor Working Party (2001) Randomized trial of procarbazine, lomustine, and vincristine in the adjuvant treatment of high-grade astrocytoma: a Medical Research Council trial. *J Clin Oncol* **19**: 509–518.

Medlock MD, Madsen JR, Barnes PD, Anthony DS, Cohen LE, Scott RM (1997) Optic chiasm astrocytomas of childhood. 1. Long-term follow-up. *Pediatr Neurosurg* **27**: 121–128.

Medlock MD, Scott RM (1997) Optic chiasm astrocytomas of childhood. 2. Surgical management. *Pediatr Neurosurg* **27**: 129–136.

Mitchell AE, Elder JE, Mackey DA, Waters KD, Ashley DM (2001) Visual improvement despite radiologically stable disease after treatment with carboplatin in children with progressive low-grade optic/thalamic gliomas. *J Pediatr Hematol Oncol* **23**: 572–577.

Nelson DF, Curran WJ, Scott C, Nelson JS, Weinstein AS, Ahmad K, Constine LS, Murray K, Powlis WD, Mohiuddin M, et al. (1993) Hyperfractionated radiation therapy and bis-chlorethyl nitrosourea in the treatment of malignant glioma—possible advantage observed at 72.0 Gy in 1.2 Gy B.I.D. fractions: report of the Radiation Therapy Oncology Group Protocol 8302. *Int J Radiat Oncol Biol Phys* **25**: 193–207.

Newton HB, Junck L, Bromberg J, Page MA, Greenberg HS (1990) Procarbazine chemotherapy in the treatment of recurrent malignant astrocytomas after radiation and nitrosourea failure. *Neurology* **40**: 1743–1746.

Nicholson HS, Krailo M, Ames MM, Seibel NL, Reid JM, Liu-Mares W, Vezina LG, Ettinger AG, Reaman GH (1998) Phase I study of temozolomide in children and adolescents with recurrent solid tumors: a report from the Children's Cancer Group. *J Clin Oncol* **16**: 3037–3043.

Orr LC, Fleitz J, McGavran L, Wyatt-Ashmead J, Handler M, Foreman NK (2002) Cytogenetics in pediatric low-grade astrocytomas. *Med Pediatr Oncol* **38**: 173–177.

Packer RJ, Ater J, Allen J, Phillips P, Geyer R, Nicholson HS, Jakacki R, Kurczynski E, Needle M, Finlay J, Reaman G, Boyett JM (1997) Carboplatin and vincristine chemotherapy for children with newly diagnosed progressive low-grade gliomas. *J Neurosurg* **86**: 747–754.

Packer RJ, Sutton LN, Bilaniuk LT, Radcliffe J, Rosenstock JG, Siegel KR, Bunin GR, Savino PJ, Bruce DA, Schut L (1988) Treatment of chiasmatic/hypothalamic gliomas of childhood with chemotherapy: an update. *Ann Neurol* **23**: 79–85.

Pollack IF, Claassen D, al-Shboul Q, Janosky JE, Deutsch M (1995) Low-grade gliomas of the cerebral hemispheres in children: an analysis of 71 cases. *J Neurosurg* **82**: 536–547.

Pollack IF, Finkelstein SD, Burnham J, Holmes EJ, Hamilton RL, Yates AJ, Finlay JL, Sposto R; Children's Cancer Group (2001) Age and TP53 mutation frequency in childhood malignant gliomas: results in a multi-institutional cohort. *Cancer Res* **61**: 7404–7407.

Pollack IF, Finkelstein SD, Woods J, Burnham J, Holmes EJ, Hamilton RL, Yates AJ, Boyett JM, Finlay JL, Sposto R; Children's Cancer Group (2002a) Expression of p53 and prognosis in children with malignant gliomas. *N Engl J Med* **346**: 420–427.

Pollack IF, Hamilton RL, Burnham J, Holmes EJ, Finkelstein SD, Sposto R, Yates AJ, Boyett JM, Finlay JL (2002b) Impact of proliferation index on outcome in childhood malignant gliomas: results in a multi-institutional cohort. *Neurosurgery* **50**: 1238–1244; discussion 1244–1245.

Prados M, Mamelak AN (1994) Metastasizing low grade gliomas in children. Redefining an old disease. *Cancer* **73**: 2671–2673.

Prados MD, Edwards MS, Rabbitt J, Lamborn K, Davis RL, Levin VA (1997) Treatment of pediatric low-grade gliomas with a nitrosourea-based multiagent chemotherapy regimen. *J Neurooncol* **3**: 235–241.

Prados MD, Scott C, Curran WJ, Nelson DF, Leibel S, Kramer S (1999) Procarbazine, lomustine, and vincristine (PCV) chemotherapy for anaplastic astrocytoma: A retrospective review of radiation therapy oncology group protocols comparing survival with carmustine or PCV adjuvant chemotherapy. *J Clin Oncol* **17**: 3389–3395.

Raffel C (1996) Molecular biology of pediatric gliomas. *J Neurooncol* **28**: 121–128.

Raffel C, Frederick L, O'Fallon JR, Atherton-Skaff P, Perry A, Jenkins RB, James CD (1999) Analysis of oncogene and tumor suppressor gene alterations in pediatric malignant astrocytomas reveals reduced survival for patients with PTEN mutations. *Clin Cancer Res* **5**: 4085–4090.

Rampling R, Cruickshank G, Papanastassiou V, Nicoll J, Hadley D, Brennan D, Petty R, MacLean A, Harland J, McKie E, Mabbs R, Brown M (2000) Toxicity evaluation of replication-competent herpes simplex virus (ICP 34.5 null mutant 1716) in patients with recurrent malignant glioma. *Gene Ther* **7**: 859–866.

Reddy AT, Packer RJ (1999) Chemotherapy for low-grade gliomas. *Child's Nerv Syst* **15**: 506–513.

Sandberg-Wollheim M, Malmstrom P, Stromblad LG, Anderson H, Borgstrom S, Brun A, Cronqvist S, Hougaard K, Salford LG (1991) A randomized study of chemotherapy with procarbazine, vincristine, and lomustine with and without radiation therapy for astrocytoma grades 3 and/or 4. *Cancer* **68**: 22–29.

Sanson M, Ameri A, Monjour A, Sahmoud T, Ronchin P, Poisson M, Delattre JY (1996) Treatment of recurrent malignant supratentorial gliomas with ifosfamide, carboplatin and etoposide: a phase II study. *Eur J Cancer* **32A**: 2229–2235.

Shapiro WR, Young DF (1976) Treatment of malignant glioma. A controlled study of chemotherapy and irradiation. *Arch Neurol* **33**: 494–450.

Smith JS, Perry A, Borell TJ, Lee HK, O'Fallon J, Hosek SM, Kimmel D, Yates A, Burger PC, Scheithauer BW, Jenkins RB (2000) Alterations of chromosome arms 1p and 19q as predictors of survival in oligo-dendrogliomas, astrocytomas, and mixed oligoastrocytomas. *J Clin Oncol* **18**: 636–645.

Sneed PK, Gutin PH, Larson DA, Malec MK, Phillips TL, Prados MD, Scharfen CO, Weaver KA, Wara WM (1994) Patterns of recurrence of glioblastoma multiforme after external irradiation followed by implant boost. *Int J Radiat Oncol Biol Phys* **29**: 719–727.

Sposto R, Ertel IJ, Jenkin RD, Boesel CP, Venes JL, Ortega JA, Evans AE, Wara W, Hammond D (1989) The effectiveness of chemotherapy for treatment of high grade astrocytoma in children: results of a randomized trial. A report from the Childrens Cancer Study Group. *J Neurooncol* **7**: 165–177.

Subach BR, Witham TF, Kondziolka D, Lunsford LD, Bozik M, Schiff D (1999) Morbidity and survival after 1,3-bis(2-chloroethyl)-1-nitrosourea wafer implantation for recurrent glioblastoma: a retrospective case-matched cohort series. *Neurosurgery* **45**: 17–22; discussion 22–23.

Tao ML, Barnes PD, Billett AL, Leong T, Shrieve DC, Scott RM, Tarbell NJ (1997) Childhood optic chiasm gliomas: radiographic response following radiotherapy and long-term clinical outcome. *Int J Radiat Oncol Biol Phys* **39**: 579–587.

Tfayli A, Hentschel P, Madajewicz S, Manzione J, Chowhan N, Davis R, Roche P, Iliya A, Roque C, Meek A, Shady M (1999) Toxicities related to intraarterial infusion of cisplatin and etoposide in patients with brain tumors. *J Neurooncol* **42**: 73–77.

Thomas HD, Lind MJ, Ford J, Bleehen N, Calvert AH, Boddy AV (2000) Pharmacokinetics of carboplatin administered in combination with the bradykinin agonist Cereport (RMP-7) for the treatment of brain tumours. *Cancer Chemother Pharmacol* **45**: 284–290.

Tihan T, Fisher PG, Kepner JL, Godfraind C, McComb RD, Goldthwaite PT, Burger PC (1999) Pediatric astrocytomas with monomorphous pilomyxoid features and a less favorable outcome. *J Neuropathol Exp Neurol* **58**: 1061–1068.

Walker DA, Taylor RE, Perilongo G, Zanetti I, Gnekow AK, Garre ML, Kühl J, Robinson K (2000) Vincristine and carboplatin in low grade glioma: an interim report of the International Consortium on Low Grade Glioma. Paper presented at the 9th International Symposium on Paediatric Neuro-Oncology (ISPNO), San Francisco.

Walker MD, Alexander E, Hunt WE, MacCarty CS, Mahaley MS, Mealey J, Norrell HA, Owens G, Ransohoff J, Wilson CB, Gehan EA, Strike TA (1978) Evaluation of BCNU and/or radiotherapy in the treatment of anaplastic gliomas. A cooperative clinical trial. *J Neurosurg* **49**: 333–343.

Walker MD, Strike TA, Sheline GE (1979) An analysis of dose-effect relationship in the radiotherapy of malignant gliomas. *Int J Radiat Oncol Biol Phys* **5**: 1725–1731.

Walker MD, Green SB, Byar DP, Alexander E, Batzdorf U, Brooks WH, Hunt WE, MacCarty CS, Mahaley MS, Mealey J, Owens G, Ransohoff J, Robertson JT, Shapiro WR, Smith KR, Wilson CB, Strike TA (1980) Randomized comparisons of radiotherapy and nitrosoureas for the treatment of malignant glioma after surgery. *N Engl J Med* **303**: 1323–1329.

Wedge SR, Newlands ES (1996) O^6-benzylguanine enhances the sensitivity of a glioma xenograft with low O6-alkylguanine-DNA alkyltransferase activity to temozolomide and BCNU. *Br J Cancer* **73**: 1049–1052.

Wisoff JH, Boyett JM, Berger MS, Brant C, Li H, Yates AJ, McGuire-Cullen P, Turski PA, Sutton LN, Allen JC, Packer RJ, Finlay JL (1998) Current neurosurgical management and the impact of the extent of resection in the treatment of malignant gliomas of childhood: a report of the Children's Cancer Group trial no. CCG-945. *J Neurosurg* **89**: 52–59.

Wolff JE, Gnekow AK, Kortmann RD, Pietsch T, Urban C, Graf N, Kuhl J (2002) Preradiation chemotherapy for pediatric patients with high-grade glioma. *Cancer* **94**: 264–271.

Yule SM, Hide TA, Cranney M, Simpson E, Barrett A (2001) Low grade astrocytomas in the West of Scotland 1987–96: treatment, outcome, and cognitive functioning. *Arch Dis Child* **84**: 61–64.

Yung WK, Albright RE, Olson J, Fredericks R, Fink K, Prados MD, Brada M, Spence A, Hohl RJ, Shapiro W, Glantz M, Greenberg H, Selker RG, Vick NA, Rampling R, Friedman H, Phillips P, Bruner J, Yue N, Osoba D, Zaknoen S, Levin VA (2000) A phase II study of temozolomide vs. procarbazine in patients with glioblastoma multiforme at first relapse. *Br J Cancer* **83**: 588–593.

Zucchetti M, Boiardi A, Silvani A, Parisi I, Piccolrovazzi S, D'Incalci M (1999) Distribution of daunorubicin and daunorubicinol in human glioma tumors after administration of liposomal daunorubicin. *Cancer Chemother Pharmacol* **44**: 173–176.

11
EPENDYMOMA

Ute Bartels, Douglas J Hyder, Annie Huang and Eric Bouffet

Ependymoma is the third most common brain tumour in children, accounting for 6–12% of all brain tumours in the paediatric population (Duffner et al. 1985, Nazar et al. 1990, Horn et al. 1999). The tumour is predominantly a disease of young children with nearly 50% of patients diagnosed under the age of 5 years (Nazar et al. 1990, Grill et al. 2001).

Ependymomas may arise in relation to any part of the ventricular system, the posterior fossa being the most common site (50–60%). Supratentorial ependymomas are less frequent (30–40%), while, unlike in adults, intraspinal ependymomas are exceptional in childhood (0–10%) (Wiestler et al. 2000).

The mainstay of treatment in ependymoma is surgery aiming for maximal resection, as the extent of resection is the primary determinant of outcome. Complete resection, which is influenced by the site and the characteristics of the tumour, is, however, only possible in 50–60% of the children (Merchant 2002). The benefit of aggressive surgery at the expense of neurological function is unclear, especially when the tumour involves the brainstem or the lower cranial nerves. Postoperative adjuvant therapy with radiation and/or chemotherapy varies according to the age of the patient, the extent of surgery, and, in some protocols, the tumour location and grading.

Although ependymoma has sometimes been considered as a benign neoplasm, data from the SEER (Surveillance, Epidemiology and End Result) registry reported by Ries et al. (2002) suggest that survival in paediatric ependymomas is worse than in medulloblastomas. The overall 10-year survival rate of the tumour is 30–50% and this poor overall survival has not significantly changed in the last decade (Ikezaki et al. 1993, Pollack et al. 1995, Bouffet et al. 1998, Merchant 2002).

Histopathological features
Ependymomas originate from the ependymal lining of the cerebral ventricles, the central canal of the spinal cord, and ependymal rests in the subcortical white matter. According to the most recent criteria of the World Health Organization, ependymoma is currently classified into three grades (Table 11.1):
- Myxopapillary ependymoma and subependymoma, corresponding to WHO grade I (exceptional in childhood)
- Ependymomas with cellular, papillary or tancytic differentiation, and the clear cell variant, corresponding to WHO grade II
- Anaplastic ependymoma, corresponding to WHO grade III.

Myxopapillary ependymomas, most exclusively occurring in the conus–cauda–filium terminale region, are slowly growing tumours with a favourable prognosis; they are described

TABLE 11.1
World Health Organization classification of ependymal tumours*

WHO grade	WHO designation
I	Myxopapillary ependymoma
I	Subependymoma
II	Ependymoma
	Cellular ependymoma
	Papillary ependymoma
	Clear cell ependymoma
	Tancytic ependymoma
III	Anaplastic ependymoma

*Wiestler et al. (2000).

in more detail in Chapter 18. Subependymomas are rare tumours arising most frequently in middle-aged and elderly males. Most often they remain asymptomatic and are often found incidentally.

In children the majority of ependymomas are WHO grade II, histologically characterized by perivascular pseudorosettes and ependymal rosettes with occasional mitoses and foci of necrosis. The tumour is usually delineated from adjacent brain structures. Tumour cells are positive for GFAP, S100 protein and vimentin by immunohistochemistry.

Anaplastic ependymomas have a higher mitotic activity, with microvascular proliferation and perivascular rosettes; ependymal rosettes are rare or absent. They remain mostly well demarcated, but may occasionally be invasive. Their immunoprofiles resemble those of conventional ependymoma, but GFAP expression may be reduced (Wiestler et al. 2000).

The classification of ependymoma has been revised several times since Bailey and Cushing's first description in 1926. For example, for many years ependymoblastoma was classified as a malignant ependymoma. The revision of the WHO system in 1993 (Kleihues et al. 1993) reclassified ependymoblastoma as an embryonal tumour like medulloblastoma and PNET. As a consequence, the results and conclusions of studies reported before the 1990s should be interpreted cautiously.

As with other brain tumours, there are discrepancies in tumour grading between pathologists (Schiffer et al. 1991, Gerszten et al. 1996). Studies involving independent pathology reviews have shown interobserver discrepancies in a range of 24–31% (Horn et al. 1999, Timmermann et al. 2000). In a prospective randomized trial by the Children's Cancer Group, there was a 69% discrepancy rate between institutional and central pathology review (Robertson et al. 1998). So far no consensus in classifying ependymomas has been achieved, and comparisons between series remain difficult.

In addition to routine histology and immunohistochemistry, other prognostic indicators in ependymomas have been reported. Monoclonal antibodies such as Ki-67 and MIB-1 are markers of the proliferative potential and predict the tumour's growth fraction. Prayson (1999) found that MIB-1 labelling index does not provide reliable correlation with clinical outcome or recurrence. Conversely, Bennetto et al. (1998) evaluated the Ki-67 labelling index (LI) as an independent prognostic indicator for survival in a retrospective study with 74 cases of childhood ependymoma. Gilbertson et al. (2002) studied the expression of ERBB2 and ERBB4 (receptors of the tyrosine kinase type 1 family) in childhood ependymomas and found that a high level of coexpression was associated with increased tumour proliferation and poor clinical outcome. These findings correlated significantly with Ki-67 LI.

Molecular biology and cytogenetic studies

Comparative genomic hybridization (CGH) provides information on genomic imbalance using in situ hybridization to metaphase chromosomes. Series that have reviewed adult and some paediatric ependymomas have reported imbalances on chromosomes 1, 6, 10, 13, 14, 17 and 22, and mutations in the neurofibromatosis 2 (NF2) gene. Most abnormalities are observed in adult tumours and are less frequent in childhood (Kramer et al. 1998). No chromosomal imbalances are seen in 40–45 % of childhood ependymomas (Reardon et al. 1999, Ward et al. 2001, Carter et al. 2002). However, in a study involving paediatric ependymomas, Grill et al. (2002) described 22q loss as the most frequent copy number abnormality. Other authors have postulated the presence of a putative ependymoma tumour suppressor gene located on chromsome 22, independent of the NF2 gene (Vagner-Capodano et al. 1999, Rousseau-Merck et al. 2000). In the study by Carter et al. (2002), gain of 1q was significantly correlated with posterior fossa ependymoma in children and aggressive behaviour. Dyer et al. (2002) used CGH in 53 paediatric ependymomas and identified three distinct patterns of genomic imbalances, which significantly correlated with clinical outcome. Ependymomas with six or less chromosome imbalances had a significantly worse outcome, showed more aggressive behaviour and recurred more frequently in children older than 3 years. Ependymomas arising in children less than 3 years old usually did not show any genomic imbalances, suggesting that they are biologically different from those occurring in older children.

P53 mutations do not seem to play a role in the pathogenesis or the behaviour of pediatric ependymoma (Fink et al. 1996, Suzuki and Iwaki 2000), although Korshunov et al. (2002) reported evidence of overexpression of p53 protein in high-grade ependymomas and association with poor outcome.

Unlike some other paediatric brain tumours, there are no known syndromes that predispose children to develop ependymoma. In adults there is a known association of NF2 and intramedullary spinal cord ependymomas.

Diagnostic features of intracranial ependymomas

Whilst most childhood ependymomas are located in the posterior fossa, supratentorial tumours are predominant in young infants (Comi et al. 1998). Clinical presentation of intracranial ependymomas is not specific and, like other brain tumours, depends on tumour location and the size and age of the patient. Since most tumours grow along the ventricles, signs and symptoms of increased intracranial pressure following hydrocephalus are common. Posterior fossa ependymomas may present with cranial nerve deficits and problems with balance, coordination and gait.

Imaging characteristics of ependymoma are similarly nonspecific. Calcifications and cystic areas in variable sizes are usual. Haemorrhage is less common, whereas obstructive hydrocephalus is a mostly prominent accompanying feature.

On computed tomography (CT) the tumour mass has increased density and shows calcification in up to 80% of cases (Comi et al. 1998, Warmuth-Metz and Kühl 2002). On T_1-weighted magnetic resonance imaging (MRI), ependymomas are usually hypointense or isointense to grey matter and enhance heterogeneously after gadolinium injection. The enhancement is more intense along the cyst walls, leading to a grape-like appearance. On T_2-weighted, proton density and FLAIR (fluid attenuated inversion recovery) imaging, ependymomas are hyperintense (Lefton et al. 1998). Extension through the foramina of Luschka and Magendie is suggestive of ependymoma (Tortori-Donati et al. 1995).

Risk factors and prognostic considerations

EXTENT OF RESECTION

The extent of surgical resection has been shown by both prospective and retrospective studies to be a major prognostic factor in ependymoma (Perilongo et al. 1997, Horn et al. 1999, Timmermann et al. 2000, Grill et al. 2001). The critical role of surgery was clarified when routine postoperative imaging was introduced as part of the standard management of paediatric brain tumours. Studies in which the extent of resection was based on surgical notes or the surgeon's appreciation were inconsistent in their conclusions.

Imaging-confirmed complete surgical resection leads to improved event-free and overall survival. Conversely incomplete resection increases the likelihood of recurrence. For posterior fossa tumours, brainstem invasion or extension to the cranial nerves significantly reduces the chance of a complete resection. Some surgeons advocate more aggressive resection, which may include the sacrifice of the lower cranial nerves and/or the risk of permanent bulbar deficit. The long-term benefit of aggressive surgical approaches is unproven. Foreman et al. (1996) have suggested a role for second-look surgery, and there are currently ongoing cooperative studies assessing the feasibility and long-term benefits of this strategy.

DISSEMINATION AT THE TIME OF DIAGNOSIS

It is unclear whether tumour dissemination influences survival in ependymoma since the incidence of dissemination in paediatric ependymoma is largely unknown. No large study has prospectively assessed the incidence of seeding at the time of diagnosis with systematic CSF cytology and spinal MRI. The reported overall incidence of leptomeningeal disease at the time of diagnosis varies between 5% and 18% (Goldwein et al. 1990, Rezai et al. 1996, Perilongo et al. 1997, Scheurlen and Kühl 1998). Metastatic spread along the CSF pathway is observed more frequently in posterior fossa tumours with anaplastic features (Duffner et al. 1985, Rezai et al. 1996).

Dissemination at presentation was not associated with a significantly worse outcome in a retrospective review conducted by Pollack et al. (1995). In contrast, in two multicentre German prospective trials (HIT 88/89 and HIT 91), 5 of 55 children with anaplastic ependymoma showed dissemination at time of diagnosis either by CSF cytology or MRI, and none of these 5 children lived beyond 2 years from diagnosis (Timmermann et al. 2000).

AGE

Younger children (3 years and below) seem to do worse than older children (Pollack et al.

1995, Perilongo et al. 1997, Hukin et al. 1998, Horn et al. 1999). Several factors, such as posterior fossa location and the reluctance to use radiotherapy in young children, may affect the survival rates in young children. Whether the behaviour of ependymoma in infants and young children is more aggressive than in older children is still unclear. The size of ependymoma is inversely correlated to age. Children under 1 year of age most often present with tumour sizes >5 cm (Comi et al. 1998).

TUMOUR LOCATION

There is some evidence that the tumour site influences the resection of the tumour and therefore the outcome. Up to 50% of posterior fossa ependymomas infiltrate the brainstem and/or grow laterally in the cerebellopontine angle. In a retrospective analysis of posterior fossa ependymomas, tumours arising from the vestibular area or the lateral recess showed a significantly lower mean survival time (40 months) when compared with tumours originating from the caudal half of the fourth ventricular floor (170 months) (Ikezaki et al. 1993). About 30% of paediatric ependymomas are located in the supratentorial compartment, where a total resection is more likely (Ernestus et al. 1997, Palma et al. 2000).

GRADING

To date, histology has not been a consistent prognostic factor: some studies have not demonstrated a significant association between anaplastic features and outcome (Pollack et al. 1995, Robertson et al. 1998), whereas others have (Ernestus et al. 1996, Paulino et al. 2002). In North America, there is a trend towards considering tumour anaplasia as an independent prognostic factor following the preliminary data from CCG 9941 and the retrospective review conducted by Merchant et al. (2002a). Merchant and co-workers reported 50 paediatric patients with localized ependymomas and found a significant correlation of the tumour grade with progression free survival (PFS): a 3 year PFS of 28% ± 14% for patients with anaplastic ependymoma compared to 84% ± 7% for those with differentiated ependymoma. However, most ongoing cooperative studies do not take histology into account in treatment stratification.

Treatment

SURGERY

Many children with ependymomas present with signs and symptoms of raised intracranial pressure (ICP). Management of raised ICP will depend on the individual needs of each child: some may improve with dexamethasone, whereas others may need external drainage, third ventriculostomy or some combination of these treatments (Sainte-Rose et al. 2001).

Surgery is the mainstay of treatment of ependymoma, aiming at maximal resection with preservation of neurological function. The risk of transient or permanent morbidity of aggressive debulking may limit the surgical resection in ependymoma (Khan et al. 2001). Tumour site and extent may influence the degree of resection: supratentorial ependymomas are more likely to be completely resected than posterior fossa tumours. In a prospective study postoperative imaging demonstrated residual tumour in 53% of cases of posterior fossa ependymomas (Robertson et al. 1998), whereas series focusing on supratentorial ependy-

TABLE 11.2
Extent of resection by site

Study	Patients	TR	Suprat	TR	Infrat	TR
Pierre-Kahn et al. (1983)	47	18	15	10	32	8
Ross and Rubinstein (1989)	15	3	4	4	10	7
Nazar et al. (1990)	35	10	0	0	35	10
Undjian and Marinov (1990)	60	15	23	7	37	8
Pollack et al. (1995)	40	23	12	8	25	15
Foreman et al. (1996)	31	7	11	5	20	2
Evans et al. (1996)	36	8	0	0	36	8
Perilongo et al. (1997)	92	53	32	18	60	35
Horn et al. (1999)	83	35	19	15	64	20
Palma et al. (2000)	23	15	23	15	0	0
Total	462	187 (39%)	139	82 (64%)	319	113 (36%)

TR = total resection; Suprat = supratentorial; Infrat = infratentorial.

momas report significantly higher resection rates (Hukin et al. 1998, Palma et al. 2000). The range of the extent of resection rates by site is shown in Table 11.2.

Because of the impact of resection on survival, some authors advocate a second surgical procedure when the postoperative imaging shows a significant residual mass. In a pilot experience reported by Foreman et al. (1997), chemotherapy followed by second-look surgery facilitated gross total resection in posterior fossa ependymomas with little additional morbidity. Merchant (2002) reported successful second-look surgery in 10 of 12 patients, with only one patient suffering significant postoperative morbidity.

RADIOTHERAPY

Postoperative radiotherapy was introduced in the management of ependymomas in the 1950s. Many reports suggest an increased survival with postoperative radiotherapy (reviewed by Bouffet et al. 1998). However, many of those studies were non-randomized, and there are controversies regarding the need, volume and dose of postoperative radiation for ependymoma.

Some reports have questioned the necessity of postoperative radiotherapy following a gross total resection. Two studies have suggested that it might be possible to defer radiation for patients with completely resected supratentorial ependymomas with favourable histological features (Hukin et al. 1998, Palma et al. 2000). The Children's Oncology Group is currently assessing the feasibility of such a strategy for patients with completely resected non-anaplastic supratentorial ependymoma (Merchant 2002).

Strategies using chemotherapy to delay radiation have been developed for infants who are more likely to suffer severe long-term cognitive effects from radiation. Duffner et al. (1993) reported 48 children less than 3 years of age with intracranial ependymomas treated with prolonged postoperative chemotherapy and delayed radiation and found that earlier radiation was associated with better short-term event-free survival. In this study, differences in survivals were seen between age-groups, suggesting an optimal timing of radiation following chemotherapy. The authors concluded that future treatment trials should emphasize a delay in radiation of no more than 1 year. In contrast, Grill et al. (2001) reported the experience of the French Society of Pediatric Oncology (SFOP) and concluded that deferring radiotherapy until the time of relapse did not compromise the overall survival. Overall the strategy to use chemotherapy to delay radiation may have a detrimental effect on overall survival (Fisher et al. 1998). Some cooperative groups are currently revisiting the role and time of radiation in this group of children.

With regard to radiation volume, the trend has been toward a decrease. Early use of craniospinal radiation was based on reports of dissemination in ependymoma from autopsies (Salazar et al. 1975, 1983). However, it is increasingly clear that most ependymoma relapses occur at the primary site and that seeding is often a late event (Rezai et al. 1996, Humpl et al. 2001, Paulino et al. 2002). Craniospinal and whole brain radiation in patients with localized ependymoma does not improve the overall or event-free survival (Timmermann et al. 2000, Paulino 2001) or prevent neuraxis dissemination even for high-grade ependymoma (Horn et al. 1999, Oya et al. 2002). Due to the lack of proven benefit of prophylactic craniospinal irradiation in ependymoma, most studies currently use local field radiation (Timmermann et al. 2000, Merchant et al. 2002b). Some still consider craniospinal radiation as the standard radiation technique for patients with anaplastic ependymoma. Pilot studies are now assessing the feasibility and safety of reduced field radiation using conformal techniques.

The standard dose of radiation is 54 Gy in 30 fractions given 5 days each week (standard fractionation). For patients who have undergone subtotal resection, higher local doses of radiotherapy may be necessary (Merchant et al. 1997). Preliminary results in 5 infants and children with anaplastic ependymoma treated with a boost of stereotactic radiosurgery have indicated good local control without acute side-effects (Aggarwal et al. 1997). Hyperfractionation has been reported in a recent prospective study, but its benefit remains to be proven (Massimino et al. 2004).

CHEMOTHERAPY
Chemotherapy has not been correlated with improvements in event-free or overall survival in pilot studies or randomized trials of childhood ependymomas (Evans et al. 1996, Bouffet et al. 1998, Robertson et al. 1998). Therefore, the role of chemotherapy remains unclear and should ideally be investigated prospectively in pilot studies for newly diagnosed patients and phase II studies for recurrent ependymomas. The response rate to single agents in phase II studies is disappointing. Cisplatin is reported to be the most active agent. Etoposide given orally at low doses also has some efficacy (Needle et al. 1997, Chamberlain 2001). There are as yet no published data documenting the activity of temozolomide in childhood ependymoma. Multi-agent combinations with drugs such as vincristine, carboplatin/cisplatin, cyclophosphamide, ifosfamide, CCNU, procarbazin and etoposide have been used either in newly diagnosed patients or at relapse. No drug or drug combination has been shown to have superior value in ependymomas. This lack of proven efficacy gives little rationale to the baby brain protocols, which aim to use chemotherapy in order to delay or avoid radiation. In a prospective, multicentre trial using a 6 drug chemotherapy regimen after surgery, all children (27) with postoperative residual tumour showed progression within 2 years from

TABLE 11.3

Current protocols in cooperative study groups in non-metastatic intracranial ependymoma

Study group	Surgery	Second-look surgery	Irradiation (local)	Chemotherapy	Eligibility
SFOP (Société Française d'Oncologie Pédiatrique)	Incomplete		66 Gy (HF)	No	>5yr
	Complete		60 Gy (HF)	No	
SIOP (Société Internationale d'Oncologie Pédiatrique)	Incomplete	Recommended after chemotherapy	54 Gy (C) or 72 Gy (HF)	VCR, CPM, VP16 (2 or 4 cycles)	>3yr
	Complete		54 Gy (C) or 72 Gy (HF)	No	
HIT 2000 (German group)	Incomplete	Recommended after first surgery and/or radiation	72 Gy (HF)	Cisplatin/VCR Carbo/VP16 (each cycle 5 times) following radiation*	>4yr
	Complete		72 Gy (HF)	Cisplatin/VCR Carbo/VP16 (each cycle 5 times) following radiation*	
COG (Children's Oncology Group)	Incomplete	Recommended after chemotherapy	59.4 Gy (C)	Carbo, VCR, CPM, VP16 (7 weeks) following surgery	>1yr
	Complete**		59.4 Gy (C)	No	
	Complete***		No	No	

HF = hyperfractionation; C = conformal radiation; VCR = vincristine; CPM = cyclophosphamid; Carbo = carboplatin; VP16 = etoposid.
*Only in patients with anaplastic ependymoma.
**Including supratentorial anaplastic ependymoma.
***Gross total resection of supratentorial ependymoma (WHO grade II).

228

initial surgery, and no radiological response to chemotherapy was observed (Grill et al. 2001). The Paediatric Oncology Group has reported an impressive 48% response rate in infants with ependymoma using a combination of vincristine and cyclophosphamide (Duffner et al. 1993). Unfortunately responses did not translate into survival benefit, and these results have not been confirmed in subsequent studies.

Chemotherapy has been used by some authors in order to facilitate a second surgical attempt after an incomplete initial resection (Foreman et al. 1997, Merchant 2002). Prospective studies conducted by the International Society of Paediatric Oncology (SIOP) and the Children's Oncology Group (COG) are currently evaluating the role of chemotherapy prior to second-look surgery. International differences in cooperative study protocols and therapeutic strategies for ependymoma by various centres in Europe and North America are outlined in Table 11.3.

Recurrent ependymoma
Most ependymomas recur, and the 5-year event-free survival in most series is less than 50%. The majority of the recurrences occur within the first 2 years following initial resection. However, late relapses are possible. The site of relapse is the primary tumour site in more than 90% of patients. Neuraxis dissemination is less common and often a late event (Pollack et al. 1995, Gilles et al. 1995, Perilongo et al. 1997, Horn et al. 1999) and isolated neuraxis failure is rare (Merchant 2002).

Reoperation is once again the mainstay of treatment for recurrent ependymoma. The role of surgery at the time of relapse justifies intensive surveillance imaging during follow-up (Steinbok et al. 1996, Good et al. 2001).

Treatment options after recurrence include postoperative treatment with chemotherapy, particularly when resection was incomplete (Goldwein et al. 1990). However, pilot data have provided some interesting results using radiosurgery. The Mayo Clinic has reported a 3-year local control of 68% in a series of 17 patients with recurrent ependymoma (Stafford et al. 2000). In another study (Hodgson et al. 2001), 28 children with recurrent ependymoma treated with radiosurgery showed a 3 year local control rate of 29%. Some patients with radionecrosis and progressive neurologic symptoms may require reoperation following radiosurgery. Factors predicting the success of radiosurgery are the site and the size of the lesion, with small (<3 cm) posterior fossa recurrences showing the best results. Eventually many children will develop a second or third recurrence. Surgery is usually considered again if the recurrence is local and the risks of repeat resection acceptable. Chemotherapy is often used as adjuvant treatment for second and subsequent recurrences. The choice of the drugs is limited due to prior therapy and the paucity of effective agents.

Conclusions and further directions
Previous reports have pointed out the lack of cooperative studies in paediatric ependymoma. Over the last decade an increasing number of pilot studies have been conducted, mainly in young children. These studies have contributed to a reconsideration of the initial principle of avoidance of radiotherapy in children under the age of 3 years. We may hope that this decade will see the outcome of studies conducted in older children. With these studies, the

respective roles of second-look surgery, chemotherapy and modern techniques of radio-therapy may be better understood. One of the main challenges in ependymomas concerns the histological grading, its reliability and reproducibility, precluding accurate comparisons between series. The development of new molecular markers may contribute to a better understanding of the biological behaviour of ependymomas.

REFERENCES

Aggarwal R, Yeung D, Kumar P, Muhlbauer M, Kun LE (1997) Efficacy and feasibility of stereotactic radio-surgery in the primary management of unfavorable pediatric ependymoma. *Radiother Oncol* **43**: 269–273.

Bailey P, Cushing H (1926) *A Classification of the Tumors of the Glioma Group on a Histogenetic Basis with a Correlated Study of Prognosis*. Philadelphia: JB Lippincott.

Bennetto L, Foreman N, Harding B, Hayward R, Ironside J, Love S, Ellison D (1998) Ki-67 immunolabelling index is a prognostic indicator in childhood posterior fossa ependymomas. *Neuropathol Appl Neurobiol* **24**: 434–440.

Bouffet E, Perilongo G, Canete A, Massimino M (1998) Intracranial ependymomas in children: a critical review of prognostic factors and a plea for cooperation. *Med Pediatr Oncol* **30**: 319–329.

Carter M, Nicholson J, Ross F, Crolla J, Allibone R, Balaji V, Perry R, Walker D, Gilbertson R, Ellison DW (2002) Genetic abnormalities detected in ependymomas by comparative genomic hybridisation. *Br J Cancer* **86**: 929–939.

Chamberlain MC (2001) Recurrent intracranial ependymoma in children: salvage therapy with oral etoposide. *Pediatr Neurol* **24**: 117–121.

Comi AM, Backstrom JW, Burger PC, Duffner PK (1998) Clinical and neuroradiologic findings in infants with intracranial ependymomas. Pediatric Oncology Group. *Pediatr Neurol* **18**: 23–29.

Duffner PK, Cohen ME, Freeman AI (1985) Pediatric brain tumors: an overview. *CA Cancer J Clin* **35**: 287–301.

Duffner PK, Horowitz ME, Krischer JP, Friedman HS, Burger PC, Cohen ME, Sanford RA, Mulhern RK, James HE, Freeman CR (1993) Postoperative chemotherapy and delayed radiation in children less than three years of age with malignant brain tumors. *N Engl J Med* **328**: 1725–1731.

Dyer S, Prebble E, Davison V, Davies P, Ramani P, Ellison D, Grundy R (2002) Genomic imbalances in pediatric intracranial ependymomas define clinically relevant groups. *Am J Pathol* **161**: 2133–2141.

Ernestus RI, Schröder R, Stützer H, Klug N (1996) Prognostic relevance of localization and grading in intracranial ependymomas of childhood. *Child's Nerv Syst* **12**: 522–526.

Ernestus RI, Schröder R, Stützer H, Klug N (1997) The clinical and prognostic relevance of grading in intracranial ependymomas. *Br J Neurosurg* **11**: 421–428.

Evans AE, Anderson JR, Lefkowitz-Boudreaux IB, Finlay JL (1996) Adjuvant chemotherapy of childhood posterior fossa ependymoma: cranio-spinal irradiation with or without adjuvant CCNU, vincristine, and prednisone: a Children's Cancer Group study. *Med Pediatr Oncol* **27**: 8–14.

Fink KL, Rushing EJ, Schold SC, Jr., Nisen PD (1996) Infrequency of p53 gene mutations in ependymomas. *J Neurooncol* **27**: 111–115.

Fisher PG, Needle MN, Cnaan A, Zhao H, Geyer JR, Molloy PT, Goldwein JW, Herman-Liu AB, Phillips PC (1998) Salvage therapy after postoperative chemotherapy for primary brain tumors in infants and very young children. *Cancer* **83**: 566–574.

Foreman NK, Love S, Thorne R (1996) Intracranial ependymomas: analysis of prognostic factors in a popula-tion-based series. *Pediatr Neurosurg* **24**: 119–125.

Foreman NK, Love S, Gill SS, Coakham HB (1997) Second-look surgery for incompletely resected fourth ventricle ependymomas: technical case report. *Neurosurgery* **40**: 856–860.

Gerszten PC, Pollack IF, Martinez AJ, Lo KH, Janosky J, Albright AL (1996) Intracranial ependymomas of childhood. Lack of correlation of histopathology and clinical outcome. *Pathol Res Pract* **192**: 515–522.

Gilbertson RJ, Bentley L, Hernan R, Junttila TT, Frank AJ, Haapasalo H, Connelly M, Wetmore C, Curran T, Elenius K, Ellison DW (2002) ERBB receptor signaling promotes ependymoma cell proliferation and represents a potential novel therapeutic target for this disease. *Clin Cancer Res* **8**: 3054–3064.

Gilles FH, Sobel EL, Tavaré CJ, Leviton A, Hedley-Whyte ET (1995) Age-related changes in diagnoses, histological features, and survival in children with brain tumors: 1930–1979. The Childhood Brain Tumor

Consortium. *Neurosurgery* **37**: 1056–1068.

Goldwein J, Glauser T, Packer R, Finlay JL, Sutton L, Curran T, Laehy JM, Rorke LB, Schut L, D'Angio GJ (1990) Recurrent intracranial ependymomas in children. Survival, patterns of failure and prognostic factors. *Cancer* **66**: 557–563.

Good CD, Wade AM, Hayward RD, Phipps KP, Michalski AJ, Harkness WF, Chong WK (2001) Surveillance neuroimaging in childhood intracranial ependymoma: how effective, how often, and for how long? *J Neurosurg* **94**: 27–32.

Grill J, Le Deley MC, Gambarelli D, Raquin MA, Couanet D, Pierre-Kahn A, Habrand JL, Doz F, Frappaz D, Gentet JC, Edan C, Chastagner P, Kalifa C (2001) Postoperative chemotherapy without irradiation for ependymoma in children under 5 years of age: a multicenter trial of the French Society of Pediatric Oncology. *J Clin Oncol* **19**: 1288–1296.

Grill J, Avet-Loiseau H, Lellouch-Tubiana A, Sévenet N, Terrier-Lacombe MJ, Vénuat AM, Doz F, Sainte-Rose C, Kalifa C, Vassal G (2002) Comparative genomic hybridization detects specific cytogenetic abnormalities in pediatric ependymomas and choroid plexus papillomas. *Cancer Genet Cytogenet* **136**: 121–125.

Hodgson DC, Goumnerova LC, Loeffler JS, Dutton S, Black PM, Alexander E, Xu R, Kooy H, Silver B, Tarbell NJ (2001) Radiosurgery in the management of pediatric brain tumors. *Int J Radiat Oncol Biol Phys* **50**: 929–935.

Horn B, Heideman R, Geyer R, Pollack I, Packer R, Goldwein J, Tomita T, Schomberg P, Ater J, Luchtman-Jones L, Rivlin K, Lamborn K, Prados M, Bollen A, Berger M, Dahl G, McNeil E, Patterson K, Shaw D, Kubalik M, Russo C (1999) A multi-institutional retrospective study of intracranial ependymoma in children: identification of risk factors. *J Pediatr Hematol Oncol* **21**: 203–211.

Hukin J, Epstein F, Lefton D, Allen J (1998) Treatment of intracranial ependymoma by surgery alone. *Pediatr Neurosurg* **29**: 40–45.

Humpl T, Neuser H, Brühl K, Bartels U, Schwarz M, Gutjahr P (2001) Clinical aspects and prognosis of ependymoma in infants and children. A single institution experience. *Child's Nerv Syst* **17**: 246–251.

Ikezaki K, Matsushima T, Inoue T, Yokoyama N, Kaneko Y, Fukui M (1993) Correlation of microanatomical localization with postoperative survival in posterior fossa ependymomas. *Neurosurgery* **32**: 38–44.

Khan RB, Sanford RA, Kun LE, Thompson SJ (2001) Morbidity of second-look surgery in pediatric central nervous system tumors. *Pediatr Neurosurg* **35**: 225–229.

Kleihues P, Burger PC, Scheithauer BW (1993) *Histological Typing of Tumours of the Central Nervous System. World Health Organization International Histological Classification of Tumours*, 2nd edn. Berlin, Heidelberg: Springer-Verlag.

Korshunov A, Golanov A, Timirgaz V (2002) Immunohistochemical markers for prognosis of ependymal neoplasms. *J Neurooncol* **58**: 255–270.

Kramer DL, Parmiter AH, Rorke LB, Sutton LN, Biegel JA (1998) Molecular cytogenetic studies of pediatric ependymomas. *J Neurooncol* **37**: 25–33.

Lefton DR, Pinto RS, Martin SW (1998) MRI features of intracranial and spinal ependymomas. *Pediatr Neurosurg* **28**: 97–105.

Massimino M, Gandola L, Giangaspero F, Sandri A, Valagussa P, Perilongo G, Garre ML, Ricardi U, Forni M, Genitori L, Scarzello G, Spreafico F, Barra S, Mascarin M, Pollo B, Gardiman M, Cama A, Navarria P, Brisigotti M, Collini P, Balter R, Fidani P, Stefanelli M, Burnelli R, Potepan P, Podda M, Sotti G, Madon E (2004) Hyperfractionated radiotherapy and chemotherapy for childhood ependymoma: Final results of the first prospective AIEOP (Associazione Italiana di Ematologia-Oncologia Pediatrica) study. *Int J Radiat Oncol Biol Phys* **58**: 1336–1345.

Merchant TE (2002) Current management of childhood ependymoma. *Oncology* **16**: 629–642.

Merchant TE, Haida T, Wang MH, Finlay JL, Leibel SA (1997) Anaplastic ependymoma: treatment of pediatric patients with or without craniospinal radiation therapy. *J Neurosurg* **86**: 943–949.

Merchant TE, Jenkins JJ, Burger PC, Sanford RA, Sherwood SH, Jones-Wallace D, Heideman RL, Thompson SJ, Helton KJ, Kun LE (2002a) Influence of tumor grade on time to progression after irradiation for localized ependymoma in children. *Int J Radiat Oncol Biol Phys* **53**: 52–57.

Merchant TE, Zhu Y, Thompson SJ, Sontag MR, Heideman RL, Kun LE (2002b) Preliminary results from a Phase II trail of conformal radiation therapy for pediatric patients with localised low-grade astrocytoma and ependymoma. *Int J Radiat Oncol Biol Phys* **52**: 325–332.

Nazar GB, Hoffman HJ, Becker LE, Jenkin D, Humphreys RP, Hendrick EB (1990) Infratentorial ependymomas in childhood: prognostic factors and treatment. *J Neurosurg* **72**: 408–417.

231

Needle MN, Molloy PT, Geyer JR, Herman-Liu A, Belasco JB, Goldwein JW, Sutton L, Phillips PC (1997) Phase II study of daily oral etoposide in children with recurrent brain tumors and other solid tumors. *Med Pediatr Oncol* **29**: 28–32.

Oya N, Shibamoto Y, Nagata Y, Negoro Y, Hiraoka M (2002) Postoperative radiotherapy for intracranial ependymoma: analysis of prognostic factors and patterns of failure. *J Neurooncol* **56**: 87–94.

Palma L, Celli P, Mariottini A, Zalaffi A, Schettini G (2000) The importance of surgery in supratentorial ependymomas. Long-term survival in a series of 23 cases. *Child's Nerv Syst* **16**: 170–175.

Paulino AC (2001) The local field in infratentorial ependymoma: does the entire posterior fossa need to be treated? *Int J Radiat Oncol Biol Phys* **49**: 757–761.

Paulino AC, Wen BC, Buatti JM, Hussey DH, Zhen WK, Mayr NA, Menezes AH (2002) Intracranial ependymomas: an analysis of prognostic factors and patterns of failure. *Am J Clin Oncol* **25**: 117–122.

Perilongo G, Massimino M, Sotti G, Belfontali T, Masiero L, Rigobello L, Garre L, Carli M, Lombardi F, Solero C, Sainati L, Canale V, del Prever AB, Giangaspero F, Andreussi L, Mazza C, Madon E (1997) Analyses of prognostic factors in a retrospective review of 92 children with ependymoma: Italian Pediatric Neuro-oncology Group. *Med Pediatr Oncol* **29**: 79–85.

Pierre-Kahn A, Hirsch JF, Renier D, Sainte-Rose C, Roux FX, Pfister A (1983) Intracranial ependymoma in children. Prognosis and therapeutic perspectives. *Arch Fr Pediatr* **40**: 5–9.

Pollack IF, Gerszten PC, Martinez AJ, Lo KH, Shultz B, Albright AL, Janosky J, Deutsch M (1995) Intracranial ependymomas of childhood: long-term outcome and prognostic factors. *Neurosurgery* **37**: 655–666.

Prayson RA (1999) Clinicopathologic study of 61 patients with ependymoma including MIB-1 immunohisto-chemistry. *Ann Diagn Pathol* **3**: 11–18.

Reardon DA, Entrekin RE, Sublett J, Ragsdale S, Li H, Boyett J, Kepner JL, Look AT (1999) Chromosome arm 6q loss is the most common recurrent autosomal alteration detected in primary pediatric ependymoma. *Genes Chromosomes Cancer* **24**: 230–237.

Rezai AR, Woo HH, Lee M, Cohen H, Zagzag D, Epstein FJ (1996) Disseminated ependymomas of the central nervous system. *J Neurosurg* **85**: 618–624.

Ries LAG, Eisner MP, Kosary CL, Hankey BF, Miller BA, Clegg L, Edwards BK (2002) *SEER Cancer Statistics Review, 1973–1999*. Bethesda, MD: National Cancer Institute.

Robertson PL, Zeltzer PM, Boyett JM, Rorke LB, Allen JC, Geyer JR, Stanley P, Li H, Albright AL, McGuire-Cullen P, Finlay JL, Stevens KR, Milstein JM, Packer RJ, Wisoff J (1998) Survival and prognostic factors following radiation therapy and chemotherapy for ependymomas in children: a report of the Children's Cancer Group. *J Neurosurg* **88**: 695–703.

Ross GW, Rubinstein LJ (1989) Lack of histopathological correlation of malignant ependymomas with post-operative survival. *J Neurosurg* **70**: 31–36.

Rousseau-Merck M, Versteege I, Zattara-Cannoni H, Figarella D, Lena G, Aurias A, Vagner-Capodano AM (2000) Fluorescence in situ hybridization determination of 22q12–q13 deletion in two intracerebral ependymomas. *Cancer Genet Cytogenet* **121**: 223–227.

Sainte-Rose C, Cinalli G, Roux FE, Maixner R, Chumas PD, Mansour M, Carpentier A, Bourgeois M, Zerah M, Pierre-Kahn A, Renier D (2001) Management of hydrocephalus in pediatric patients with posterior fossa tumors: the role of endoscopic third ventriculostomy. *J Neurosurg* **95**: 791–797.

Salazar OM, Castro-Vita H, VanHoutte P, Rubin P, Aygun C (1983) Improved survival in cases of intracranial ependymoma after radiation therapy. Late report and recommendations. *J Neurosurg* **59**: 652–659.

Salazar OM, Rubin P, Bassano D, Marcial VA (1975) Improved survival of patients with intracranial ependymomas by irradiation: doseselection and field extension. *Cancer* **35**: 1563–1573.

Scheurlen W, Kühl J (1998) Current diagnostic and therapeutic management of CNS metastasis in childhood primitive neuroectodermal tumors and ependymomas. *J Neurooncol* **38**: 181–185.

Schiffer D, Chio A, Giordana MT, Migheli A, Palma L, Pollo B, Soffietti R, Tribolo A (1991) Histologic prognostic factors in ependymoma. *Child's Nerv Syst* **7**: 177–182.

Stafford SL, Pollock BE, Foote RL, Gorman DA, Nelson DF, Schomberg PJ (2000) Stereotactic radiosurgery for recurrent ependymoma. *Cancer* **88**: 870–875.

Steinbok P, Hentschel S, Cochrane DD, Kestle JR (1996) Value of postoperative surveillance imaging in the management of children with some common brain tumors. *J Neurosurg* **84**: 726–732.

Suzuki SO, Iwaki T (2000) Amplification and overexpression of mdm2 gene in ependymomas. *Mod Pathol* **13**: 548–553.

Timmermann B, Kortmann RD, Kühl J, Meisner C, Slavc I, Pietsch T, Bamberg M (2000) Combined postoperative irradiation and chemotherapy for anaplastic ependymomas in childhood: results of the German prospective trials HIT 88/89 and HIT 91. *Int J Radiat Oncol Biol Phys* **46**: 287–295.

Tortori-Donati P, Fondelli MP, Cama A, Garre ML, Rossi A, Andreussi L (1995) Ependymomas of the posterior cranial fossa: CT and MRI findings. *Neuroradiology* **37**: 238–243.

Undjian S, Marinov M (1990) Intracranial ependymomas in children. *Child's Nerv Syst* **6**: 131–134.

Vagner-Capodano AM, Zattara-Cannoni H, Gambarelli D, Figarella-Branger D, Lena G, Dufour H, Grisoli F, Choux M (1999) Cytogenetic study of 33 ependymomas. *Cancer Genet Cytogenet* **115**: 96–99.

Ward S, Harding B, Wilkins P, Harkness W, Hayward R, Darling JL, Thomas DG, Warr T (2001) Gain of 1q and loss of 22 are the most common changes detected by comparative genomic hybridisation in paediatric ependymoma. *Genes Chromosomes Cancer* **32**: 59–66.

Warmuth-Metz M, Kühl J (2002) Neuroradiological differential diagnosis in medulloblastomas and ependymomas: results of the HIT'91-study. *Klin Pädiatr* **214**: 162–166.

Wiestler OD, Schiffer D, Coons SW, Prayson RA, Rosenblum MK (2000) Ependymal tumours. In: Kleihues P, Cavenee WK, eds. *Pathology and Genetics of Tumours of the Nervous System*. Lyon: IARC Press, pp. 71–82.

12
BRAINSTEM TUMOURS

Carolyn R Freeman and Jean-Pierre Farmer

The brainstem, comprising the midbrain, pons and medulla oblongata, is a compact, highly organized region of the brain, which, in addition to conveying ascending and descending tracts, contains the nuclei of cranial nerves III to XII and is responsible for a number of complex functions, including control of respiratory and cardiovascular activity and regulation of the level of consciousness.

Magnetic resonance imaging (MRI) is the imaging modality of choice for all patients in whom a brainstem lesion is suspected. MRI alone or in combination with newer techniques such as spectroscopy offers the potential for differentiating between non-neoplastic lesions of the brainstem (e.g. vascular malformations such as angiomas, which may be a cause of spontaneous haemorrhage; infectious diseases such as tuberculosis; and demyelinating diseases such as multiple sclerosis) and tumours (Zimmerman 1996).

Tumours arising in the brainstem are of several distinct types. Collectively, they account for approximately 10–15% of all CNS tumours occurring in the paediatric age-group. Boys and girls are approximately equally affected. The median age at presentation is between 5 and 10 years. There are no known predisposing factors, although it is of note that patients with neurofibromatosis type I (NF1) have a rather high frequency of abnormalities of the brainstem, some of which (4–9% of all patients) are brainstem gliomas (Molloy et al. 1995, Pollack et al. 1996, Bilaniuk et al. 1997).

Clinical presentation and imaging findings

Tumours arising in the brainstem can be broadly grouped as low grade (favourable) or unfavourable (Table 12.1). Each type has a unique clinical presentation that is based on the location of the tumour, its histology, and its rate and pattern of growth.

Focal intrinsic tumours can arise at any level in the brainstem but are most commonly seen in the midbrain and medulla oblongata. They are also seen, albeit much less frequently, in the pons. Although originally defined as small in size (<2 cm) (Epstein and McCleary 1986) or limited in extent (less than half of a single involved segment of the brainstem) (Barkovich et al. 1990–91), a more important characteristic is that they grow in a predictable fashion that depends on their origin in the brainstem, displace rather than invade adjacent tissues, and on imaging are well marginated (Epstein and Constantini 1996, Fischbein et al. 1996, Farmer et al. 2001). They are slowly growing tumours that usually present with a long history. Those arising in the tectal region of the midbrain obstruct the aqueduct of Sylvius and cause hydrocephalus. Young children typically present with macrocephaly, older children with symptoms and signs of raised intracranial pressure. In contrast, focal tumours

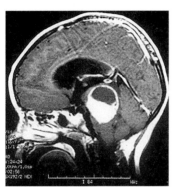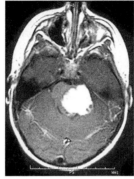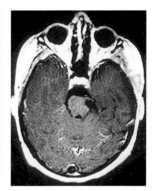

Fig. 12.1. Typical appearance of a pilocytic astrocytoma arising in the midbrain in a 3-year-old girl who presented with a long-standing right hemiparesis. Axial T_1-weighted MRI shows a well-marginated mass with uniform bright enhancement after gadolinium injection. There is an associated cyst. Subtotal resection was performed and followed with conformal radiotherapy at time of progression 6 months following surgery. Five years later she remains well with a residual right hemiparesis and no evidence of tumour on MRI.

at other levels in the brainstem almost always present with localized findings such as an isolated cranial nerve deficit and a contralateral hemiparesis.

Most focal intrinsic tumours are pilocytic astrocytomas that have a characteristic appearance on MRI. They are well circumscribed and enhance brightly and uniformly after gadolinium injection (Fig. 12.1). There may be a cystic component, which may be quite large relative to the size of the solid, biologically active, component of the tumour. In contrast, focal lesions in the tectal region are often iso-intense and non-enhancing (Fig. 12.2); many are likely glial hamartomas.

Dorsal exophytic tumours arise from subependymal tissue in the floor of the IVth ventricle and grow exophytically along the path of least resistance through the floor into the ventricle but do not invade the brainstem. They present, therefore, with non-localizing findings, commonly intractable vomiting (due to area postrema irritation) and failure to thrive in younger children and symptoms and signs of raised intracranial pressure due to obstruction of CSF flow in older patients. Cranial nerve deficits (VI if there is hydrocephalus, otherwise

235

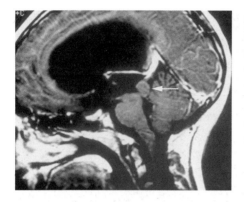

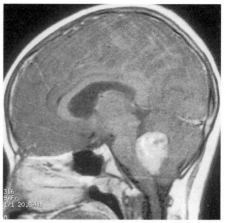

Fig. 12.2. Sagittal T_1-weighted MRI of an 11-year-old girl who presented with ataxia. Note marked hydrocephalus due to a small lesion in the tectal region (arrow) that did not enhance after contrast injection. CSF diversion was performed. The patient remains well without any evidence of progression nearly 9 years later.

Fig. 12.3. This 11-year-old girl was followed in GI clinic for intractable vomiting. Sagittal T_1-weighted MRI shows a typical dorsal exophytic brainstem tumour. Surgical resection was performed leaving a thin layer of tumour on the brainstem. Such patients will require frequent MRIs (every 3–4 months) during the first 12–18 months following surgery.

IX–XII) are seen in about half of the patients but long tract signs are unusual. On MRI, dorsal exophytic tumours are well circumscribed and well delineated from surrounding structures (Fig. 12.3). They are hypointense on T_1-weighted images and hyperintense on T_2-weighted images, and enhance uniformly and brightly after gadolinium injection. They may have a cystic component. These features point towards the usual histologic diagnosis, namely pilocytic astrocytoma.

Cervicomedullary tumours are in reality tumours of the spinal cord that arise in the upper cervical region and grow rostrally beyond the foramen magnum to involve the brainstem. They are usually low-grade lesions (pilocytic astrocytoma or ganglioglioma) whose axial growth is limited by the pyramidal decussations located ventrally at the junction of the cervical cord and medulla, at which point the tumour grows posteriorly, distorting the dorsal aspect of the medulla (Epstein and Farmer 1993). The clinical presentation is typically with lower cranial nerve deficits (IX–XII), long tract signs and torticollis. Hydrocephalus is unusual. On MRI, the findings are quite characteristic (Fig. 12.4). There is often an associated syrinx in the cord.

Diffuse intrinsic tumours, which account for approximately 70% of all brainstem tumours, typically arise in the pons. At presentation they usually involve the whole pons, which is expanded, and often extend axially to involve the midbrain and medulla oblongata as well. Ventral exophytic growth, encasing the basilar artery, is common. Diffuse intrinsic tumours present with a short duration of symptoms (median 1 month) consisting of multiple, bilateral cranial nerve deficits (especially VI and VII), long tract signs and ataxia.

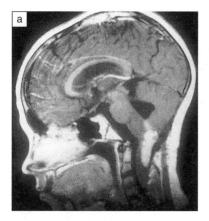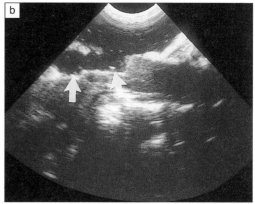

Fig. 12.4. Sagittal MRI of a 7-year-old boy who presented with pain on swallowing and unilateral lower cranial nerve deficits. (a) The growth of the tumour that originated at the cervicomedullary junction is limited by the pyramidal decussations (arrow). (b) Intraoperative ultrasound confirmed that complete resection had been achieved (arrows).

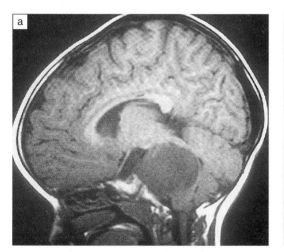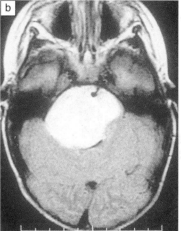

Fig. 12.5. Diffuse intrinsic pontine tumour in a 2.5-year-old girl who presented with bilateral cranial nerve deficits and ataxia. (a) The tumour was hypointense and non-enhancing on T_1-weighted MRI. The extent of the tumour is only fully appreciated on T_2-weighted MRI, which is consequently a better study for radiotherapy treatment planning purposes.

On MRI, diffuse intrinsic tumours are hypointense on T_1-weighted images and hyperintense on T_2-weighted images and enhance little if at all after contrast injection (Fig. 12.5). Such findings are compatible with a histological diagnosis of fibrillary astrocytoma (WHO grade II). Some, however, show patchy or even ring enhancement, suggestive of higher grade histology.

237

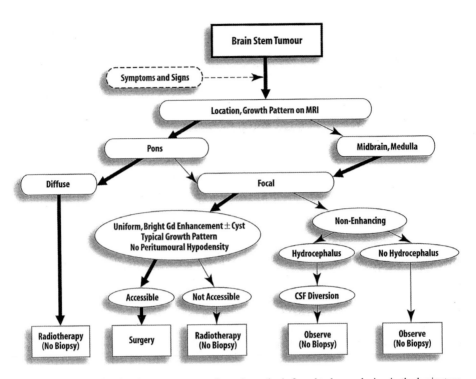

Fig. 12.6. An algorithm for the management of a patient who is found to have a lesion in the brainstem, based on location and growth pattern. Heavier arrows show the more frequent clinical situations. In general, any patient with an atypical clinical presentation and/or imaging findings should undergo biopsy prior to definitive treatment.

Other types of tumour that may rarely arise in the brainstem include *primitive neuro-ectodermal tumours* and *atypical teratoid/rhabdoid tumours*. Patients with these tumour types are typically younger (<3 years of age) than those with other tumour types, and on imaging have relatively well circumscribed tumours that could be considered focal but with characteristics otherwise more typical of diffuse intrinsic tumours, that is, hypointense on T_1-weighted and hyperintense in T_2-weighted MRI, with little or no enhancement after contrast injection (Zagzag et al. 2000). Many patients already have leptomeningeal spread at diagnosis. Such a presentation mandates the use of biopsy for histopathological diagnosis, since the management of these patients will differ substantially from that for patients with other types of tumour arising in the brainstem. Aggressive treatment that includes both chemotherapy and radiotherapy, as for similar tumours at other location in the CNS, is required for any chance of survival. These tumours will not be discussed further here.

Management
Management decisions are based on the clinical presentation and MRI findings, according to the algorithm shown in Figure 12.6.

OBSERVATION ONLY

Observation only, without any tumour-directed treatment, is appropriate in two situations. As noted, patients with NF1 are not infrequently found to have lesions in the brainstem, and it is essential to differentiate the 'unidentified bright objects' (UBOs) found incidentally on MRI from tumours. Even lesions with MRI findings otherwise characteristic for tumour may behave differently in patients with NF1 (Pollack et al. 1996, Bilaniuk et al. 1997). Spontaneous regression as well as stability of imaging findings over months and even years is well described. While patients with hydrocephalus at diagnosis or subsequently will require a CSF diversionary procedure, tumour-directed intervention of any type (surgery, radiotherapy or chemotherapy) should be limited to patients with lesions that exhibit clear evidence of progression on serial imaging and/or cause significant clinical deterioration. Results of treatment at this point are generally very good to excellent (Pollack et al. 1996, Broniscer et al. 1997).

Patients with small, well circumscribed, tectal tumours that are iso-intense and non-enhancing on MRI are best managed initially by CSF diversion, usually IIIrd ventriculostomy, followed by close observation. Most such lesions, which as noted may in fact be glial hamartomas, remain stable over long periods of time without any tumour-specific treatment (Boydston et al. 1991–92, May et al. 1992, Pollack et al. 1994, Robertson et al. 1995, Grant et al. 1999, Bowers et al. 2000, Farmer et al. 2001). This is an important point since surgery (even biopsy) for lesions in this location is associated with a substantial risk of morbidity and mortality (Lapras et al. 1994).

SURGERY

In general, all other favourable, low-grade, tumour types will be best managed surgically if feasible. This is certainly the case for patients with typical cervicomedullary tumours. In these patients, microscopically complete resection can be achieved in approximately 80% of cases and subtotal removal in most of the remainder. As for spinal cord astrocytomas at other levels the probability of long-term tumour control after such treatment is excellent (Epstein and McCleary 1986, Epstein and Wisoff 1987).

In patients with dorsal exophytic tumours, however, the fact that there is no clear tumour–brainstem interface means that even an optimal tumour resection will leave a thin layer of tumour on the floor of the IVth ventricle. While most patients (70–80%) do well following surgery alone, close follow-up is necessary for the first 2–3 years in order to identify patients who will progress and institute appropriate treatment, since the probability of permanent tumour control after further treatment consisting of surgery alone, surgery followed by radiotherapy, or radiotherapy alone appears to be excellent (Pollack et al. 1993, Khatib et al. 1994).

Surgery for intrinsic focal tumours requires special expertise and availability of the required technology such as neuronavigation and electrophysiological monitoring. Judgement is required with respect to selection of patients for surgery (Epstein and McCleary 1986, Pendl et al. 1990, Bricolo et al. 1991, Pierre-Khan et al. 1993). The tumours must be surgically accessible, meaning that they extend to the surface of the brainstem or can be approached above or below the facial colliculus. They should have imaging characteristics suggestive of pilocytic histology, specifically well-defined borders, uniform bright enhancement with contrast material, and possibly an associated cyst. There should be no peritumoural hypodensity or oedema. Patients with bulkier lesions and/or less favourable imaging characteristics are likely to fare less well in terms of tumour control. Patients with tumours in the medulla, and particularly those with preoperative symptoms and signs such as an impaired gag reflex, difficulty swallowing, or voice change as a result of vocal cord paresis, are at significantly higher risk of serious postoperative morbidity (Epstein and Constantini 1996).

Over the past decade it has been generally accepted that surgery has no role in the management of patients with diffuse intrinsic brainstem tumours. Even biopsy is thought to be unnecessary because in the context of a typical clinical presentation and characteristic MRI findings, histology obtained by biopsy (which may or may not be representative of the tumour as a whole) does not influence treatment (Albright 1996). More extensive surgery for these highly invasive tumours is associated with a prohibitive risk of morbidity without any realistic expectation of improved outcome (Epstein and Constantini 1996).

RADIOTHERAPY

Indications for treatment with radiotherapy in patients with favourable tumour types include progression following surgical resection and definitive treatment of surgically inaccessible tumours. In both situations, the standard approach consists of external beam irradiation to a target volume that includes the macroscopic disease as demonstrated by T_1-weighted gadolinium enhanced MRI at time of treatment plus a margin of 0.5–1 cm depending on the type of immobilization device used and the reproducibility of patient positioning from day to day (Kortmann et al. 1998). A total dose of the order of 54 Gy is given in once-daily fractions, 5 days each week, over a period of 6 weeks. Other approaches have been used in patients with low-grade brainstem tumours including radiosurgery (Kondziolka et al. 1993, Hadjipanayis et al. 2002), stereotactic irradiation with large fraction sizes (Freeman et al. 1994), and interstitial irradiation using iodine-125 (Mundinger et al. 1991, Kreth et al. 1995, Voges and Sturm 1999). However, the risks of such treatments outside the context of a clinical trial cannot be justified in the absence of any established benefit over conventional external beam irradiation, which in the setting of progression after surgery is associated with tumour control in 80–100% of cases and in the setting of surgically inaccessible focal lesions in at least 50–70% of cases (Stroink et al. 1986, Farmer et al. 2001).

Radiotherapy is the treatment of choice for patients with diffuse intrinsic brainstem tumours. These patients are often treated on a semi-urgent basis because of rapidly worsening neurological status. Because they are of higher histological grade, wider margins of 1.5–2 cm around the lesion, which is usually best seen on T_2-weighted or FLAIR MRI, are used. A dose of 54 Gy given in once daily fractions, 5 days each week, over a total of 6 weeks constitutes standard practice. Treated in this way, the majority of patients show significant improvement by 2–3 weeks into treatment, allowing steroids if used to be tapered and discontinued even well before the end of treatment. The prognosis is very poor, however, with a median time to progression of only 5–6 months and a median survival time of only approximately 11 months. Survival at 2 years is less than 20%. Features that correlate with a particularly adverse outcome include short duration of clinical history, presence of a VIth nerve deficit at diagnosis, pontine location, greater volume of tumour and degree of brainstem enlargement, and encasement of the basilar artery on MRI, as well as other imaging findings such as a poorly circumscribed tumour, presence of peritumoural hypointensity and ring enhancement, suggestive of high-grade histology.

The dismal prognosis for children with diffuse intrinsic gliomas has been the impetus for the development of active research programs that during the 1980s and early 1990s in North America focused on the use of hyperfractionated radiotherapy (HFRT) that allows the use of higher doses of radiotherapy (Freeman 1996). Large numbers of children were accrued to series of phase I/II studies that tested HFRT at doses ranging from 64.8 to 78 Gy. At intermediate dose levels of 70.2 Gy and 72 Gy there was a suggestion of increased efficacy when compared with lower doses of HFRT and with historical controls treated with conventional radiotherapy to doses of 54 Gy, but this was not confirmed in a subsequent study that randomized patients between HFRT to a dose of 70.2 Gy and conventional radiotherapy to 54 Gy, with cisplatin given by infusion on weeks 1, 3 and 5 of the radiotherapy in both arms (Freeman et al. 2000). There was no evidence of benefit at higher doses of HFRT of 75.6 Gy and 78 Gy, and morbidity was considerable. This included steroid dependency, vascular events, and white matter changes outside the radiation field, as well as hearing loss, hormonal deficiencies, and late developing seizure disorders in the small number of long-term survivors (Freeman et al. 1993, 1996; Packer et al. 1994; Prados et al. 1995).

Accelerated radiotherapy to a total dose of 50.4 Gy given in 28 twice daily fractions of 1.8 Gy over 3 weeks was tested by the UK Children's Cancer Study Group. Progression-free and overall survival rates were similar to those seen in the HFRT studies (Lewis et al. 1997).

CHEMOTHERAPY

The role, if any, for chemotherapy in brainstem tumours remains undefined. As for low-grade gliomas at other locations in the CNS, chemotherapy might be considered in young patients with progressive disease after surgical resection and in patients with surgically inaccessible lesions in order to delay radiotherapy. However, the risks associated with the use of radiotherapy for tumours in the brainstem are relatively low so that, in practice, chemotherapy, with its attendant risk that the tumour will be larger and associated with a further deteriorated neurological status, will rarely be the treatment of choice for such patients.

Chemotherapy has no established role either in the management of diffuse intrinsic brainstem tumours. Many agents have been studied, alone and in combination, and in all possible sequences – that is, prior to radiotherapy, concurrent with radiotherapy, and as adjuvant treatment following radiotherapy – all with disappointing results (Freeman and Perilongo 1999, Walker et al. 1999). Response rates are low, and no agent or combination has been shown to have a significant impact on outcome. Other agents such as tamoxifen, given at high doses, have also been tried with similarly disappointing results (Broniscer et al. 2000). New agents and novel chemotherapy/radiotherapy combinations are presently under investigation by the paediatric cooperative groups in North America and in Europe.

Prognosis

The prognosis for children with low-grade brainstem tumours in terms of progression-free and overall survival is very good to excellent. What is perhaps less clear is the prognosis with respect to functional outcome and quality of life. Mulhern et al. (1994) have shown that quality of survival for patients with lesions in the brainstem depends largely on the degree of neurological impairment. In general, patients with surgically accessible tumours, especially the dorsal exophytic tumours, can be expected to have an excellent likelihood for normal quality of life. However, surgery for focal lesions intrinsic to the brainstem is not without risk, and good judgement is required to determine the best strategy for a given patient. Overall, it appears that patients successfully treated with surgery will have the best quality of life, while those with significant neurological deficits as a result of surgery or those that recur after surgery and subsequently require radiotherapy fare less well. Similarly, while the risks associated with use of radiotherapy for tumours in the brainstem are relatively low (Mulhern et al. 1994), patients who fail radiotherapy and need surgery for salvage are at much greater risk for sequelae that affect the quality of survival (Farmer et al. 2001).

Quality of life is also an issue in patients with diffuse intrinsic brainstem gliomas. Even though the prognosis overall for children with these tumours is dismal, the majority (more than 80%) do very well in the months following radiotherapy up until time of tumour progression. This period of time when the child is almost back to normal is usually very much appreciated by the family, so that although experimental regimens are clearly justified they should avoid, if at all possible, significant jeopardy to quality of life.

Controversies

For the favourable tumour types, there are few controversies. The issues revolve rather around the availability of the surgical expertise required for their optimal management. For young patients with surgically inaccessible lesions and those who progress after surgery, the issue will be whether to use chemotherapy to delay or avoid radiotherapy, although it seems likely that the gains, if any, will be small and possibly outweighed by the risks of delaying effective treatment with radiotherapy.

For patients with diffuse intrinsic tumours the dismal prognosis that has not improved at all despite two decades of very active research argues for continued investigation. One question that keeps resurfacing in this patient population is whether biopsy, which is not necessary for diagnosis, should be performed for better evaluation of the biology of the tumour that may in the future lead to targeted therapy. Another issue, given the normally very good quality of life after standard treatment consisting of radiotherapy alone, is the degree of acceptable risk associated with aggressive experimental regimens. This is usually much debated among members of the treating team but is obviously a matter in which the parents should be involved as well. This may become an even greater issue at time of progression after radiotherapy. The results of any treatment at this point are usually so limited that supportive care will usually be the best option but may be possible only in the context of a close working relationship between members of the treating team, the palliative care service, the primary care physician, and the parents.

242

REFERENCES

Albright AL (1996) Diffuse brainstem tumors: when is a biopsy necessary? *Pediatr Neurosurg* **24**: 252–255.

Barkovich AJ, Krischer J, Kun LE, Packer R, Zimmerman RA, Freeman CR, Wara WM, Albright L, Allen JC, Hoffman HJ (1990–91) Brain stem gliomas: a classification system based on magnetic resonance imaging. *Pediatr Neurosurg* **16**: 73–83.

Bilaniuk LT, Molloy PT, Zimmerman RA, Phillips PC, Vaughan SN, Liu GT, Sutton LN, Needle M (1997) Neurofibromatosis type 1: brain stem tumours. *Neuroradiology* **39**: 642–653.

Bowers DC, Georgiades C, Aronson LJ, Carson BS, Weingart JD, Wharam MD, Melhem ER, Burger PC, Cohen KJ (2000) Tectal gliomas: natural history of an indolent lesion in pediatric patients. *Pediatr Neurosurg* **32**: 24–29.

Boydston WR, Sanford RA, Muhlbauer MS, Kun LE, Kirk E, Dohan FC, Schweitzer JB (1991–92) Gliomas of the tectum and periaqueductal region of the mesencephalon. *Pediatr Neurosurg* **17**: 234–238.

Bricolo A, Turazzi S, Cristofori L, Talacchi A (1991) Direct surgery for brainstem tumours. *Acta Neurochirurgica* Suppl. 53: 148–158.

Broniscer A, Gajjar A, Bhargava R, Langston JW, Heideman R, Jones D, Kun LE, Taylor J (1997) Brain stem involvement in children with neurofibromatosis type 1: role of magnetic resonance imaging and spectroscopy in the distinction from diffuse pontine glioma. *Neurosurgery* **40**: 331–338.

Broniscer A, da Costa Leite C, Lanchote VL, Machado TMS, Cristófani LM (2000) Radiation therapy and high-dose tamoxifen in the treatment of patients with diffuse brainstem gliomas: results of a Brazilian cooperative study. Brainstem Glioma Cooperative Group. *J Clin Oncol* **18**: 1246–1253.

Epstein F, Constantini S (1996) Practical decisions in the treatment of pediatric brain stem tumors. *Pediatr Neurosurg* **24**: 24–34.

Epstein FJ, Farmer J-P (1993) Brain-stem glioma growth patterns. *J Neurosurg* **78**: 408–412.

Epstein F, McCleary EL (1986) Intrinsic brain-stem tumors of childhood: surgical indications. *J Neurosurg* **64**: 11–15.

Epstein F, Wisoff J (1987) Intra-axial tumors of the cervicomedullary junction. *J Neurosurg* **67**: 483–487.

Farmer J-P, Montes JL, Freeman CR, Meagher-Villemure K, Bond MC, O'Gorman AM (2001) Brainstem gliomas: a 10-year institutional review. *Pediatr Neurosurg* **34**: 206–214.

Fischbein NJ, Prados MD, Wara W, Russo C, Edwards MSB, Barkovich AJ (1996) Radiologic classification of brain stem tumors: correlation of magnetic resonance imaging appearance with clinical outcome. *Pediatr Neurosurg* **24**: 9–23.

Freeman CR (1996) Hyperfractionated radiotherapy for diffuse intrinsic brain stem tumors in children. *Pediatr Neurosurg* **24**: 103–110.

Freeman CR, Perilongo,G (1999) Chemotherapy for brain stem gliomas. *Child's Nerv Syst* **15**: 545–553.

Freeman CR, Krischer JP, Sanford RA, Cohen ME, Burger PC, del Carpio R, Halperin EC, Munoz L, Friedman HS, Kun LE (1993) Final results of a study of escalating doses of hyperfractionated radiotherapy in brain stem tumors in children: a Pediatric Oncology Group study. *Int J Radiat Oncol Biol Phys* **27**: 197–206.

Freeman CR, Souhami L, Caron J-L, Villemure J-G, Olivier A, Montes J, Farmer J-P, Podgorsak EB (1994) Stereotactic external beam irradiation in previously untreated brain tumors in children and adolescents. *Med Pediatr Oncol* **22**: 173–180.

Freeman CR, Bourgouin PM, Sanford RA, Cohen ME, Friedman HS, Kun LE (1996) Long term survivors of childhood brain stem gliomas treated with hyperfractionated radiotherapy. *Cancer* **77**: 555–562.

Freeman CR, Kepner J, Kun LE, Sanford RA, Kadota R, Mandell L, Friedman H (2000) A detrimental effect of a combined chemotherapy–radiotherapy approach in children with diffuse intrinsic brain stem gliomas? *Int J Radiat Oncol Biol Phys* **47**: 561–564.

Grant GA, Avellino AM, Loeser JD, Ellenbogen RG, Berger MS, Roberts TS (1999) Management of intrinsic gliomas of the tectal plate in children. *Pediatr Neurosurg* **31**: 170–176.

Hadjipanayis CG, Kondziolka D, Gardner P, Niranjan A, Dagam S, Flickinger JC, Lunsford LD (2002) Stereotactic radiosurgery for pilocytic astrocytomas when multimodal therapy is necessary. *J Neurosurg* **97**: 56–64.

Khatib ZA, Heideman RL, Kovnar EH, Langston JA, Sanford RA, Douglass EC, Ochs J, Jenkins JJ, Fairclough DL, Greenwald C, Kun LE (1994) Predominance of pilocytic histology in dorsally exophytic brain stem tumors. *Pediatr Neurosurg* **20**: 2–10.

Kondziolka D, Lunsford LD, Flickinger JC (1993) Intraparenchymal brain stem radiosurgery. *Neurosurg Clin N Am* **4**: 469–479.

243

Kortmann R-D, Timmermann B, Becker G, Kühl J, Bamberg M (1998) Advances in treatment techniques and time/dose schedules in external radiation therapy of brain tumours in children. *Klin Pädiatr* **210**: 220–226.

Kreth FW, Faist M, Warnke PC, Robner R, Volk B, Ostertag CB (1995) Interstitial radiosurgery of low-grade gliomas. *J Neurosurg* **82**: 418–429.

Lapras CI, Bognar L, Turjman F, Villanyi E, Mottolese C, Fischer C, Jouvet A, Guyotat J (1994) Tectal plate gliomas. *Acta Neurochir* **126**: 76–83.

Lewis J, Lucraft H, Gholkar A (1997) UKCCSG study of accelerated radiotherapy for pediatric brain stem gliomas. *Int J Radiat Oncol Biol Phys* **38**: 925–929.

May PL, Blaser SI, Hoffman HJ, Humphreys RP, Harwood-Nash DC (1992) Benign intrinsic tectal "tumors" in children. *J Neurosurg* **74**: 867–871.

Molloy PT, Bilaniuk LT, Vaughan SN, Needle MN, Liu GT, Zackai EH, Phillips PC (1995) Brainstem tumors in patients with neurofibromatosis type 1: a distinct clinical entity. *Neurology* **45**: 1897–1902.

Mulhern RK, Heideman RL, Khatib ZA, Kovnar EH, Sanford RA, Kun LE (1994) Quality of survival among children treated for brain stem glioma. *Pediatr Neurosurg* **20**: 226–232.

Mundinger F, Braus DF, Krauss JK, Birg W (1991) Long-term outcome of 89 low-grade brain-stem gliomas after interstitial radiation therapy. *J Neurosurg* **75**: 740–746.

Packer RJ, Boyett JM, Zimmerman RA, Albright AL, Kaplan AM, Rorke LB, Selch MT, Cherlow JM, Findlay JC, Wara WM (1994) Outcome of children with brain stem gliomas after treatment with 7800 cGy of hyperfractionated radiotherapy. *Cancer* **74**: 1827–1834.

Pendl G, Vorkapic P, Koniyama M (1990) Microsurgery of midbrain lesions. *Neurosurgery* **26**: 641–648.

Pierre-Kahn A, Hirsch J-F, Vinchon M, Payan C, Sainte-Rose C, Renier D, Lelouch-Tubiana A, Fermanian J (1993) Surgical management of brain-stem tumors in children: results and statistical analysis of 75 cases. *J Neurosurg* **79**: 845–852.

Pollack IF, Hoffman HJ, Humphreys RP, Becker L (1993) The long-term outcome after surgical treatment of dorsally exophytic brain-stem gliomas. *J Neurosurg* **78**: 859–863.

Pollack IF, Pang D, Albright AL (1994) The long-term outcome in children with late-onset aqueductal stenosis resulting from benign intrinsic tectal tumors. *J Neurosurg* **80**: 681–688.

Pollack IF, Shultz B, Mulvihill JJ (1996) The management of brainstem gliomas in patients with neurofibromatosis 1. *Neurology* **46**: 1652–1660.

Prados MD, Wara WM, Edwards MSB, Larson DA, Lamborn K, Levin VA (1995) The treatment of brain stem and thalamic gliomas with 78 Gy of hyperfractionated radiation therapy. *Int J Radiat Oncol Biol Phys* **32**: 85–91.

Robertson P, Muraszko KM, Brunberg JA, Axtell RA, Dauser RC, Turrisi AT (1995) Pediatric midbrain tumors: a benign subgroup of brainstem gliomas. *Pediatr Neurosurg* **22**: 65–73.

Stroink AR, Hoffman HJ, Hendrick EB, Humphreys RP (1986) Diagnosis and management of pediatric brain-stem gliomas. *J Neurosurg* **65**: 745–750.

Voges J, Sturm VV (1999) Interstitial irradiation with stereotactically implanted I-125 seeds for the treatment of cerebral glioma. *Crit Rev Neurosurg* **9**: 223–233.

Walker DA, Punt JAG, Sokal M (1999) Clinical management of brain stem glioma. *Arch Dis Child* **80**: 558–564.

Zagzag D, Miller DC, Knopp E, Farmer J-P, Lee M, Biria S, Pellicer A, Epstein FJ, Allen JC (2000) Primitive neuroectodermal tumors of the brainstem: investigation of seven cases. *Pediatrics* **106**: 1045–1053.

Zimmerman RA (1996) Neuroimaging of primary brainstem gliomas: diagnosis and course. *Pediatr Neurosurg* **25**: 45–53.

13
PRIMITIVE NEUROECTODERMAL TUMOURS

Stephen Lowis

Primitive neuroectodermal tumours (PNETs) are the most common malignant primary brain tumour of childhood, constituting 30–40% of such tumours, and affecting 0.5 per 100,000 children each year. The peak incidence is at the age of 7 years, although cases are reported up to late adult life. There is a slight male preponderance. The most common site is in the posterior fossa: tumours at this site are referred to as medulloblastoma or PNET-MB.

The WHO classification of brain tumours groups PNET and PNET-MB with other embryonal tumours, medulloepithelioma, ependymoma and atypical teratoid–rhabdoid tumour, although PNET-MB makes up the largest proportion of this group (Kleihues and Cavanee 2000). There is some evidence to suggest falling incidence of PNET-MB, and of increasing incidence of supratentorial PNET (Lannering et al. 1990, Thorne et al. 1994, Linet et al. 1999).

A predisposition to PNET-MB, and in particular the desmoplastic histological subtype, is seen in families affected with Gorlin syndrome, in which there is mutation of the PTCH gene. Mutation of PTCH is seen in approximately 8% of cases of sporadic PNET-MB, and loss of heterozygosity for the PTCH locus (9q22.3–q310) is reported in some PNET-MB.

Medulloblastoma is one of the diagnostic features of Gorlin syndrome (Schofield et al. 1995, Cowan et al. 1997, Kimonis et al. 1997), and approximately 5% of patients with Gorlin syndrome develop PNET-MB (Schofield et al. 1995, Cowan et al. 1997). Such patients will typically present around the age of 2 years, and it seems advisable that patients with Gorlin syndrome undergo regular developmental and neurological surveillance. There is no evidence at present that repeated neuroimaging is of value for such patients, and repeated CT examination is contraindicated, given the marked hypersensitivity of these patients to ionizing radiation.

Pathology
PNET is a highly malignant embryonal tumour of the CNS, with the capacity for differentiation along diverse pathways. The cell of origin is debated, but the precursor for a proportion may be the external granule cell layer of the cerebellum. Cells appear as undifferentiated round cells, but may mark with antibodies to synaptophysin, vimentin, GFAP, N-CAM, retinal S-antigen and p75NTR. The patterns of expression of genes such as SOX and ZIC in medulloblastoma is similar to that seen in granule cell precursors (Yokota et al. 1996, Lee et al. 2002).

The presence of desmoplasia is said to be associated with a more favourable prognosis than classical PNET, possibly because it is more lobulated and therefore more readily removed, although this is not in itself used to stratify therapy. Expression of p75NTR (the low-affinity NGF receptor) is seen in the external granule cell layer of fetal cerebellum, and is also significantly correlated with the desmoplatic subtype of medulloblastoma. Expression of p75NTR was also correlated with older age at presentation, and with tumours originating in the lateral cerebellar hemispheres in a series of 167 tumours, and has been taken as evidence for a distinct subtype derived from the external granule cell layer (Bühren et al. 2000).

Presentation

For all primary CNS tumours, clinical features relate to the site of the tumour. The majority of PNETs arise in the posterior fossa, involving the cerebellar vermis. Obstruction of the fourth ventricle or the aqueduct of Sylvius will give rise to obstructive hydrocephalus, and this may be the precipitant of admission. Symptoms and signs of acutely raised intracranial pressure (ICP) prompt urgent neurosurgical referral in a patient with symptoms of ataxia or headaches for several months.

Spread of posterior fossa PNET is by local invasion, to the cerebellar peduncle, floor of the fourth ventricle, and cervical spine. Occasionally, rostral extension is seen. Involvement of the brainstem may give rise to cranial nerve palsies. Diplopia or nystagmus may be attributable to raised ICP, cerebellar or cranial nerve involvement.

Spread of PNET-MB occurs to distant sites in approximately 15% of patients. Leptomeningeal deposits may be asymptomatic, but cord compression may lead to symptoms including pain and motor loss.

Supratentorial tumours may present with symptoms and signs of raised ICP, but may also cause epileptic convulsions. sPNET is often highly vascular, and haemorrhage may also lead to acute presentation. PNET may arise rarely within the spinal cord, and present with neurological symptoms (pain) and signs (loss of function). Metastatic spread may have occurred for any PNET at presentation, and leptomeningeal deposits may lead to similar signs (see Figs. 3.67, 3.68, pp. 84, 85).

Assessment and staging

A patient presenting with acutely raised ICP must be assessed rapidly and measures taken to reduce ICP immediately. Initial management of raised ICP should include administration of dexamethasone with or without mannitol prior to urgent CNS imaging. Management of the acute treatment of patients with raised ICP is discussed in Chapter 9.

Rapid assessment of hydrocephalus may be obtained by CT, and this may also allow imaging of the primary tumour. MRI, although indicated preoperatively, may require sedation or general anaesthesia, which may not be appropriate for all patients at presentation.

It may be felt appropriate to relieve obstructive hydrocephalus before proceeding to biopsy or resection. External ventricular drainage, third ventriculostomy or ventriculo-peritoneal shunting may allow this, and enable a planned resection to be performed when the patient has recovered neurologically.

246

TABLE 13.1
Chang classification of tumour and metastasis stage for medulloblastoma*

T stage

T1   Tumour <3cm in diameter and limited to the classic midline position in the vermis, the roof of the fourth ventricle, and less frequently to the cerebellar hemispheres

T2   Tumour >3cm and invading one adjacent structure or partially filling the fourth ventricle

T3a Tumour further invading two adjacent structures or completely filling the fourth ventricle with extension into the aqueduct of Sylvius, foramen of Magendie or foramen of Luschka, thus producing marked internal hydrocephalus

T3b Tumour arising from floor of the fourth ventricle and filling fourth ventricle

T4   Tumour spread throughout aqueduct of Sylvius to involve third ventricle and midbrain, or down into upper cervical cord

M stage

M0   No gross subarachnoid or haematogenous metastasis

M1   Microscopic tumour cells found in CSF

M2   Gross nodular seeding

M3   Gross nodular seeding in spinal subarachnoid space

M4   Extraneuraxial metastasis

*Chang et al. (1969).

All patients should have imaging of the spinal cord and whole brain by gadolinium enhanced MRI: the entire spine must be imaged in at least two planes. Preoperative assessment is preferred to postoperative, but an interval of no more than 72 hours after a first operation is generally agreed to be acceptable in the assessment of metastatic disease. Lumbar puncture has been shown to have a higher diagnostic value than ventricular CSF sampling, and an attempt to obtain lumbar CSF should be made before treatment commences. Both MRI and lumbar CSF should be used, as the use of either alone will miss approximately 15% of patients with metastatic disease (Fouladi et al. 1999). Initial tumour assessment is of importance in stratification of patients into standard or high-risk groups, for which outcome is significantly different. Leptomeningeal disease will be seen in 15–20% of children, and this significantly affects surgical approach, chemotherapy, radiotherapy and eventual outcome. The importance of early neuraxis imaging cannot be emphasized strongly enough.

MRI appearances of PNET are often of a solid, homogeneously enhancing mass, but there may be cystic or lobulated areas, and portions of the tumour may not enhance. Typical appearances of PNET are shown in Fig. 3.1 (p. 23).

Staging of PNET-MB is according to the Chang staging system (Table 13.1), which was initially developed in 1969, and includes both pre- and intraoperative findings. Tumour size and brainstem invasion are no longer prognostic. The identification of microscopic (M1) or nodular (M2–3) metastatic disease does identify high risk groups, but there is no difference in outcome for M2 or M3 disease. Extraneural metastasis (M4) is most uncommon. In contrast, postoperative residual disease significantly affects outcome, but is not part of the current Chang system. It is clear that a revised staging system is needed.

Prognostic factors

The prognosis for patients with unresected PNET is clearly significantly worse than for those

247

with complete or near-complete surgical clearance (Evans et al. 1990, Jenkin et al. 1990, Tait et al. 1990, Albright et al. 1996). A significantly better outcome with chemotherapy was seen in those patients with complete or near-complete resection, compared to those with gross macroscopic residual disease in the first SIOP study (Tait et al. 1990), and in general, an attempt at radical resection should always be made. Brainstem involvement has been reported to carry an adverse outcome, relating to the difficulty in attaining a complete surgical excision (Tait et al. 1990, Carrie et al. 1993, Chan et al. 2000).

Tumour dissemination has been known as a powerful adverse prognostic marker for many years, and this has been reported in numerous series (Geyer et al. 1991, Schofield et al. 1992, Zerbini et al. 1993, Bouffet et al. 1994, Albright et al. 1996, Miralbell et al. 1999, Zeltzer et al. 1999). In addition, a supratentorial tumour and younger age at diagnosis indicate a likely poor outcome (Packer et al. 1985, Evans et al. 1990).

Not all reported data for clinical studies separate sPNET from PNET-MB, but the prognosis for sPNET is significantly worse. In the CCG 921 study, which treated both sPNET and PNET-MB with craniospinal radiotherapy and chemotherapy with vincristine, CCNU and prednisone or '8 in 1' chemotherapy, progression-free survival (PFS) at 3 years was reported to be 45% for sPNET, compared with 54% at 5 years for PNET-MB (Albright et al. 1995, Zeltzer et al. 1999). In most current strategies, sPNET patients are regarded as having high-risk disease.

Treatment of children under the age of 3 years has for many tumours differed from that for older children, because of the perceived need to avoid radiotherapy. In the UKCCSG 'Baby Brain' protocol, the outcome with this strategy was extremely poor for PNET, with an event-free survival (EFS) at 2 years of only 4%. Young age has been reported to be associated with a worse outcome in several larger series (Albright et al. 1996, Zeltzer et al. 1999, Jenkin et al. 2000). Although lack or delay of radiation therapy is in part identified as a cause of adverse outcome, a greater proportion of patients may have spinal metastatic disease. These data are reviewed extensively by Saran et al. (1998).

There is now increasing recognition that biological characteristics influence outcome for patients with PNET. For example, the most common cytogenetic abnormality associated with PNET-MB is a deletion of chromosome 17p, seen in 40–50% of patients, and this has been reported to carry an adverse prognostic effect (Cogen 1991), although not in all series (Emadian et al. 1996, Biegel et al. 1997). The region most commonly deleted is 17p13.3, which includes the Hypermethylated in Cancer gene. The TP53 gene is located at 17p13.1, and this gene seems to be relatively infrequently mutated in PNET.

Gene amplification is also seen in PNET, and of those identified to date, Myc-C appears to be of greatest prognostic value (Herms et al. 2000). Amplification seems to be present more commonly in high-risk tumours: no survivors with Myc-C amplification were reported from four patients in the series of Badiali et al. (1991) and Batra et al. (1995).

In medulloblastoma cell lines in vitro, loss of caspase 8 expression correlates with increased cellular resistance to pro-apoptotic stimuli such as TRAIL, and both expression and sensitivity are restored by demethylation or pre-treatment with IFN gamma. Differential expression of genes is also of prognostic value in vivo. For example, high expression of Trk-C is seen more commonly in survivors of PNET-MB (Grotzer et al. 2000a,b). The pattern

248

of gene array expression for some genes such as PTCH, Myc-N, Gli-1 and IGF-2 may distinguish the desmoplastic variant of medulloblastoma (for which a better overall prognosis is expected) from other PNETs.

The importance of ErbB2 in both tumorigenesis and prognosis has been reported by Gilbertson and others, and is reviewed extensively in Chapter 5. ErbB2 is the central member of the class I receptor tyrosine kinase (RTK I) family. Dysregulation of both ErbB2 and ErbB4 is seen in medulloblastoma, and elevated levels of ErbB2 receptor expression were associated with reduced patient survival in a series of 55 patients treated by radiotherapy with or without chemotherapy (Gilbertson et al. 1995). In a series of 86 patients selected by availability of tissue, ErbB2 expression was associated with a 5 year overall survival of only 54%, compared to 100% without (Gajjar et al. 2004). The possibility of stratification of therapy based upon biological characteristics is close, and reducing the overall morbidity of this tumour appears to be an achievable goal.

Therapy

Initial therapy for PNET involves stabilization of the patient, which may require external ventricular drainage, and surgical resection. Complete surgical resection is a positive feature, but aggressive resection is not recommended where this would lead to increased morbidity. The first SIOP study did not identify residual disease as a prognostic factor (Tait et al. 1990), but in the CCG 921 study, postoperative residual $<1.5\,cm^3$ was predictive of improved PFS (Zeltzer et al. 1999). For supratentorial tumours, PFS was 40% for residual $<1.5\,cm^3$ vs 13% for $>1.5\,cm^3$, although this difference was not statistically significant because of small numbers. This has, however, become the appropriate cut off for neurosurgical resection wherever attainable.

Survival with surgery alone is unlikely, and radiation therapy has been standard for many years. Local and distant recurrence is seen, and the entire neuraxis is included in the radiation field. Conventional treatment involves craniospinal radiation (craniospinal radiotherapy, CSRT) to 36 Gy with a boost to the tumour bed to a total of 50–55 Gy. With this strategy, PFS of around 55–70% for children with standard risk MB can be anticipated at 5 years (Kun and Constine 1991, Packer et al. 1994).

Attempts to avoid radiotherapy completely in 'at risk' groups such as infants have been associated with poor outcomes, and hence postoperative craniospinal radiotherapy is almost always recommended.

CHEMOTHERAPY

The value of chemotherapy for patients with localized, completely resected disease was for many years uncertain. PNET is clearly able to respond to chemotherapy, and agents shown to have activity include alkylating drugs (CCNU, BCNU, cyclophosphamide, temozolomide), cisplatin and carboplatin. Combinations of chemotherapy agents used have included the so-called '8 in 1' (eight drugs administered in one day) regime, Vincristine and CCNU, and carboplatin and etoposide.

The SIOP first study (CCNU, vincristine) showed no benefit of chemotherapy for patients with localized disease, although a benefit for chemotherapy was seen for patients with partial or subtotal resection, brainstem involvement (p=0.001), and stage T3 and T4 disease (Tait et al. 1990).

In the second SIOP study, no benefit from pre-radiotherapy chemotherapy (with vincristine, procarbazine, and methotrexate given in a 6-week module) was seen for any group. In addition, a particularly poor outcome was seen for those children receiving chemotherapy and reduced dose radiotherapy (Bailey et al. 1995).

More recently, the results of the third SIOP study, PNET-3, have been reported (Taylor et al. 2003). PNET-3 ran between 1992 and 2000. Patients were randomized to receive immediate radiotherapy alone or 'sandwich chemotherapy' consisting of a 12-week regimen of four pulses of chemotherapy, followed by CSRT and a boost to the tumour bed. Despite poor recruitment to the randomization (n=179 patients with standard risk medulloblastoma) a significant difference in PFS was seen for patients treated by chemo- and radiotherapy (EFS of 78.7% and 73.4% at 3 and 5 years respectively) compared with radiotherapy alone (64.2% and 60.0%, p=0.04). Overall survival at 5 years was 76.1% for patients treated with chemo- and radiotherapy vs 66.5% for radiotherapy alone (p=0.17). For patients who had undergone a total resection, EFS was significantly better with chemo- plus radiotherapy than with radiotherapy alone (p=0.035).

The best series so far reported was from the CCG, who reported 5 year disease-free survival of 90% for 'good risk' patients treated with standard radiotherapy and a prolonged (48 week) course of chemotherapy with cisplatin, CCNU and vincristine (Packer et al. 1994). Only patients with no evidence of residual disease, or ambiguity regarding staging were included in this group, but clearly, such results indicate that progress can be made.

In poor-risk disease, chemotherapy also improves survival, and in recent years there has been increasing acceptance of chemotherapy for patients with metastatic disease. In the CCG-942 study comparing radiotherapy alone (craniospinal dose 35–40 Gy) with radiotherapy followed by chemotherapy (vincristine, CCNU and prednisolone), patients with high-stage disease who received chemotherapy had a PFS of 46% and an overall survival of 57% compared to a PFS of zero and overall survival of 19% in those treated with RT alone (Packer et al. 1985, Evans et al. 1990, Packer 1990).

CURRENT 'STANDARD' TREATMENT
The current recommended strategy in the United Kingdom for patients with 'standard risk' disease – those children over the age of 3 years with posterior fossa tumours without evidence of metastasis – is to offer surgical resection followed by CSRT and then the cisplatin/CCNU/vincristine regimen first described by Packer et al. (1988). For older children the recommended CSRT dose is 36 Gy, but in younger children it is increasingly preferred to use a dose of 23.4 Gy.

CHANGES IN TREATMENT STRATEGY
The adverse neurological sequelae of high-dose CSRT are potentially severe, and are a function of age at irradiation, total radiation dose, the site and extent of the radiation field (Silber et al. 1992, Mulhern et al. 1998). These effects are potentially profound, particularly in young children: children may be left with severe intellectual deficits, hearing loss and pituitary

deficiency, and attempts have been made to reduce overall radiation doses used (Packer et al. 1985, Deutsch et al. 1991, Bailey et al. 1995, Goldwein et al. 1996, Packer 1999).

Whilst some studies have found nonsignificant differences when patients received reduced dose radiotherapy, more generally, there is a trend towards increasing rates of relapse. A combined CCSG/POG study (POG 8631/CCG 923) of CSRT to a dose of 23.4 Gy vs 36 Gy (without chemotherapy) was halted prematurely because a statistically significant difference in early relapse of good prognosis patients (Deutsch et al. 1996). PFS rates for these patients were 67% with standard dose, and 52% with reduced dose radiotherapy (Thomas et al. 2000).

The second SIOP study concluded that reduction of radiation dose to 25 Gy with pre-radiotherapy chemotherapy should not be made (Bailey et al. 1995), but more encouraging results have been reported by others. Reduced dose radiotherapy with adjuvant chemotherapy may avoid an increased rate of relapse, and this has been the focus of recent strategies in the US and Europe. Packer reported a series of 65 patients treated with CSRT at 23.5 Gy, with a posterior fossa boost to 55.8 Gy. PFS at 5 years was 79%. This compares favourably with other series, and is significantly better than CSRT alone at a dose of 36 Gy (Packer et al. 1999). It is, however, less than that reported in the original group of patients, for whom a PFS of 90±6% was reported at 5 years in non-disseminated patients (Packer et al. 1994).

Goldwein and co-workers reported the results of a small study in children under 5 years with medulloblastoma, using "very low dose" CSRT (18 Gy), and a boost to the posterior fossa to 50.4–55.8 Gy (Goldwein et al. 1996, Packer 1999). Post-radiotherapy chemotherapy as reported by Packer was administered for 48 weeks. Only 10 patients were treated in this study, but 7 remained disease free at 6 years. Three relapses occurred outside the posterior fossa, and one patient developed simultaneous deposits within the boost irradiation field. Neuropsychological sequelae appeared to be minimal for most, although one survivor suffered a brainstem infarct. Although these findings are encouraging, further patients need to be treated at this dose level to identify whether a significant increase in relapse frequency will be seen.

HYPERFRACTIONATED RADIOTHERAPY (HFRT)

Hyperfractionation of radiotherapy – administration of twice daily therapy, each with a smaller radiation dose, but with a greater daily and cumulative dose – has been suggested as a way of reducing long term sequelae in young patients, while maintaining efficacy. Limited data exist to support this approach, but in theory the technique may offer the possibility of improvement in patients able to tolerate twice daily treatment (Allen et al. 1996, Prados et al. 1999). A pilot study has been reported from the Italian National Cancer Institute (Gandola et al. 2002), and a second pilot study in standard risk PNET-MB is in progress in SIOP. It seems likely that HFRT may offer some improvement in efficacy of radiotherapy given the reported poorer outcome for patients for whom radiotherapy is prolonged beyond the planned 6 week interval (del Charco et al. 1998). This concept has been developed further, and the current strategy for patients with supratentorial tumours in the UKCCSG study involves hyperfractionation and acceleration of radiotherapy, followed by chemotherapy with cisplatin, CCNU and vincristine.

It is clear that PNET is a chemosensitive tumour, and that chemotherapy contributes to the cure of a proportion of patients. It is also clear that for the majority of patients, radiotherapy is necessary for cure, but for infants and children under 3 years, the long-term sequelae may be considered unacceptable. Reports of IQ tests in children who received radiotherapy for brain tumours when less than 3 years of age indicate potentially profound loss. A dose effect was reported by Grill et al. (1999), with mean FSIQ scores of 84.5, 76.9 and 63.7 respectively for children receiving no craniospinal radiation (local, posterior fossa alone), and doses of 25 Gy and 35 Gy to the craniospinal axis. These results have been echoed by other authors (Duffner et al. 1983).

The management of very young children with PNET is not straightforward, and high dose, and high dose intensity, strategies have been adopted by some groups in an attempt to eliminate radiotherapy, or at least to reduce the overall radiation dose. In the UK, a strategy of high dose intensity chemotherapy with stem cell support, followed by local radiotherapy and maintenance chemotherapy has been adopted: preliminary data indicate a reasonable outcome for localized PNET-MB, but supratentorial or pineal tumours continue to fare badly (Dr A Michalski, personal communication 2004).

The role of high-dose therapy and autologous stem cell rescue is unproven, but limited evidence is available for such an approach. In the setting of the very young patient, high dose therapy may allow radiotherapy to be avoided, thereby potentially improving neuro-psychological outcome. A high response rate of medulloblastoma to high-dose cyclophos-phamide was reported by Allen and Helson (1981) (8/8 patients) and by Lachance et al. (1995) (8/9 patients). Studies of high-dose therapy with busulphan and thioTEPA, followed by local radiotherapy to the posterior fossa, has been reported to achieve cure for some patients, albeit with severe toxicity (Dupuis-Girod et al. 1996, 1997).

Supratentorial PNET

Despite the morphological and immunophenotypic similarity of supratentorial and pineal PNET to PNET-MB, the prognosis has been repeatedly shown to be worse (Zeltzer et al. 1999, Kortmann et al. 2000, Timmermann et al. 2002). Whether this is due to a reduced likelihood of complete surgical resection, or to differing biological characteristics, is unclear. For older children, the prognosis for pineal PNET is better than for sPNET although again the reasons for this are not clear (Cohen et al. 1995, Jakacki et al. 1995, Timmermann et al. 2002). In contrast, for infants, the prognosis for pineal PNET is bleak, with no survivors of 11 reported from the infant POG study (Duffner et al. 1995) or from a CCG study (Geyer et al. 1994).

Relapsed PNET

Recurrent PNET is rarely curable, and median survival is generally less than 1 year (Torres et al. 1994, Bouffet et al. 1998). In older patients who relapse after previous CSRT, further radiotherapy cannot be administered, except in small doses to palliate locally symptomatic disease. High-dose therapy may offer an alternative for some patients, although once again, severe toxicity is often reported. Combinations of chemotherapy including thioTEPA, etoposide and carboplatin, or BCNU (Dunkel et al. 1998, Guruangan et al. 1998), and busulphan plus thioTEPA (Dupuis-Girod et al. 1996, 1997) have provided durable remissions in such high-risk patients, although generally this is provided tumour remission can be achieved (Graham et al. 1997, Dunkel et al. 1998).

The majority of tumour recurrences occur at the primary site, and local disease control is dependent upon both surgical resection and the radiotherapy dose (Hughes et al. 1988, Tarbell et al. 1991). Extraneural dissemination is also seen, but seems to be decreased in patients receiving reduced dose craniospinal radiotherapy with chemotherapy. Despite the ability of medulloblastoma to seed intraspinally, there is little evidence of benefit, and indeed, significant risk of harm from myelopathy associated with intrathecal chemotherapy (Cohen et al. 1983, Watterson et al. 1993). Metastatic recurrence has a particularly poor prognosis.

REFERENCES

Albright AL, Wisoff JH, Zeltzer P, Boyett J, Rorke LB, Stanley P, Geyer JR, Milstein JM (1995) Prognostic factors in children with supratentorial (nonpineal) primitive neuroectodermal tumors. A neurosurgical perspective from the Children's Cancer Group. *Pediatr Neurosurg* **22**: 1–7.

Albright AL, Wisoff JH, Zeltzer PM, Boyett JM, Rorke LB, Stanley P (1996) Effects of medulloblastoma resections on outcome in children: a report from the Children's Cancer Group. *Neurosurgery* **38**: 265–271.

Allen JC, Donahue B, DaRosso R, Nirenberg A (1996) Hyperfractionated craniospinal radiotherapy and adjuvant chemotherapy for children with newly diagnosed medulloblastoma and other primitive neuro-ectodermal tumors. *Int J Radiat Oncol Biol Phys* **36**: 1155–1161.

Allen JC, Helson L (1981) High-dose cyclophosphamide chemotherapy for recurrent CNS tumors in children. *J Neurosurg* **55**: 749–756.

Badiali M, Pession A, Basso G, Andreini L, Rigobello L, Galassi E, Giangaspero F (1991) N-myc and c-myc oncogenes amplification in medulloblastomas. Evidence of particularly aggressive behavior of a tumor with c-myc amplification. *Tumori* **77**: 118–121.

Bailey CC, Gnekow A, Wellek S, Jones M, Round C, Brown J, Phillips A, Neidhardt MK (1995) Prospective randomised trial of chemotherapy given before radiotherapy in childhood medulloblastoma. International Society of Paediatric Oncology (SIOP) and the (German) Society of Paediatric Oncology (GPO): SIOP II. *Med Pediatr Oncol* **25**: 166–178.

Batra SK, McLendon RE, Koo JS, Castelino-Prabhu S, Fuchs HE, Krischer JP, Friedman HS, Bigner DD, Bigner SH (1995) Prognostic implications of chromosome 17p deletions in human medulloblastomas. *J Neurooncol* **24**: 39–45.

Biegel JA, Janss AJ, Raffel C, Sutton L, Rorke LB, Harper JM, Phillips PC (1997) Prognostic significance of chromosome 17p deletions in childhood primitive neuroectodermal tumors (medulloblastomas) of the central nervous system. *Clin Cancer Res* **3**: 473–478.

Bouffet E, Gentet JC, Doz F, Tron P, Roche H, Plantaz D, Thyss A, Stephan JL, Lasset C, Carrie C, et al. (1994) Metastatic medulloblastoma: the experience of the French Cooperative M7 Group. *Eur J Cancer* **10**: 1478–1483.

Bouffet E, Doz F, Demaille MC, Tron P, Roche H, Plantaz D, Thyss A, Stephan JL, Lejars O, Sariban E, Buclon M, Zucker JM, Brunat-Mentigny M, Bernard JL, Gentet JC (1998) Improving survival in recurrent medulloblastoma: earlier detection, better treatment or still an impasse? *Br J Cancer* **77**: 1321–1326.

Buhren J, Christoph AH, Buslei R, Albrecht S, Wiestler OD, Pietsch T (2000) Expression of the neurotrophin receptor p75NTR in medulloblastomas is correlated with distinct histological and clinical features: evidence for a medulloblastoma subtype derived from the external granule layer. *J Neuropath Exp Neurol* **59**: 229–240.

Carrie C, Lasset C, Blay JY, Negrier S, Bouffet E, Barbet N, Montbarbon X, Wagner JP, Lapras C, Deruty R, et al. (1993) Medulloblastoma in adults: survival and prognostic factors. *Radiother Oncol* **29**: 301–307.

Chan AW, Tarbell NJ, Black PM, Louis DN, Frosch MP, Ancukiewicz M, Chapman P, Loeffler JS (2000) Adult medulloblastoma: prognostic factors and patterns of relapse. *Neurosurgery* **47**: 623–631; discussion 631–632.

Chang CH, Housepian EM, Herbert C (1969) An operative staging system and a megavoltage radiotherapeutic technic for cerebellar medulloblastomas. *Radiology* **93**: 1351–1359.

Cogen PH (1991) Prognostic significance of molecular genetic markers in childhood brain tumors. *Pediatr Neurosurg* **17**: 245–250.

Cohen BH, Zeltzer PM, Boyett JM, Geyer JR, Allen JC, Finlay JL, McGuire-Cullen P, Milstein JM, Rorke LB, Stanley P, et al. (1995) Prognostic factors and treatment results for supratentorial primitive neuro-ectodermal tumors in children using radiation and chemotherapy: a Children's Cancer Group randomized trial. *J Clin Oncol* **13**: 1687–1696.

Cohen ME, Duffner PK, Terplan KL (1983) Myelopathy with severe structural derangement associated with combined modality therapy. *Cancer* **52**: 1590–1596.

Cowan R, Hoban P, Kelsey A, Birch JM, Gattamaneni R, Evans DG (1997) The gene for the naevoid basal cell carcinoma syndrome acts as a tumour-suppressor gene in medulloblastoma. *Br J Cancer* **76**: 141–145.

del Charco JO, Bolek TW, McCollough WM, Maria BL, Kedar A, Braylan RC, Mickle JP, Buatti JM, Mendenhall NP, Marcus RB (1998) Medulloblastoma: time–dose relationship based on a 30-year review. *Int J Radiat Oncol Biol Phys* **42**: 147–154.

Deutsch M, Thomas P, Boyett J, Krischer JP, Finlay J, Kun L (1991) Low stage medulloblastoma: a Children's Cancer Study Group (CCSG) and Pediatric Oncology Group (POG) randomized study of standard vs reduced neuraxis radiation. *Proc Am Soc Clin Oncol* **10**: A363 (abstract).

Deutsch M, Thomas PR, Krischer J, Boyett JM, Albright L, Aronin P, Langston J, Allen JC, Packer RJ, Linggood R, Mulhern R, Stanley P, Stehbens JA, Duffner P, Kun L, Rorke L, Cherlow J, Freidman H, Finlay JL, Vietti T (1996) Results of a prospective randomized trial comparing standard dose neuraxis irradiation (3,600 cGy/20) with reduced neuraxis irradiation (2,340 cGy/13) in patients with low-stage medulloblastoma. A Combined Children's Cancer Group–Pediatric Oncology Group Study. *Pediatr Neurosurg* **24**: 167–176; discussion 176–177.

Duffner PK, Cohen ME, Thomas P (1983) Late effects of treatment on the intelligence of children with posterior fossa tumors. *Cancer* **51**: 233–237.

Duffner PK, Cohen ME, Sanford RA, Horowitz ME, Krischer JP, Burger PC, Friedman HS, Kun LE (1995) Lack of efficacy of postoperative chemotherapy and delayed radiation in very young children with pineoblastoma. Pediatric Oncology Group. *Med Pediatr Oncol* **25**: 38–44.

Dunkel IJ, Boyett JM, Yates A, Rosenblum M, Garvin JH, Bostrom BC, Goldman S, Sender LS, Gardner SL, Li H, Allen JC, Finlay JL (1998) High-dose carboplatin, thiotepa, and etoposide with autologous stem-cell rescue for patients with recurrent medulloblastoma. Children's Cancer Group. *J Clin Oncol* **16**: 222–228.

Dupuis-Girod S, Hartmann O, Benhamou E, Doz F, Mechinaud F, Bouffet E, Coze C, Kalifa C (1996) Will high dose chemotherapy followed by autologous bone marrow transplantation supplant cranio-spinal irradiation in young children treated for medulloblastoma? *J Neurooncol* **27**: 87–98.

Dupuis-Girod S, Hartmann O, Benhamou E, Doz F, Mechinaud F, Bouffet E, Coze C, Kalifa C (1997) [High-dose chemotherapy in relapse of medulloblastoma in young children]. *Bull Cancer* **84**: 264–272 (in French).

Emadian SM, McDonald JD, Gerken SC, Fults D (1996) Correlation of chromosome 17p loss with clinical outcome in medulloblastoma. *Clin Cancer Res* **2**: 1559–1564.

Evans AE, Jenkin RD, Sposto R, Ortega JA, Wilson CB, Wara W, Ertel IJ, Kramer S, Chang CH, Leikin SL, et al. (1990) The treatment of medulloblastoma. Results of a prospective randomized trial of radiation therapy with and without CCNU, vincristine, and prednisone. *J Neurosurg* **72**: 572–582.

Fouladi M, Gajjar A, Boyett JM, Walter AW, Thompson SJ, Merchant TE, Jenkins JJ, Langston JW, Liu A, Kun LE, Heideman RL (1999) Comparison of CSF cytology and spinal magnetic resonance imaging in the detection of leptomeningeal disease in pediatric medulloblastoma or primitive neuroectodermal tumor. *J Clin Oncol* **17**: 3234–3237.

Gajjar A, Hernan R, Kocak M, Fuller C, Lee Y, McKinnon PJ, Wallace D, Lau C, Chintagumpala M, Ashley DM, Kellie SJ, Kun L, Gilbertson RJ (2004) Clinical, histopathologic, and molecular markers of prognosis: toward a new disease risk stratification system for medulloblastoma. *J Clin Oncol* **22**: 971–974.

Gandola L, Cefalo G, Massimino M, Navarria P, Spreafico F, Pignoli E, Luksch R, Giombini S, Poggi G, Ferrari A, Casanova M, Polastri D, Terenziani M, Fossati-Bellani F (2002) Hyperfractionated accelerated radiotherapy (HART) after intensive postoperative sequential chemotherapy for metastatic medulloblastoma. *Med Pediatr Oncol* **39**: 248 (O115).

Geyer JR, Zeltzer PM, Boyett JM, Rorke LB, Stanley P, Albright AL, Wisoff JH, Milstein JM, Allen JC,

Finlay JL, et al. (1994) Survival of infants with primitive neuroectodermal tumors or malignant ependy-momas of the CNS treated with eight drugs in 1 day: a report from the Children's Cancer Group. *J Clin Oncol* **12**: 1607–1615.

Geyer R, Levy M, Berger MS, Milstein J, Griffin B, Bleyer WA (1991) Infants with medulloblastoma: a single institution review of survival. *Neurosurgery* **29**: 707–710; discussion 710–711.

Gilbertson RJ, Pearson AD, Perry RH, Jaros E, Kelly PJ (1995) Prognostic significance of the c-erbB-2 oncogene product in childhood medulloblastoma. *Br J Cancer* **71**: 473–477.

Goldwein JW, Radcliffe J, Johnson J, Moshang T, Packer RJ, Sutton LN, Rorke LB, D'Angio GJ (1996) Updated results of a pilot study of low dose craniospinal irradiation plus chemotherapy for children under five with cerebellar primitive neuroectodermal tumors (medulloblastoma). *Int J Radiat Oncol Biol Phys* **34**: 899–904.

Graham ML, Herndon JE, Casey JR, Chaffee S, Ciocci GH, Krischer JP, Kurtzberg J, Laughlin MJ, Longee DC, Olson JF, Paleologus N, Pennington CN, Friedman HS (1997) High-dose chemotherapy with autologous stem-cell rescue in patients with recurrent and high-risk pediatric brain tumors. *J Clin Oncol* **15**: 1814–1823.

Grill J, Renaux VK, Bulteau C, Viguier D, Levy-Piebois C, Sainte-Rose C, Dellatolas G, Raquin MA, Jambaque I, Kalifa C (1999) Long-term intellectual outcome in children with posterior fossa tumors according to radiation doses and volumes. *Int J Radiat Oncol Biol Phys* **45**: 137–145.

Grotzer MA, Janss AJ, Fung K, Biegel JA, Sutton LN, Rorke LB, Zhao H, Cnaan A, Phillips PC, Lee VM, Trojanowski JQ (2000a) TrkC expression predicts good clinical outcome in primitive neuroectodermal brain tumors. *J Clin Oncol* **18**: 1027–1035.

Grotzer, MA, Janss, AJ, Phillips, PC and Trojanowski, JQ (2000b) Neurotrophin receptor TrkC predicts good clinical outcome in medulloblastoma and other primitive neuroectodermal brain tumors. *Klin Pädiatr* **212**: 196–199.

Guruangan S, Dunkel IJ, Goldman S, Garvin JH, Rosenblum M, Boyett JM, Gardner S, Merchant TE, Gollamudi S, Finlay JL (1998) Myeloablative chemotherapy with autologous bone marrow rescue in young children with recurrent malignant brain tumors. *J Clin Oncol* **16**: 2486–2493.

Herms J, Neidt I, Luscher B, Sommer A, Schurmann P, Schroder T, Bergmann M, Wilken B, Probst-Cousin S, Hernaiz-Driever P, Behnke J, Hanefeld F, Pietsch T, Kretzschmar HA (2000) C-MYC expression in medulloblastoma and its prognostic value. *Int J Cancer* **89**: 395–402.

Hughes EN, Shillito J, Sallan SE, Loeffler JS, Cassady JR, Tarbell NJ (1988) Medulloblastoma at the joint center for radiation therapy between 1968 and 1984. The influence of radiation dose on the patterns of failure and survival. *Cancer* **61**: 1992–1998.

Jakacki RI, Zeltzer PM, Boyett JM, Albright AL, Allen JC, Geyer JR, Rorke LB, Stanley P, Stevens KR, Wisoff J, et al. (1995) Survival and prognostic factors following radiation and/or chemotherapy for primitive neuroectodermal tumors of the pineal region in infants and children: a report of the Children's Cancer Group. *J Clin Oncol* **13**: 1377–1383.

Jenkin D, Goddard K, Armstrong D, Becker L, Berry M, Chan H, Doherty M, Greenberg M, Hendrick B, Hoffman H, et al. (1990) Posterior fossa medulloblastoma in childhood: treatment results and a proposal for a new staging system. *Int J Radiat Oncol Biol Phys* **19**: 265–274.

Jenkin D, Shabanah MA, Shail EA, Gray A, Hassounah M, Khafaga Y, Kofide A, Mustafa M, Schultz H (2000) Prognostic factors for medulloblastoma. *Int J Radiat Oncol Biol Phys* **47**: 573–584.

Kimonis VE, Goldstein AM, Pastakia B, Yang ML, Kase R, DiGiovanna JJ, Bale AE, Bale SJ (1997) Clinical manifestations in 105 persons with nevoid basal cell carcinoma syndrome. *Am J Med Genet* **69**: 299–308.

Kleihues P, Cavanee WP (2000) *Pathology and Genetics of Tumors of the Central Nervous System*. World Health Organization Classification of Tumours. Lyon: IARC Press.

Kortmann RD, Kuhl J, Timmermann B, Mittler U, Urban C, Budach V, Richter E, Willich N, Flentje M, Berthold F, Slavc I, Wolff J, Meisner C, Wiestler O, Sorensen N, Warmuth-Metz M, Bamberg M (2000) Postoperative neoadjuvant chemotherapy before radiotherapy as compared to immediate radiotherapy followed by maintenance chemotherapy in the treatment of medulloblastoma in childhood: results of the German prospective randomized trial HIT '91. *Int J Radiat Oncol Biol Phys* **46**: 269–279.

Kun LE, Constine LS (1991) Medulloblastoma—caution regarding new treatment approaches. *Int J Radiat Oncol Biol Phys* **20**: 897–899.

Lachance DH, Oette D, Schold SC Jr, Brown M, Kurtzberg J, Graham ML, Tien R, Felsberg G, Colvin OM, Moghrabi A, et al. (1995) Dose escalation trial of cyclophosphamide with Sargramostim in the treatment of central nervous system (CNS) neoplasms. *Med Pediatr Oncol* **24**: 241–247.

Lannering B, Marky I, Nordborg C (1990) Brain tumors in childhood and adolescence in west Sweden 1970–1984. Epidemiology and survival. *Cancer* **66**: 604–609.

Lee CJ, Appleby VJ, Orme AT, Chan WI, Scotting PJ (2002) Differential expression of SOX4 and SOX11 in medulloblastoma. *J Neurooncol* **57**: 201–214.

Linet MS, Ries LA, Smith MA, Tarone RE, Devesa SS (1999) Cancer surveillance series: recent trends in childhood cancer incidence and mortality in the United States. *J Natl Cancer Inst* **91**: 1051–1058.

Miralbell R, Bieri S, Huguenin P, Feldges A, Morin AM, Garcia E, Wagner HP, Wacker P, von der Weid N (1999) Prognostic value of cerebrospinal fluid cytology in pediatric medulloblastoma. Swiss Pediatric Oncology Group. *Ann Oncol* **10**: 239–241.

Mulhern RK, Kepner JL, Thomas PR, Armstrong FD, Friedman HS, Kun LE (1998) Neuropsychologic functioning of survivors of childhood medulloblastoma randomized to receive conventional or reduced-dose craniospinal irradiation: a Pediatric Oncology Group study. *J Clin Oncol* **16**: 1723–1728.

Packer RJ (1990) Chemotherapy for medulloblastoma/primitive neuroectodermal tumors of the posterior fossa. *Ann Neurol* **28**: 823–828.

Packer RJ (1999) Childhood medulloblastoma: progress and future challenges. *Brain Dev* **21**: 75–81.

Packer RJ, Sutton LN, D'Angio G, Evans AE, Schut L (1985) Management of children with primitive neuroectodermal tumors of the posterior fossa/medulloblastoma. *Pediatr Neurosci* **12**: 272–282.

Packer RJ, Siegel KR, Sutton LN, Evans AE, D'Angio G, Rorke LB, Bunin GR, Schut L (1988) Efficacy of adjuvant chemotherapy for patients with poor-risk medulloblastoma: a preliminary report. *Ann Neurol* **24**: 503–508.

Packer RJ, Sutton LN, Elterman R, Lange B, Goldwein J, Nicholson HS, Mulne L, Boyett J, D'Angio G, Wechsler-Jentzsch K, et al. (1994) Outcome for children with medulloblastoma treated with radiation and cisplatin, CCNU, and vincristine chemotherapy. *J Neurosurg* **81**: 690–698.

Packer RJ, Goldwein J, Nicholson HS, Vezina LG, Allen JC, Ris MD, Muraszko K, Rorke LB, Wara WM, Cohen BH, Boyett JM (1999) Treatment of children with medulloblastomas with reduced-dose craniospinal radiation therapy and adjuvant chemotherapy: A Children's Cancer Group Study. *J Clin Oncol* **17**: 2127–2136.

Prados MD, Edwards MS, Chang SM, Russo C, Davis R, Rabbitt J, Page M, Lamborn K, Wara WM (1999) Hyperfractionated craniospinal radiation therapy for primitive neuroectodermal tumors: results of a Phase II study. *Int J Radiat Oncol Biol Phys* **43**: 279–285.

Saran FH, Driever PH, Thilmann C, Mose S, Wilson P, Sharpe G, Adamietz IA, Bottcher HD (1998) Survival of very young children with medulloblastoma (primitive neuroectodermal tumor of the posterior fossa) treated with craniospinal irradiation. *Int J Radiat Oncol Biol Phys* **42**: 959–967.

Schofield D, West DC, Anthony DC, Marshal R, Sklar J (1995) Correlation of loss of heterozygosity at chromosome 9q with histological subtype in medulloblastomas. *Am J Pathol* **146**: 472–480.

Schofield DE, Yunis EJ, Geyer JR, Albright AL, Berger MS, Taylor SR (1992) DNA content and other prognostic features in childhood medulloblastoma. Proposal of a scoring system. *Cancer* **69**: 1307–1314.

Silber JH, Radcliffe J, Peckham V, Perilongo G, Kishnani P, Fridman M, Goldwein JW, Meadows AT (1992) Whole-brain irradiation and decline in intelligence: the influence of dose and age on IQ score. *J Clin Oncol* **10**: 1390–1396.

Tait DM, Thornton-Jones H, Bloom HJ, Lemerle J, Morris-Jones P (1990) Adjuvant chemotherapy for medulloblastoma: the first multi-centre control trial of the International Society of Paediatric Oncology (SIOP I). *Eur J Cancer* **26**: 464–469.

Tarbell NJ, Loeffler JS, Silver B, Lynch E, Lavally BL, Kupsky WJ, Scott RM, Sallan SE (1991) The change in patterns of relapse in medulloblastoma. *Cancer* **68**: 1600–1604.

Taylor RE, Bailey CC, Robinson K, Weston CL, Ellison D, Ironside J, Lucraft H, Gilbertson R, Tait DM, Walker DA, Pizer BL, Imeson J, Lashford LS; International Society of Paediatric Oncology; United Kingdom Children's Cancer Study Group (2003) Results of a randomized study of preradiation chemotherapy versus radiotherapy alone for nonmetastatic medulloblastoma: The International Society of Paediatric Oncology/United Kingdom Children's Cancer Study Group PNET-3 Study. *J Clin Oncol* **21**: 1581–1591.

Thomas PR, Deutsch M, Kepner JL, Boyett JM, Krischer J, Aronin P, Albright L, Allen JC, Packer RJ, Linggood R, Mulhern R, Stehbens JA, Langston J, Stanley P, Duffner P, Rorke L, Cherlow J, Friedman HS, Finlay JL, Vietti TJ, Kun LE (2000) Low-stage medulloblastoma: final analysis of trial comparing standard-dose with reduced-dose neuraxis irradiation. *J Clin Oncol* **18**: 3004–3011.

Thorne RN, Pearson AD, Nicoll JA, Coakham HB, Oakhill A, Mott MG, Foreman NK (1994) Decline in incidence of medulloblastoma in children. *Cancer* **74**: 3240–3244.

Thorne RN, Pearson AD, Nicoll JA, Coakham HB, Oakhill A, Mott MG, Foreman NK (2002) Role of radiotherapy in the treatment of supratentorial primitive neuroectodermal tumors in childhood: results of the prospective German brain tumor trials HIT 88/89 and 91. *J Clin Oncol* **20**: 842–849.

Torres CF, Rebsamen S, Silber JH, Sutton LN, Bilaniuk LT, Zimmerman RA, Goldwein JW, Phillips PC, Lange BJ (1994) Surveillance scanning of children with medulloblastoma. *N Engl J Med* **330**: 892–895.

Watterson J, Simonton SC, Rorke LB, Packer RJ, Kim TH, Spiegel RH, Priest JR (1993) Fatal brain stem necrosis after standard posterior fossa radiation and aggressive chemotherapy for metastatic medulloblastoma. *Cancer* **71**: 4111–4117.

Yokota N, Aruga J, Takai S, Yamada K, Hamazaki M, Iwase T, Sugimura H, Mikoshiba K (1996) Predominant expression of human zic in cerebellar granule cell lineage and medulloblastoma. *Cancer Res* **56**: 377–383.

Zeltzer PM, Boyett JM, Finlay JL, Albright AL, Rorke LB, Milstein JM, Allen JC, Stevens KR, Stanley P, Li H, Wisoff JH, Geyer JR, McGuire-Cullen P, Stehbens JA, Shurin SB, Packer RJ (1999) Metastasis stage, adjuvant treatment, and residual tumor are prognostic factors for medulloblastoma in children: conclusions from the Children's Cancer Group 921 randomized phase III study. *J Clin Oncol* **17**: 832–845.

Zerbini C, Gelber RD, Weinberg D, Sallan SE, Barnes P, Kupsky W, Scott RM, Tarbell NJ (1993) Prognostic factors in medulloblastoma, including DNA ploidy. *J Clin Oncol* **11**: 616–622.

14
INTRACRANIAL GERM CELL TUMOURS

Susanne J Rogers and Frank H Saran

Tumours of the central nervous system (CNS) are highly heterogeneous with regard to pathology and prognosis. A rare subtype is the primary intracranial germ cell tumour (GCT). In America and Europe, intracranial GCTs represent approximately 3% of paediatric brain tumours (Fuller et al. 1994). Between 1972 and 1993, 125 cases of intracranial GCT were recorded in the United Kingdom population under 15 years of age (Kiltie and Gattamaneni 1995). In Japan and Taiwan the incidence can be as high as 9–15% (Jennings et al. 1985). These tumours occur in infancy through to adolescence with predominance in the second decade, and only 10% of cases are diagnosed after the age of 20. Analyses of large histopathological series have shown a predilection for midline structures, namely the pineal gland (50–60%) and suprasellar location (30–40%) (Jennings et al. 1985). Rarely the basal ganglia and non-midline structures are involved (Wong 1995). In 15–20% of cases, concurrent, non-metastatic pineal and either suprasellar, cavernous sinus, optic chiasm or wall of third ventricle lesions are detected. These are termed bifocal or multiple midline GCTs (Sawamura et al. 1998). Approximately 5–10% of patients present with metastatic spread in the cerebrospinal fluid (CSF) at diagnosis.

Aetiology

The germ cells giving rise to these tumours are thought to be primordial germ cells from the yolk sac endoderm that become misplaced on their migration to the gonadal folds and survive immune surveillance by acquiring neoplastic properties (Takei and Pearl 1981). If these cells do not differentiate they give rise to germinomas, but if further differentiation occurs, non-germinomas develop (Fig. 14.1). This germ cell theory remains controversial, as the least differentiated germinomas have an excellent outcome following treatment, while the more differentiated tumours have a poorer prognosis. This phenomenon counters oncological experience in other cancers (Sano 1995). Some authors believe that choriocarcinoma is the least differentiated tumour as it arises from trophoblastic tissue, with germinoma being the most highly differentiated as it arises from embryonic primordial cells (Diez et al. 1999). These debates reflect persisting uncertainties regarding the nature of the cells of origin and their place in embryogenesis and tumour pathogenesis.

An excess of CNS GCT occurs in patients with Klinefelter syndrome, which is associated with high levels of gonadotrophins (Arens et al. 1988). Along with the increased incidence in peripubertal patients and the site of origin near the diencephalic nuclei regulating gonadotrophin activity, this association has formed the basis for a link to gonadotrophins (Jennings et al. 1985). The presence of a characteristic lymphocytic infiltrate in germinomas has led

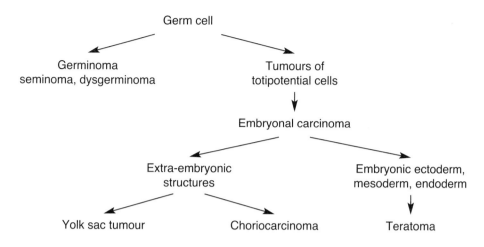

Fig. 14.1. The germ cell theory (modified from Sano et al. 1989).

to speculation that geographical variation in incidence between East and West may parallel a difference in viral infection rates, e.g. human T-cell lymphocytic virus (HTLV).

Few data are available regarding critical genetic mutations in the pathogenesis of intracranial GCTs. Speculation regarding a genetic link has arisen due to case reports of CNS GCTs occurring in children with Down syndrome (Hashimoto et al. 1995) and siblings (Wakai et al. 1980). Cytogenetic studies have repeatedly demonstrated abnormalities of chromosomes 1 and 12 that mirror the changes seen in extracranial germ cell tumours (Chaganti et al. 1993). Very rarely, patients with intracranial GCTs have been reported to subsequently develop gonadal germ cell tumours, perhaps indicating an as yet unidentified genetic predisposition (Hashimoto et al. 1992, Watanabe et al. 1995).

Clinical presentation
Presenting signs and symptoms depend on the neuroanatomical site of disease and patient-specific factors such as the developmental and biological age of the child or adolescent.

PINEAL TUMOURS
The classical presentation of a pineal tumour involving the tectal plate is Parinaud syndrome. The defining features are failure of upward gaze, headache and abnormal pupil responses (impaired constriction to light with preservation of accommodation). The location of the pineal gland in the floor of the third ventricle frequently leads to compression of the adjacent sylvian aqueduct resulting in obstructive hydrocephalus. The clinical manifestations of raised intracranial pressure (ICP) range from nonspecific, non-localizing signs and symptoms to the classical triad of morning headache with associated vomiting and papilloedema.

SUPRASELLAR TUMOURS
Whereas pineal tumours tend to present more commonly in adolescent males, suprasellar

lesions, particularly germinomas, present in the first two decades of life with equal sex incidence. Patients commonly present with obstructive hydrocephalus and/or endocrine deficits. The latter can develop over a prolonged period, starting with the development of diabetes insipidus. Over time, this will progress to the full clinical picture of panhypo-pituitarism, and at some stage a suprasellar or pituitary stalk mass lesion will be detectable on imaging. The proximity of the tumour to the optic chiasm gives rise to visual field defects or loss of visual acuity. Precocious puberty or delayed sexual development, anorexia or weight gain, somnolence, mood swings and failure to thrive are seen less frequently as manifestations of hypothalamic damage. If the primary tumour arises in an atypical location such as the basal ganglia, hemiparesis, ocular palsies, speech disturbance and hemi-anopia may be the first presentation.

Diagnosis and staging

RADIOLOGY

When a primary CNS tumour or raised ICP is suspected, computerized tomography (CT) is frequently the first radiological investigation performed. Magnetic resonance imaging (MRI) with intravenous contrast enhancement represents the gold standard in this setting. The multiplanar images allow better evaluation of the tumour extent and its relationship with normal tissues.

The ability of intracranial GCTs to disseminate via the CSF pathways makes it imperative to obtain MRI images of both the brain and spine for staging purposes. This is to exclude macroscopic intraventricular, leptomeningeal and spinal seeding that may not be demonstrated on the initial CT scan. With the exception of teratomas, the neuroradiological appearance of GCTs on MRI is of iso- or hyperdense solid masses that enhance brightly with contrast medium. Germinomas show the characteristic features of a well-defined homogeneous mass and may demonstrate subependymal spread around the ventricles. The mixed density of non-germinomas facilitates differentiation from optic chiasm gliomas at a suprasellar location. Teratomas typically contain both low-density regions, representing fat and cysts, and high-density calcified areas. The radiological appearance, in conjunction with the clinical symptoms and the age of the patient, can strongly suggest a diagnosis of CNS GCT and guide the clinician with respect to further staging investigations required prior to any neurosurgical intervention.

Post-therapy, some enhancement tends to persist, predominantly in the region of the pineal gland; this is not considered to be evidence of residual tumour if there is no concomitant mass lesion.

CYTOLOGY AND TUMOUR MARKERS

If clinically and/or radiologically a primary CNS GCT is part of the differential diagnosis, serum tumour marker levels (AFP, ß-HCG) should be obtained. Examination of the CSF should be performed in all patients, to confirm or refute microscopic tumour dissemination and establish the presence or absence of tumour marker expression in the CSF. A lumbar puncture should be performed at diagnosis if the ventricles are not obstructed. If there is raised ICP and urgent surgery is required, ventricular CSF can be analysed intraoperatively.

TABLE 14.1
Secretion of tumour markers by histological subtype

Tumour marker	Histological subtype				
	Germinoma	Teratoma	Yolk sac tumour	Chorio-carcinoma	Embryonal carcinoma
ß-HCG	+/–	–	–	+++	+/–
AFP	–	–	+++	–	+/–

Alternatively a lumbar puncture should be performed within 1–2 days of surgery for assessment of tumour markers, as the half-life of ß-HCG is only 5 days after macroscopic complete or near-complete resection. To complete staging, CSF analysis for cytology should be performed 14 days after surgical intervention to avoid false positive results. In germinomas, M1 (CSF positive) disease is a risk factor for spinal seeding; however, it does not predict recurrence (Brada and Rajan 1990).

CSF analysis is also a prerequisite in the differentiation of secreting and non-secreting GCTs (Table 14.1). CSF tumour marker levels are mandatory, as they may be elevated in isolation thus establishing the diagnosis of a secreting GCT and subsequently defining the appropriate management strategy, particularly if initially serum markers are negative. In the presence of a typical clinical presentation, neuroimaging and positive tumour markers in either serum or CSF, it is currently accepted practice that therapy commences without histopathological verification (Nicholson et al. 2002). In all tumour types, serum and CSF tumour marker levels (AFP, ß-HCG) and CSF cytology must be documented as a baseline prior to therapy to enable the clinician to assess response to treatment and follow-up.

TISSUE DIAGNOSIS

If a CNS GCT is suspected and tumour marker assays do not yield a diagnosis of a secreting intracranial GCT, histopathological verification is required. Initial concerns regarding tumour seeding secondary to tumour biopsy have not been substantiated (Rao et al. 1981). The differential diagnosis of a pineal mass includes pinealoblastoma, pineocytoma, glioma and benign cysts. At a suprasellar location, the possible differential diagnosis includes predominantly optic chiasm and hypothalamic gliomas and craniopharyngioma. The standard diagnostic neurosurgical procedure is an open biopsy of the mass lesion. There is, however, increasing use of less invasive techniques such as stereotactic and endoscopic biopsy. Modern neurosurgical techniques using a stereotactic approach are deemed safe and mortality is in the region of 0.5% in experienced hands (Sawamura et al. 1997). The advantages of less morbid approaches must be balanced against the potential for sampling error as GCTs can be mixed in approximately 30% of cases (Weiner and Finlay 1999).

Histological subtypes

The main distinctions to be made are between localized and metastatic disease and between secreting and non-secreting intracranial GCTs, as these two factors determine the management strategy. Histological category is the single most important prognostic factor for outcome,

TABLE 14.2
Histological classification of germ cell tumours*

Germinomas	Pure
	ß-HCG producing
Teratomas	Mature
	Immature
	Mixed with germinoma
GCT with a highly malignant component	Teratoma with malignant transformation
	Choriocarcinoma
	Embryonal carcinoma mixed with immature tumour
	Yolk sac tumour

*Rosenblum and Ng (1997).

TABLE 14.3
Therapeutic categorization of intracranial germ cell tumours*

Good risk	Pure germinoma
	Mature teratoma
Intermediate risk	Germinoma with raised ß-HCG
	Extensive (>4 cm) or multifocal germinoma
	Immature teratoma
	Germinoma ± mature or immature teratoma
Poor risk	Teratoma with malignant transformation
	Embryonal carcinoma
	Yolk sac tumour
	Choriocarcinoma
	Mixed germ cell tumour with elements of embryonal carcinoma, yolk sac tumour, choriocarcinoma or teratoma with malignant transformation

*Matsutani et al. (1997).

as the natural history and treatment of the two histopathological subtypes are quite distinct (Matsutani et al. 1997). Table 14.2 shows the WHO classification according to histological subtype, and Table 14.3 stratifies tumour type by risk level.

GERMINOMA

Extragonadal GCTs are histologically identical to their gonadal counterparts but whereas a non-secreting testicular GCT is referred to as a seminoma, and an ovarian primary as a dysgerminoma, in the CNS these histological appearances are termed germinoma. Germinomas represent 60–70% of intracranial GCTs (Bjornsson et al. 1985; unpublished SIOP CNS GCT 96 trial data). Light microscopy reveals large uniform cells with abundant clear cytoplasm. Septae infiltrated by lymphocytes form the cells into lobules in a fibrovascular stroma. If syncytiotrophoblastic cells are present, the tumour may secrete low levels (up to 50 IU/l) of ß-HCG.

NON-GERMINOMAS

The non-germinomatous GCTs are divided into non-secreting intra-embryonic mature and immature teratomas, secreting extra-embryonic yolk sac tumour, embryonal carcinoma and choriocarcinoma.

TERATOMAS

Mature teratomas are histologically benign tumours derived from ecto-, endo- and mesoderm and may contain ectopic normal tissues such as skin, bone and epithelial tissue.

Immature teratomas consist of less well-differentiated elements that resemble fetal tissues, in a mitotically active stroma. Particularly common are peripheral neuroectodermal (PNET) like tissues, which may form neuroepithelial rosettes and aberrant retinal melanotic neuroepithelium. They are of varying malignant potential according to the nature and proportion of immature elements.

SECRETING TUMOURS

Yolk sac elements are frequently found in mixed GCTs; however, pure tumours are found in the pineal gland and are myxoid and gelatinous in consistency. Diagnostic features of yolk sac tumours on light microscopy include Schiller–Duval bodies (tumour cells collected around a central vessel in a pattern resembling a renal glomerulus). The detection of AFP indicates the presence of yolk sac elements. Serum AFP is naturally raised in infants up to 8 months old and therefore must be age-corrected. Outside this age range, serum levels above 25 ng/ml are diagnostic of a secreting GCT, and prognosis is related to the level of AFP (unpublished SIOP CNS GCT 96 trial data: Gabriele Calaminus, personal communication 2004).

Choriocarcinoma is very rare in its pure form but characteristically contains cytotrophoblast and syncytiotrophoblast elements, with ectatic vessels and areas of haemorrhagic necrosis. The syncytiotrophoblasts produce ß-HCG, and, by convention, a tumour is labelled as secreting when levels exceed 50 IU/ml (in Europe) or 100 IU/ml (in the USA) either in serum or in CSF. High levels of ß-HCG may account for alternative clinical presentations such as gynaecomastia and a positive pregnancy test in the absence of a conceptus.

Embryonal carcinoma cells are large and form nests and sheets. 'Embryoid bodies' may occasionally form, mimicking embryonic features such as amniotic cavities.

Treatment and outcome

Most of the evidence to date regarding intracranial GCTs is limited to retrospective, single institution series where data have been collected over decades with heterogeneous staging and treatment.

When a CNS GCT is suspected, referral to a specialist centre with experience in the management of paediatric oncology patients (patients under the age of 16 years) is recommended. In the UK this will be a United Kingdom Children's Cancer Study Group (UKCCSG) affiliated centre (Nicholson et al. 2002). Here, treatment will be planned and delivered in a multidisciplinary fashion. The core members of the team include the paediatric oncologist, paediatric neurosurgeon, neuropathologist, paediatric radiotherapist, paediatric endocrinologist, paediatric ophthalmologist, paediatric neuropsychologist, paediatric anaesthetist, specialist nurses in the hospital and community, play therapist, physiotherapist, occupational therapist and social worker. Children will usually be offered treatment according to a current national or international trial protocol allowing prospective data collection guiding future practice.

GERMINOMA

Surgery

In an emergency situation, an endoscopic ventriculostomy or ventriculoperitoneal shunt will serve to alleviate raised ICP secondary to obstructive hydrocephalus and/or to obtain diagnostic tissue. Otherwise, histological verification is obtained via a stereotactic or open biopsy.

Germinomas are curable with low morbidity by radiotherapy alone, regardless of the extent of surgery at diagnosis (Sawamura et al. 1997). Neurosurgery, particularly around the pineal gland, is associated with a degree of morbidity (3% mortality in the series reported by Sawamura et al. 1997). Surgical cure should therefore not be attempted in these cases as it does not alter subsequent management or improve outcome. Radical surgery is reserved for large residual masses after completion of treatment. At 'second look' surgery, usually either fibrotic tissue or mature teratoma is recovered, reflecting the relative frequency of mixed histopathology tumours (Weiner and Finlay 1999).

Radiotherapy and chemotherapy

Approximately 90% of germinomas are radiocurable (Sano 1995, Sawamura et al. 1998, Bamberg et al. 1999). Prior to modern neurosurgical advances, when biopsies of central midline tumours were rarely performed, empirical radiotherapy with 20 Gy was recommended for a radiologically suspected GCT (Abay et al. 1981). If the mass substantially regressed, the diagnosis of a germinoma was assumed and a complete course of radiotherapy was delivered. Today, a tissue diagnosis is perceived as mandatory for a non-secreting tumour given the low morbidity and mortality of modern neurosurgery and the impact of histology on management. Historically, the gold standard treatment for intracranial germinomas has been craniospinal radiotherapy (CSRT) followed by a boost to the primary tumour area. However, irradiation of the developing brain is associated with late neurocognitive and endo-crinological sequelae in an age and dose dependent manner. Given that most patients are diagnosed in their teens, these fears seem unfounded in this clinical setting as there is currently no evidence that the moderate whole or partial brain doses delivered lead to notice-able neurocognitive decline compared to pre-treatment levels (Sands et al. 2001, Buckner et al. 1999, Sutton et al. 1999, Merchant et al. 2000). A further late effect of radiotherapy is a 1–2% risk of second malignancies developing over 1–2 decades post-treatment (Mertens et al. 2001, Moller et al. 2001). As cure is achievable in virtually all patients with pure germinomas, the emphasis of current clinical trials is on minimizing the late sequelae of treatment while maintaining high cure rates.

The need for routine craniospinal radiotherapy in patients with all stages of germinoma is disputed (Linstadt et al. 1988, Brada and Rajan 1990, Wolden et al. 1995). Patients with M0 disease may not require prophylactic spinal irradiation if an adequate cranial volume is treated, as it is unusual to develop isolated spinal relapses if the primary tumour is well controlled (Haddock et al. 1997, Dattoli and Newall 1990). However, CSRT must be considered when the disease extends along the ventricular walls or is bifocal (Shibamoto et al. 1988). Positive CSF cytology does not adversely affect prognosis if prophylactic spinal irradiation is delivered (Shibamoto et al. 1994).

The optimal radiotherapy volume in patients with M0 disease remains under evaluation. Given that the majority of relapses occur within the ventricles, there is a move away from craniospinal axis or whole brain to partial brain (particularly whole ventricular) irradiation plus a boost to the primary tumour (Ono et al. 1994; Claire Alapetite, personal communication 2004). A retrospective series has shown that for M0 disease, relapse-free and overall survival did not differ significantly when radiotherapy was delivered to the tumour bed, the whole brain, the entire neuraxis or the ventricles and spine (Shibamoto et al. 1988).

Over the last two decades the dose perceived to successfully treat subclinical disease has decreased from 35–36 Gy to 24 Gy. This knowledge has been derived from successive prospective studies performed by the German MAKEI group in the 1980s and '90s (Calaminus et al. 1994, Bamberg 1999) and subsequently by the SIOP CNS GCT 96 study (G Calaminus, personal communication 2004). Additionally, these studies demonstrated that the dose to the primary tumour can be safely reduced from 50–55 Gy to 40 Gy, a view supported by other prospective and retrospective data (Shibamoto et al. 2001, Bouffet et al. 1999, Buckner et al. 1999). In the presence of macroscopic metastatic disease, CSRT and boost to the primary tumour and metastases is the treatment of choice. In the European experience of the SIOP CNS GCT 96 trial, all 11 patients with macroscopic metastatic disease at diagnosis remain in continuous complete remission after radiotherapy alone (G Calaminus, personal communication 2004).

Four-fifths of germinomas are chemosensitive (Weiner et al. 1999). A further aim of current studies (SFOP, SIOP) is to explore whether using chemotherapy in combination with focal radiotherapy will maintain the high cure rates demonstrated with wide-field radiotherapy, while reducing late morbidity. Without chemotherapy, tumour recurrence is seen in 7–12% of patients, mostly at the edges of the focal radiotherapy field or in the ventricles. A prospective study of combined modality treatment using carboplatin, ifosfamide and etoposide followed by focal radiotherapy of 40 Gy has been published with good initial results (93±7% event-free survival and 100% overall survival at 5 years). Forty-six per cent of patients experienced grade 3 or 4 haematological toxicity, and all patients with diabetes insipidus developed electrolyte imbalances (Bouffet et al. 1999). With further follow-up the event-free survival has decreased to 86%, indicating that chemotherapy is likely to be less successful in treating subclinical disease particularly in the ventricular area, given the known propensity of germinomas for subependymal spread (C Alapetite, personal communication 2004). The current non-randomized SIOP CNS GCT 96 protocol compares wide-field irradiation (24 Gy to the neuroaxis followed by a 16 Gy tumour boost, total dose 40 Gy) and systemic chemotherapy (carboplatin, ifosfamide and etoposide) followed by focal radiotherapy (40 Gy) to the primary tumour, identical to the approach chosen by the SFOP group. Early reports show that at a median follow-up of 24 months, of 131 patients with M0 and M1 disease, 125 are in complete remission. Two patients have relapsed after CSRT

265

and 4 after chemotherapy and focal irradiation (G Calaminus, personal communication 2004). In the aforementioned prospective clinical trials, most patients who relapsed were successfully salvaged by second-line chemotherapy including high-dose procedures and further radiotherapy.

Additionally, a documented complete response to chemotherapy may allow a further reduction in radiation dose (Allen et al. 1994). This risk-adapted strategy is supported by Phase II data showing that after a complete response to 4 cycles of standard dose cisplatin and etoposide chemotherapy, 30.6 Gy local irradiation yielded similar results to 54 Gy delivered to the same volume when less than a complete response was achieved (Buckner et al. 1999). Radiotherapy dose has been reduced as low as 24 Gy after cisplatin and etoposide chemotherapy and reported to give 100% disease–free survival rates at 2 years (Sawamura et al. 1998) and 5 years (Aoyama et al. 2002).

Results of a multi-institutional high-dose chemotherapy approach without first-line radiotherapy have been reported (Balmaceda et al. 1996). This strategy yielded an 82% complete response rate but only an 84% overall survival at 2 year follow-up. Significant toxicity was reported along with an increase in late relapses (median time to failure 35 months, with 25% of relapses seen after 57 months) and a chemotherapy-related mortality rate of 10%. Of the 50% of patients who relapsed, the majority were successfully salvaged by radiotherapy and chemotherapy. Given the attendant morbidity and mortality, not seen with radiotherapy alone, and the large percentage of patients requiring second-line treatment, the validity of such an approach is at present questionable. The use of chemotherapy alone, especially in high-dose strategies, in the first-line treatment of germinomas therefore remains experimental. In addition, no data have been presented to date supporting or refuting the hypothesis that combined modality treatment in this patient cohort reduces late morbidity compared to wide-field radiation. The use of combined modality treatment for patients over 8–10 years of age remains controversial, given the increase in acute morbidity and the unavoidable but low risk of radiation-induced second malignancies.

Other approaches able to minimize the late sequelae of radiotherapy include the use of 3-dimensional CT planning and either conformal or stereotactic treatment delivery for the boost volume by reducing the volume of surrounding normal tissue irradiated to high doses (Zissiadis et al. 2001). Given the clear technical advantages of conformal treatment techniques and the availability in most radiotherapy units today, this should represent the standard of care for radiotherapy delivered in this setting even in the absence of confirmatory clinical data.

Relapses in the CNS can be salvaged, although further radiotherapy is often required to achieve a second durable complete remission (Sawamura et al. 1999).

TERATOMA
Surgery
Surgery is the treatment of choice in the management of mature teratomas. Its use in the management of obstructive hydrocephalus and histological verification are as described above.

Mature teratomas are not responsive to nonsurgical oncological treatment modalities, and therefore a complete surgical resection is the treatment of choice and curative. Survival is in the order of 93% at 10 years (Sano 1995, Matsutani et al. 1997). Immature teratomas also benefit from radical resection, being significantly less chemo- and radiosensitive than other non-germinomatous GCTs. The literature reports 70–75% overall survival at 10 years, reflecting a difference in behaviour according to histology (Sano 1995, Matsutani et al. 1997).

Radiotherapy and chemotherapy

For residual disease following resection of an immature teratoma, a 'watch and wait' strategy should be considered. Only in the case of unequivocal progressive and symptomatic disease should radiotherapy be considered, as immature teratomas are chemo-insensitive (Hooda and Finlay 1999). Evidence for the benefit of high-dose radiotherapy is based on single case reports and therefore remains controversial in this setting.

SECRETING TUMOURS

Surgery

Acute relief of hydrocephalus is undertaken if indicated. If serum or CSF is positive for tumour markers in a patient with a clinical and radiological mass lesion suspicious of a GCT, tumour biopsy is not indicated prior to nonsurgical oncological therapy as these are accepted as pathognomonic for a secreting GCT (Nicholson et al. 2002).

Historical series show that surgery followed by irradiation alone produces a 5 year survival rate of less than 25% (Hooda and Finlay 1999). Significant improvement of event-free and overall survival was observed only after the introduction of platinum-based chemotherapy into the treatment strategy. But although chemosensitive, these tumours respond less well to chemo- and radiotherapy than germinomas. It has been postulated that debulking surgery may enhance the efficacy of adjuvant treatment (Sawamura 1996). Current European practice is for surgery to be reserved for resection of mature and immature teratomas and the removal of any large residual mass of secreting GCT after completion of therapy if tumour markers have normalized. The reason not to recommend a radical resection at initial diagnosis in secreting GCTs is based on the documented significant peri- and postoperative morbidity (Nicholson et al. 2002). Most commonly, the histology of residual masses yields mature or immature teratoma, which may give rise to recurrence (Buckner et al. 1999). Immediate surgery is indicated if repeat imaging demonstrates progressive disease despite normalization of previously elevated tumour markers ('growing teratoma' syndrome).

Radiotherapy and chemotherapy

In contrast to its radiotherapy-sparing aim in germinomas, chemotherapy significantly contributes to an increase in survival in secreting tumours. Postoperative adjuvant radiotherapy alone resulted in a cure rate of approximately 20% in secreting CNS germ cell tumours (Jennings et al. 1985). Since the introduction of platinum-based chemotherapy, results have dramatically improved (Kida et al. 1986, Calaminus et al. 1994, Itoyama et al. 1995). Although complete responses following chemotherapy may be achieved, these tumours remain incurable by this modality alone (Calaminus et al. 1994, Schild et al. 1996, Baranzelli et al. 1998). In the French experience, 12 of 13 patients treated with surgery and chemotherapy alone (vinblastine, bleomycin, carboplatin etoposide, ifosfamide) relapsed; while in an

American series, the 3 year survival rate decreased from 46% to 11% if radiotherapy was omitted from first-line treatment (Schild et al. 1996, Baranzelli et al. 1998). The German MAKEI group reported that 20 of 27 patients given radiotherapy were event-free survivors, in contrast to only 1 of 11 patients in whom radiotherapy was omitted (Calaminus et al. 1994). This stands in contrast to a series of 26 patients treated at the Memorial Sloane Kettering Cancer Centre with carboplatin, bleomycin and etoposide chemotherapy following surgery, where 9 of these patients remained in continuous first remission at the time of publication. Sixteen patients survived at 2 years (Balmaceda et al. 1996). Further follow-up is required to be able to assess this treatment strategy given the propensity of secreting GCTs for late relapses up to 5 years after treatment.

In a Japanese series, 4 out of 10 patients with secreting GCTs were long-term survivors following combined modality treatment including a platinum-based chemotherapy protocol, while all 7 patients who were treated only with surgery and radiotherapy died (Kida et al. 1986). A further series of 8 patients treated with a cisplatin-based strategy all became long-term survivors unlike any patient treated with surgery and radiotherapy alone (Itoyama et al. 1995).

The current SIOP CNS GCT 96 trial employs 4 cycles of cisplatin, etoposide, ifosfamide (PEI) chemotherapy followed by 54 Gy focal radiotherapy or 30 Gy craniospinal irradiation followed by a 24 Gy tumour bed boost in case of metastatic disease at diagnosis. At 5 years, the event-free survival rate is 63% for localized disease and 75% for metastatic disease (G Calaminus, personal communication 2004).

At present, cisplatin-based chemotherapy followed by focal radiotherapy in localized disease or CSRT in patients with metastatic disease at diagnosis is accepted as the standard of care.

Follow-up

Recurrent germinoma is potentially curable with salvage therapy, so close follow-up is warranted. As non-secreting tumours can occasionally recur as secreting tumours, regular measurement of serum tumour markers post-treatment should be considered. Baseline neuroimaging is useful once any acute changes secondary to treatment have resolved. Also recommended are regular ophthalmological and endocrinological follow-up, particularly if any abnormalities were detected at presentation. Early neuropsychological assessment is beneficial to ascertain the educational needs of the child or adolescent and to provide career guidance where appropriate. Manifestations of neurological impairment secondary to treatment include decreased IQ, shortened attention and memory spans and processing speed (Sands et al. 2001). Neurosurgery and chemotherapy are also believed to have a mild to moderate effect on perceptual and motor skills. It has been shown that no change in cognitive function was detectable in patients with intracranial GCTs when assessed post-therapy compared to pre-treatment (Sands et al. 2001). It is apparent that fewer long-term neuro-cognitive deficits attributable to radiotherapy are seen in this group of patients, compared to those treated similarly for other tumours such as medulloblastoma. This is due to the higher median age at diagnosis in germinoma patients (approximately 12–13 years), by which time neuronal development is nearly complete.

Other potential long-term toxicities to consider include hearing impairment if the cochlea is included in the high-dose radiotherapy volume, particularly if cisplatin was administered (Duffner et al. 1985). Alkylating agents such as ifosfamide may cause infertility, and cisplatin may cause renal damage. Clinicians must remain vigilant for these late sequelae during follow-up. The spinal radiotherapy field may give a small scattered radiotherapy dose to the gonads leading to temporarily impaired fertility in males or may permanently impact on fertility in female patients if the ovaries are within or in close proximity to the field. It is hypothesized that the addition of chemotherapy to radiotherapy may double the incidence of treatment-related second malignancies, and longer follow-up is required to assess whether combined modality treatment will manifest any unanticipated late sequelae.

Summary

Intracranial GCTs are rare primary CNS malignancies in children and adolescents. Treatment should be coordinated and delivered in a centre experienced in the management of paediatric oncology patients. Significant progress in the understanding of the disease has been made over the last two decades. Adequate staging, including MRI of the brain and spine, serum and CSF tumour markers, and CSF cytology, are the key to selecting the appropriate treatment strategy.

Primary germinomas are eminently treatable and cure rates exceeding 90% are commonly reported. Currently, wide-field radiotherapy is the gold standard. Future clinical trials are aimed at reducing treatment related morbidity while maintaining high cure rates. Whether this is best achieved by modification of a radiotherapy only approach or by a combined modality approach remains controversial. Benign mature and immature teratomas are best treated by complete surgical resection. For secreting malignant CNS GCTs, the introduction of cisplatin-based chemotherapy into multimodality treatment has led to significant improvement in outcome, but radiotherapy remains a pivotal element of first-line treatment. With tumour control rates in the order of 50–65% at 3–5 years, future efforts will remain concentrated on increasing the proportion of long-term survivors through improved risk-adapted strategies.

Given the rarity of paediatric primary CNS GCTs it is evident that no single centre can run a meaningful clinical trial. Therefore participation in national and multinational studies is strongly encouraged in order to increase our understanding of tumour biology and treatment related parameters. This is the only way to continuously improve not only the outcome but also the long-term quality of life of these children and adolescents as increasing numbers survive.

REFERENCES

Abay EO, Laws ER, Grado GL, Bruckman JE, Forbes GS, Gomez MR, Scott M (1981) Pineal tumour in children and adolescents. Treatment by CSF shunting and radiotherapy. *J Neurosurg* **55**: 889–895.

Allen JC, DaRosso RC, Donahue B, Nirenberg A (1994) A phase II trial of preirradiation carboplatin in newly diagnosed germinoma of the central nervous system. *Cancer* **74**: 940–944.

Aoyama H, Shirato H, Ikedo J, Fujieda K, Miyasaka K, Sawamura Y (2002) Induction chemotherapy followed by low-dose involved-field radiotherapy for intracranial germ cell tumors. *J Clin Oncol* **20**: 857–865.

Arens R, Marcus D, Engelberg S, Findler G, Goodman RM, Passwell JH (1998) Cerebral germinomas and

Klinefelter syndrome. A review. *Cancer* 1: 1228–1231.

Balmaceda C, Heller G, Rosenblum M, Diez B, Villablanca JG, Kellie S, Maher P, Vlamis V, Walker RW, Leibel S, Finlay JL (1996) Chemotherapy without irradiation—a novel approach for newly diagnosed CNS germ cell tumors: results of an international cooperative trial. The First International Central Nervous System Germ Cell Tumor Study. *J Clin Oncol* 14: 2908–2915.

Bamberg M, Kortmann R, Calamnius G, Becker G, Meisner C, Harms D, Göbel U (1999) Radiation therapy for intracranial germinoma: results of the German cooperative prospective trials MAKEI 83/86/89. *J Clin Oncol* 17: 2585–2592.

Baranzelli MC, Patte C, Bouffet E, Portas M, Mechinaud-Lacroix F, Sariban E, Roche H, Kalifa C (1998) An attempt to treat pediatric intracranial alphaFP and betaHCG secreting germ cell tumors with chemotherapy alone. SFOP experience with 18 cases. Societé Française d'Oncologie Pédiatrique. *J Neuro-oncol* 37: 229–239.

Bjornsson J, Scheithauer BW, Okazaki H, Leech RW (1985) Intracranial germ cell tumors: pathobiological and immunohistochemical aspects of 70 cases. *J Neuropathol Exp Neurol* 44: 32–46.

Bouffet E, Baranzelli MC, Patte C, Portas M, Edan C, Chastagner P, Mechinaud-Lacroix F, Kalifa C (1999) Combined treatment modality for intracranial germinomas: results of a multicentre SFOP experience. Société Française d'Oncologie Pédiatrique. *Br J Cancer* 79: 1199–1204.

Brada M, Rajan B. (1990) Spinal seeding in cranial germinoma. *Br J Cancer* 61: 339–340.

Buckner JC, Peethambaram PP, Smithson WA, Groover RV, Schomberg PJ, Kimmel DW, Raffel C, O'Fallon JR, Neglia J, Shaw EG (1999) Phase II trial of primary chemotherapy followed by reduced-dose radiation for CNS germ cell tumors. *J Clin Oncol* 17: 933–940.

Calaminus G, Bamberg M, Baranzelli MC, Benoit Y, di Montezemolo LC, Fossati-Bellani F, Jürgens H, Kühl HJ, Lenard HG, Curto ML, Mann JR, Patte C, Pearson A, Perilongo G, Schmidt D, Schober R, Göbel U (1994) Intracranial germ cell tumors: a comprehensive update of the European data. *Neuropediatrics* 25: 26–32.

Chaganti RS, Rodriguez E, Bosl GJ (1993) Cytogenetics of male germ-cell tumours. *Urol Clin N Am* 20: 55–66.

Dattoli M, Newall J (1990) Radiation therapy for intracranial germinoma: the case for limited volume treatment. *Int J Rad Oncol Biol Phys* 19: 429–433.

Diez B, Balmaceda C, Matsutani M, Weiner H (1999) Germ cell tumours of the CNS in children: recent advances in therapy. *Child's Nerv Syst* 15: 578–585.

Duffner PK, Cohen ME, Thomas PR Lansky SB (1985) The long-term effects of cranial irradiation on the central nervous system. *Cancer* 56: 1841–1846.

Fuller BG, Kapp DS, Cox R (1994) Radiation therapy of pineal tumours. 25 new cases and review of 208 previously reported cases. *Int J Radiat Oncol Biol Phys* 28: 229–245.

Haddock MG, Schild SE, Scheithauer BW, Schomberg PJ (1997) Radiation therapy for histologically confirmed primary central nervous system germinoma. *Int J Radiat Oncol Biol Phys* 38: 915–923.

Hashimoto M, Hatasa M, Shinoda S, Masuzawa T (1992) Medulla oblongata germinoma in association with Klinefelter syndrome. *Surg Neurol* 37: 384–387.

Hooda BS, Finlay JL (1999) Recent advances in the diagnosis and treatment of central nervous system germ-cell tumours. *Cur Opin Neurol* 12: 693–696.

Hashimoto T, Sasagawa I, Ishigooka M, Kubota Y, Nakada T, Fujita T, Nakai O (1995) Down's syndrome associated with intracranial germinoma and testicular embryonal carcinoma. *Urol Int* 55: 120–122.

Itoyama Y, Kochi M, Kuratsu J, Takamura S, Kitano I, Marubayashi T, Uemura S, Ushio Y. (1995) Treatment of intracranial nongerminomatous malignant germ cell tumours producing alpha-fetoprotein. *Neurosurg* 36: 459–464; discussion 464–466.

Jennings MT, Gelman R, Hochberg F (1985) Intracranial germ cell tumours: natural history and pathogenesis. *J Neurosurg* 63: 155–167.

Kida Y, Kobayashi T, Yoshida J, Kato K, Kageyama N (1986) Chemotherapy with cisplatin in AFP-secreting germ-cell tumors of the central nervous system. *J Neurosurg* 65: 470–475.

Kiltie AE, Gattamaneni HR (1995) Survival and quality of life of paediatric intracranial germ cell tumour patients treated at the Christie Hospital, 1972–1993. *Med Pediatr Oncol* 25: 450–456.

Linstadt D, Wara WM, Edwards MS, Hudgins RJ, Sheline GE (1988) Radiotherapy of primary intracranial germinomas: the case against routine craniospinal irradiation. *Int J Radiat Oncol Biol Phys* 15: 291–297.

Matsutani M, Sano K, Takakura K, Fujimaki T, Nakamura O, Funata N, Seto T (1997) Primary intracranial germ cell tumours: a clinical analysis of 153 histologically verified cases. *J Neurosurg* 86: 446–455.

Merchant TE, Sherwood SH, Mulhern RK, Rose SR, Thompson SJ, Sanford RA, Kun LE (2000) CNS

270

germinoma: disease control and long-term functional outcome for 12 children treated with craniospinal irradiation. *Int J Radiat Oncol Biol Phys* **46**: 1171–1176.

Mertens AC, Yasui Y, Neglia JP, Potter JD, Nesbit ME, Ruccione K, Smithson WA, Robinson LL (2001) Late mortality experience in five-year survivors of childhood and adolescent cancer: the Childhood Cancer Survivor study. *J Clin Oncol* **19**: 3163–3172.

Moller TR, Garwicz S, Barlow L, Falck Winther J, Glattre E, Olafsdottir G, Olsen JH, Perfekt R, Ritvanen A, Sankila R, Tulinius H; Association of the Nordic Cancer Registries; Nordic Society for Pediatric Hematology and Oncology (2001) Decreasing late mortality among five-year survivors of cancer of childhood and adolescence: a population based studying the Nordic countries. *J Clin Oncol* **19**: 3173–3181; comment 3161–3162.

Nicholson JC, Punt J, Hale J, Saran F, Calaminus G; Germ Cell Tumour Working Groups of the United Kingdom Children's Cancer Study Group (UKCCSG) and International Society of Paediatric Oncology (SIOP) (2002) Neurosurgical management of paediatric germ cell tumours of the central nervous system—a multi-disciplinary approach for the new millennium. *Br J Neurosurg* **16**: 93–95.

Ono N, Isobe I, Uki J, Kurihara H, Shimizu T, Kohno K (1994) Recurrence of primary intracranial germinomas after complete response with radiotherapy: recurrence patterns and therapy. *Neurosurg* **35**: 615–620; discussion 620–621.

Rao YT, Medini E, Haselow RE, Jones TK, Levitt SH (1981) Pineal and ectopic pineal tumours. The role of radiation therapy. *Cancer* **48**: 708–713.

Rosenblum MK, Ng HK (1997) Germ cell tumours. In: Kleihues P, Cavanee WK, eds. *Pathology and Genetics of Tumours of the Nervous System*. Lyon: International Agency for Research on Cancer, pp. 164–169.

Sands SA, Kellie SJ, Davidow AL, Diez B, Villablanca J, Weiner HL, Pietanza MC, Balmaceda C, Finlay J. (2001) Long-term quality of life and neuropsychologic functioning for patients with CNS germ-cell tumors: from the First International CNS Germ-Cell Tumor Study. *J Neuro-oncol* **3**: 174–183.

Sano K (1995) So-called germ cell tumours: are they really of germ cell origin? *Br J Neurosurg* **9**: 391–401.

Sano K, Matsutani M, Seto T (1989) So-called intracranial germ cell tumours: personal experiences and a theory of their pathogenesis. *Neurol Res* **11**: 118–126.

Sawamura Y (1996) Current diagnosis and treatment of central nervous system germ cell tumours. *Cur Opin Neurol* **9**: 419–423.

Sawamura Y, de Tribolet N, Ishii N, Abe H (1997) Management of primary intracranial germinomas: diagnostic surgery or radical resection. *J Neurosurg* **87**: 262–266.

Sawamura Y, Ikeda J, Shirato H, Tada M, Abe H (1998) Germ cell tumours of the central nervous system: treatment considerations based on 111 cases and their long-term clinical outcomes. *Eur J Cancer* **34**: 104–110.

Sawamura Y, Ikeda J, Tada M, Shirato H (1999) Salvage therapy for recurrent germinomas in the central nervous system. *Br J Neurosurg* **13**: 376–381.

Schild SE, Haddock MG, Scheithauer BW, Marks LB, Norman MG, Burger PC, Wong WW, Lyons MK, Schomberg PJ (1996) Nongerminomatous germ cell tumours of the brain. *Int J Radiat Oncol Biol Phys* **36**: 557–563.

Shibamoto Y, Abe M, Yamashita J, Takahashi M, Hiraoka M, Ono K, Tsutsui K (1988) Treatment result of intracranial germinoma as a function of the irradiated volume. *Int J Radiat Oncol Biol Phys* **15**: 285–290.

Shibamoto Y, Oda Y, Yamashita J, Takahashi M, Kikuchi H, Abe M (1994) The role of cerebrospinal fluid cytology in radiotherapy planning for intracranial germinoma. *Int J Radiol Oncol Biol Phys* **29**: 1089–1094.

Shibamoto Y, Sasai K, Oya N, Hiraoka M (2001) Intracranial germinoma: radiation therapy with tumor volume-based dose selection. *Radiology* **218**: 452–456.

Sutton LN, Radcliffe J, Goldwein J, Philips P, Janss AJ, Packer RJ, Zhao H (1999) Quality of life of adult survivors of germinomas treated with craniospinal irradiation. *Neurosurg* **45**: 1292–1297; discussion 1297–1298.

Takei Y, Pearl GS (1981) Ultrastructural study of intracranial yolk sac tumor: with special reference to the oncologic phylogeny of germ cell tumors. *Cancer* **48**: 2038–2046.

Wakai S, Segawa H, Kitahara S, Asano T, Sano K, Ogihara R, Tomita S (1980) Teratoma in the pineal region in two brothers. Case reports. *J Neurosurg* **53**: 239–243.

Watanabe T, Makiyama Y, Nishimoto H, Matsumoto M, Kikuchi A, Tsubokawa T (1995) Metachronous ovarian dysgerminoma after a suprasellar germ-cell tumor treated by radiation therapy. Case report. *J Neurosurg* **83**: 149–153.

Weiner HL, Finlay JL (1999) Surgery in the management of primary intracranial germ cell tumors. *Child's Nerv Syst* **15**: 770–773.

Wolden SL, Wara WM, Larson DA, Prados MD, Edwards MS, Sneed PK (1995) Radiation therapy for primary intrcranial germ-cell tumors. *Int J Radiat Biol Phys* **32**: 943–949.

Wong TT, Ho DM, Chang TK, Yang DD, Lee LS. (1995) Familial neurofibromatosis 1 with germinoma involving the basal ganglion and thalamus. *Child's Nerv Syst* **11**: 456–458.

Zissiadis Y, Dutton S, Kieran M, Goumnerova L, Scott RM, Kooy HM, Tarbell NJ (2001) Stereotactic radiotherapy for pediatric intracranial germ cell tumors. *Int J Radiat Oncol Biol Phys* **51**: 108–112.

15
CHOROID PLEXUS PAPILLOMA AND CARCINOMA

Stephen Lowis

Choroid plexus tumours (CPTs) are rare, comprising approximately 0.5–0.6% of all primary CNS tumours. Greenberg (1999) reported a series of 73 patients with intraventricular tumours, of which 6 had arisen from the choroids plexus. Epidemiological data for incidence are limited, however. The SEER registry, from a population of approximately 35 million, reported only 26 such tumours between 1973 and 1996. Such rarity presents particular problems when trying to define appropriate therapy, and in recent years, attempts have been made to adopt a multinational collaborative approach. Published data indicates that the majority of CPTs arise before the age of 2 years, and 85% before 5 years; the sex distribution seems to be equal; and there are no racial, ethnic or geographic factors implicated in either the incidence or aetiology of CPTs.

Pathology

CPTs are epithelial, arising most commonly from the choroid plexus of the lateral or fourth ventricle. Papillomas have a characteristic lobulated appearance, although invasion into brain parenchyma may be seen. Tumours may show extensive differentiation and appear as almost normal choroid plexus. Cells stain with cytokeratin and transthyretin, which distinguish them from ependymoma. Other markers include glial fibrillary acidic protein (GFAP), carcinoembryonic antigen and S100.

Tumours are highly vascular and arise in close proximity to areas such as the limbic system. Invasion into brain parenchyma is more typical of choroid plexus carcinoma, and may prevent surgical clearance. More commonly, tumour expansion is into the ventricular system.

A grading system for CPT has been defined by the WHO, with grade I being papilloma and grade III carcinoma (Kleihues and Cavanee 2000). The majority (80%) of tumours are papillomas. Progression from benign to malignant tumours has been described, and there is evidence of increasing malignancy with time (Chow et al. 1999).

Aetiology

There has been considerable interest in the possible role of SV40 virus in the development of choroid plexus carcinoma, particularly following the accidental contamination of a batch of polio vaccine with the virus in the 1970s. SV40 is capable of transforming human choroid cells in vitro (Carruba et al. 1983, 1984, 1985) and can produce choroid plexus tumours in mice (Brinster et al. 1984, Small et al. 1985). Furthermore, transgenic mice which express the SV40 early region develop CPTs with high frequency (Brinster et al. 1984, Cho et al. 1989). Finally, SV40-like DNA was found in 10 of 20 tumours in the series of Bergsagel et al. (1992). Whether the virus is causative or merely a bystander able to proliferate in actively dividing tumour tissue is not certain, but there is a significant amount of evidence suggesting a role for SV40 in these tumours.

Malignant atypical teratoid/rhabdoid tumours may show areas of differentiation towards choroid plexus carcinoma, and there are reports of choroid plexus carcinoma in families with Li–Fraumeni syndrome, and with mutations in hSNF5/INI1 (Sevenet et al. 1999).

Presentation
Clinical features at presentation are not specific, but are those associated with any supra-tentorial mass in a young child. Excessive production of CSF may lead to a communicating hydrocephalus even when local anatomical distortion does not lead to obstruction of the ventricular system (Tomita et al. 1988, McEvoy et al. 2000), and symptoms and signs of raised intracranial pressure are the most common presenting features. Other features may include visual problems, failure to thrive and developmental delay. CPTs may present as a congenital neoplasm diagnosed in utero.

Imaging
CT is likely to show the tumour, even when the primary tumour is in the fourth ventricle. There is often hydrocephalus, and the tumour is typically smooth, lobulated and isodense, lying within the ventricle. Although typically in the lateral ventricle in infants, this has not been the case in my own experience. Calcification may be present, and strongly suggests CPT in this setting.

CPTs are highly vascular, and flow voids may be seen on MRI. Marked enhancement with gadolinium is expected. There may be associated haemorrhage. Images of choroid plexus carcinomas can be seen in Figures 3.29–3.32 (pp. 50–52).

Dissemination is seen in approximately 30%, and is more common, but not exclusively seen in carcinoma (Leys et al. 1986, Bennedbaek and Therkildsen 1990, Domingues et al. 1991, Enomoto et al. 1991, Peschgens et al. 1995, Kang et al. 1997). Metastasis is most commonly seen through the CSF, but extracerebral spread has been reported, to abdomen (Geerts et al. 1996), bone (Valladares et al. 1980), and lung (Sheridan and Besser 1994).

Treatment
The degree of surgical clearance seems to be of prognostic value, and where possible, complete surgical clearance should be attempted, with second-look surgery if necessary (Packer et al. 1992, Pierga et al. 1993, Berger et al. 1998). The outcome for those children with a complete surgical resection is clearly better than for those without: in the series reported by Duffner et al. (1995), three of four patients with complete remission remain alive with no evaluable disease. Berger et al. (1998) reported surgery to be the only prognostic factor in a series of 22 children treated over 11 years by the Société Française d'Oncologie Pédiatrique.

A discussion of surgical techniques is beyond the scope of this chapter, but the highly vascular nature of these tumours means that control of the vascular supply is paramount. The role of chemotherapy in modifying vascularity of such tumours is uncertain, but we have adopted this approach in one patient with a choroid plexus papilloma.

Radiotherapy appears to be associated with improved survival in completely resected carcinoma, with 5 year overall survival of 68% in those receiving radiotherapy vs 12% in those who did not, in the review of patients published by Wolff et al. (1999). For patients aged less than 3 years at diagnosis, however, this benefit was not seen. In addition, radiotherapy in very young children is associated with a risk of major neurocognitive sequelae, and may be felt to be unacceptable.

Given the relatively low frequency of complete surgical resection, and concerns regarding use of radiotherapy, chemotherapy has been used by a number of groups, although patient numbers are always small. Chemotherapy has been reported to be effective in these small series, allowing delay or even omission of radiotherapy (Gianella-Borradori et al. 1992, Duffner et al. 1995). A role may exist for chemotherapy in allowing staged surgical removal of a tumour (Souweidane et al. 1999). Potentially active agents include bleomycin, cisplatin, carboplatin, cyclophosphamide, vincristine, procarbazine and, particularly, etoposide.

Summary

The extreme rarity of CPTs means that useful data relating to treatment are difficult to obtain. Systematic overviews are of value in indicating those agents likely to be of benefit, and of these, etoposide seems to have significant beneficial effect. A working group, coordinated through International Society of Paediatric Oncology (SIOP), has now been established, and an international collaborative protocol has been developed. It is hoped that with this common approach, a rapid accumulation of useful data can be achieved in a relatively short time.

REFERENCES

Bennedbaek O, Therkildsen MH (1990) Choroid plexus carcinoma—report of a case with metastases within the central nervous system. *Acta Oncol* **29**: 241–243.
Berger C, Thiesse P, Lellouch-Tubiana A, Kalifa C, Pierre-Kahn A, Bouffet E (1998) Choroid plexus carcinomas in childhood: clinical features and prognostic factors. *Neurosurgery* **42**: 470–475.
Bergsagel DJ, Finegold MJ, Butel JS, Kupsky WJ, Garcea RL (1992) DNA sequences similar to those of simian virus 40 in ependymomas and choroid plexus tumors of childhood. *N Engl J Med* **326**: 988–993.
Brinster RL, Chen HY, Messing A, van Dyke T, Levine AJ, Palmiter RD (1984 "Transgenic mice harboring SV40 T-antigen genes develop characteristic brain tumors. *Cell* **37**: 367–379.
Carruba G, Dallapiccola B, Brinchi V, de Giuli Morghen C (1983) Ultrastructural and biological characterization of human choroid cell cultures transformed by Simian Virus 40. *In Vitro* **19**: 443–452.
Carruba G, Dallapiccola B, Mantegazza P, Garaci E, Micara G, Radaelli A, De Giuli Morghen C (1984) Transformation of human choroid cells in vitro by SV40. Ultrastructural and cytogenetic analysis of cloned cell lines. *J Submicrosc Cytol* **16**: 459–470.
Carruba G, Mantegazza P, Garaci E, Radaelli A, De Giuli Morghen C (1985) Differential expression of surface proteins, virus receptors and histocompatibility antigens in SV40-transformed human choroid cells and their clones. *J Submicrosc Cytol* **17**: 21–30.
Cho HJ, Seiberg M, Georgoff I, Teresky AK, Marks JR, Levine AJ (1989) Impact of the genetic background of transgenic mice upon the formation and timing of choroid plexus papillomas. *J Neurosci Res* **24**: 115–122.

Chow E, Jenkins JJ, Burger PC, Reardon DA, Langston JW, Sanford RA, Heideman RL, Kun LE, Merchant TE (1999) Malignant evolution of choroid plexus papilloma. *Pediatr Neurosurg* **31**: 127–130.

Domingues RC, Taveras JM, Reimer P, Rosen BR (1991) Foramen magnum choroid plexus papilloma with drop metastases to the lumbar spine. *AJNR* **12**: 564–565.

Duffner PK, Kun LE, Burger PC, Horowitz ME, Cohen ME, Sanford RA, Krischer JP, Mulhern RK, James HE, Rekate HL, et al. (1995) Postoperative chemotherapy and delayed radiation in infants and very young children with choroid plexus carcinomas. The Pediatric Oncology Group. *Pediatr Neurosurg* **22**: 189–196.

Enomoto H, Mizuno M, Katsumata T, Doi T (1991) Intracranial metastasis of a choroid plexus papilloma originating in the cerebellopontine angle region: a case report. *Surg Neurol* **36**: 54–58.

Geerts Y, Gabreels F, Lippens R, Merx H, Wesseling P (1996) Choroid plexus carcinoma: a report of two cases and review of the literature. *Neuropediatrics* **27**: 143–148.

Gianella-Borradori A, Zeltzer PM, Bodey B, Nelson M, Britton H, Marlin A (1992) Choroid plexus tumors in childhood. Response to chemotherapy, and immunophenotypic profile using a panel of monoclonal antibodies. *Cancer* **69**: 809–816.

Greenberg ML (1999) Chemotherapy of choroid plexus carcinoma. *Child's Nerv Syst* **15**: 571–577.

Kang HS, Wang KC, Kim YM, Kim IO, Kim SK, Chi JG, Cho BK (1997) Choroid plexus carcinoma in an infant. *J Korean Med Sci* **12**: 162–167.

Kleihues P, Cavanee WP (2000) *Pathology and Genetics of Tumors of the Central Nervous System. World Health Organization Classification of Tumours*. Lyon: IARC Press.

Leys D, Pasquier F, Lejeune JP, Lesoin F, Petit H, Delandsheer JM (1986) [Benign choroid plexus papilloma. 2 local recurrences and intraventricular seeding.] *Neurochirurgie* **32**: 258–261 (French).

McEvoy AW, Harding BN, Phipps KP, Ellison DW, Elsmore AJ, Thompson D, Harkness W, Hayward RD (2000) Management of choroid plexus tumours in children: 20 years experience at a single neurosurgical centre. *Pediatr Neurosurg* **32**: 192–199.

Packer RJ, Perilongo G, Johnson D, Sutton LN, Vezina G, Zimmerman RA, Ryan J, Reaman G, Schut L (1992) Choroid plexus carcinoma of childhood. *Cancer* **69**: 580–585.

Peschgens T, Stollbrink-Peschgens C, Mertens R, Volker A, Thron A, Heimann G (1995) [Therapy of choroid plexus carcinoma in childhood. Case report and review of the literature.] *Klin Pädiatr* **207**: 52–58 (German).

Pierga JY, Kalifa C, Terrier-Lacombe MJ, Habrand JL, Lemerle J (1993) Carcinoma of the choroid plexus: a pediatric experience. *Med Pediatr Oncol* **21**: 480–487.

Sevenet N, Sheridan E, Amram D, Schneider P, Handgretinger R, Delattre O (1999) Constitutional mutations of the hSNF5/INI1 gene predispose to a variety of cancers. *Am J Hum Genet* **65**: 1342–1348.

Sheridan M, Besser M (1994) Fatal pulmonary embolism by tumor during resection of a choroid plexus papilloma: case report. *Neurosurgery* **34**: 910–912; discussion 912.

Small JA, Blair DG, Showalter SD, Scangos GA (1985) Analysis of a transgenic mouse containing simian virus 40 and v-myc sequences. *Mol Cell Biol* **5**: 642–648.

Souweidane MM, Johnson JH, Lis E (1999) Volumetric reduction of a choroid plexus carcinoma using pre-operative chemotherapy. *J Neurooncol* **43**: 167–171.

Tomita T, McLone DG, Flannery AM (1988) Choroid plexus papillomas of neonates, infants and children. *Pediatr Neurosci* **14**: 23–30.

Valladares JB, Perry RH, Kalbag RM (1980) Malignant choroid plexus papilloma with extraneural metastasis. Case report. *J Neurosurg* **52**: 251–255.

Wolff JE, Sajedi M, Coppes MJ, Anderson RA, Egeler RM (1999) Radiation therapy and survival in choroid plexus carcinoma. *Lancet* **353**: 2126 (letter).

16
CRANIOPHARYNGIOMA

Eddy Estlin

Epidemiology

Craniopharyngiomas account for 3–4% of CNS tumours in all age groups and 8–9% in the paediatric population (Vernet et al. 1999). At their point of origin, craniopharyngiomas are midline tumours that arise either from the pituitary stalk or from the tuber cinereum – the floor of the third ventricle. Tumours that arise from the pituitary stalk typically extend downward into the pituitary fossa itself, or else extend out from it, and tumours arising from the tuber cinereum are more likely to extend upwards to the hypothalamus into the third ventricle (Hayward 1999). Craniopharyngioma is an epithelial tumour that is thought to originate from the embryonic remnants of Rathke's pouch, and two main histological variants are described, adamantinomatous and squamous papillary. For children, over 95% of cases are of the adamantinomatous subtype (Weiner et al. 1994).

There does not appear to be any racial or ethnic predilection for the development of craniopharyngioma, and the tumour occurs slightly more commonly in boys than in girls. The incidence of craniopharyngioma in children is greatest at age 6–10 years (Bunin et al. 1998). The location of craniopharyngioma, with the intimate association of the tumour to the visual pathways, hypothalamus and limbic system predisposes patients to significant visual, endocrine and neuropsychological deficits, both at presentation and as a result of treatment. Therefore, these tumours demand a high level of multidisciplinary skill in their diagnosis, treatment and follow-up.

Clinical presentation

The most common triad of presenting symptoms in a child with a craniopharyngioma is visual failure owing to compression of the optic chiasm, optic nerve and tracts, endocrinopathy with growth failure or diabetes insipidus and symptoms and signs of raised intracranial pressure (ICP). This last complication results from the upward expansion of the tumour into the third ventricle causing obstructive hydrocephalus. In addition, children with large tumours may show evidence of hypothalamic disturbance at the time of their presentation, with obesity or neuropsychological deficits (Hayward 1999).

Visual signs and symptoms at presentation are noted in approximately 50% of children with craniopharyngioma. Ophthalmological signs in keeping with raised ICP, such as optic atrophy and papilloedema, concomitant squint and bitemporal hemianopia are often found (Kennedy and Smith 1975). In general, prechiasmatic extension of tumour with compression of the optic nerves can lead to loss of visual acuity, and posterior tumours can result in chiasmatic compression and complex visual field defects. In a study of 30 children with

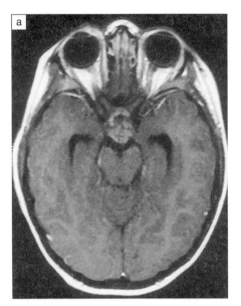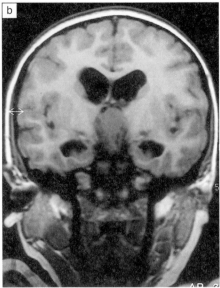

Fig. 16.1. T$_1$-weighted axial post-gadolinium (a) and T$_1$-weighted coronal (b) scans demonstrating a well-defined partly cystic suprasellar mass that obliterates the third ventricle. The coronal image shows the tumour to contain fluid of an intermediate signal intensity.

craniopharyngioma, 19 children had visual loss, and 15 had endocrine deficits (Fisher et al. 1998). Fewer than 30% of children are endocrinologically normal at diagnosis. Growth hormone deficiency is the most common finding and occurs in up to 75% of cases; gonadotrophin deficiency is observed in up to 60% of cases; and thyroid or adrenal dysfunction is present in approximately one-third of cases. Diabetes insipidus is relatively uncommon, occurring in only approximately 15% of children at presentation with craniopharyngioma (Wisoff 2001).

The preoperative assessment of children who present with suspected craniopharyngioma should include formal neuro-ophthalmologic and endocrinological evaluations. In addition, neuropsychological evaluations prior to therapy should be viewed as important. Radiological imaging is essential to define the location of any cystic, solid and calcified portions of the tumour and their relationships to the surrounding, often distorted anatomy. CT and MRI have complimentary roles in the diagnosis of craniopharyngioma. CT is superior for the detection of varied and complex calcifications, and of secondary changes in the skull base such as enlargement of the sella turcica and/or erosion of the dorsum sella. MRI provides valuable information about the relationships of the tumour to the surrounding structures (Fig. 16.1).

Craniopharyngioma cysts are uniformly bright on T2-weighted sequences; on T$_1$-weighted sequences, however, the signal intensity of the fluid may range from hypo- to hyperintense, reflecting the heterogenous cyst contents of protein, lipid and iron.

Craniopharyngiomas characteristically consist of both solid and cystic elements (Wisoff 2001). Surgery and radiotherapy are the mainstay of treatment, but there is significant variation in practice worldwide for the relative contributions of these treatment modalities to the overall management of children presenting with craniopharyngioma.

Treatment with surgery

Surgery for craniopharyngioma is performed either by the transcranial, or less commonly the trans-sphenoidal routes. The advent of high-resolution CT and MRI, the development of the ultrasonic aspirator for neurosurgical procedures, and improvements in the medical management in the postoperative period mean that gross total removal of tumour can be achieved for the majority of children when attempted (Hayward 1999); for example, Yasargil et al. (1990) described a 90% complete resection rate for 144 patients who underwent microsurgical resection of their craniopharyngioma. In other contemporary series, complete resection rates of 52% (De Vile et al. 1996c) and 77% (Weiner et al. 1994) have been reported.

Intraoperative complications and tumour adherence to major blood vessels such as the carotids and their major branches are well reported for surgery with craniopharyngioma (De Vile et al. 1996c). In addition, the radical resection of the gliotic capsule that often surrounds craniopharyngioma tumours may cause further damage to the surrounding hypothalamus, and the neuroendocrine and neuropsychological sequelae of therapy for craniopharyngiomas will be discussed later in this chapter.

Radical resection of craniopharyngioma can certainly be successful in preventing local recurrence of the disease. However, long-term event-free survival is not guaranteed, and an overall risk of recurrence of approximately 25% has been reported in many series (Habrand et al. 1999). The potential for significant visual or hypothalamic sequelae in relation to radical surgery, or the inoperability or some craniopharyngioma tumours at presentation, has led to the use of adjuvant radiotherapy for the treatment of this condition.

Radiotherapy

Although children with craniopharyngioma do not inevitably progress with their disease following subtotal resection (Weiner et al. 1994), radiotherapy has become the standard for adjuvant therapy when complete resection of tumour has not been achieved with surgery. Moreover, subtotal resection followed by radiotherapy has been advocated to confer a more favorable outcome in terms of long-term morbidity in the face of equal efficacy with radical surgery (Rajan et al. 1993). For many series where radiotherapy has been employed following subtotal resection, the overall and relapse-free survivals are at least equivalent to those for complete resection (Habrand et al. 1999). Radiotherapy is usually administered as external beam irradiation by conventional schedules. A dose–response effect for radiotherapy has been observed, with relapse rates approaching 50% being reported for patients receiving less than 50 Gy of radiotherapy vs 16% for patients receiving 55–57 Gy (Sung et al. 1981). In contemporary treatment protocols, children with craniopharyngioma generally receive radiotherapy at doses of 50–55 Gy delivered in 180 cGy fractions to maximize tumour control with the minimum of toxicity to surrounding tissue such at the hypothalamus, optic pathway and pituitary.

Stereotactic radiosurgery has also been employed for small solid tumours (<2.5 cm) with good long-term results in terms of disease control and treatment-related sequelae (Plowman et al. 1999, Wisoff 2001). The installation of radioisotopes such as ^{90}yttrium has also been successfully been employed in the intracavity therapy of recurrent cystic craniopharyngioma in a number of series (Blackburn et al. 1999, Wisoff 2001).

Chemotherapy

Intracystic chemotherapy with bleomycin has an established role in the therapy of cystic craniopharyngioma at presentation at relapse (Mottolese et al. 2001). However, the difficulties in the management of patients presenting with craniopharyngioma mirror in many ways those of children presenting with low-grade glioma that affects the hypothalamus and optic chiasm. In the latter condition, the role of chemotherapy has been advocated in younger children as a means of avoiding potentially damaging radical surgery to the area of the hypothalamus, and also to delay the use of potentially damaging radiotherapy. It is perhaps surprising that chemotherapy has not been more extensively evaluated in craniopharyngioma, but the small body of evidence that does exist suggests a potential role for chemotherapy in this non-malignant condition.

For four children who experienced their first tumour recurrence following initial surgery and radiotherapy, chemotherapy consisting of five intravenous ambulatory courses of doxorubicin (99 mg/m^2 as a continuous infusion over 72 hours) together with oral CCNU (80 mg/m^2 on day 1) was administered to the children, with an interval of 6 weeks between courses. In one patient a cystic relapse occurred after 3 years remission, but for the others a continuous remission was maintained for between 3 and 12 years post-chemotherapy (Lippins et al. 1998). Similarly, an adult case has been reported to respond to chemotherapy with vincristine, BCNU and procarbazine for treatment of relapsed disease following initial surgery and radiotherapy (Bremer et al. 1984). When the possible long-term sequelae associated with radical surgery or the use of radiotherapy at a young age in children are considered, then a case could be made for the role of chemotherapy to be investigated for children with craniopharyngioma.

Treatment of recurrent disease

In an international multicentre report of 474 children with craniopharyngioma, the overall recurrence rate was almost 30%. Following total resection, 20% of children relapsed, compared with 29% following subtotal resection plus adjuvant radiotherapy and 56.6% with subtotal resection alone. However, tumours in younger children recurred more frequently, with a recurrence rate of 37% for children who were diagnosed at less than 5 years of age (Choux et al. 1991). Most series report recurrences occurring within two to five years after primary treatment (Wisoff 2001). The treatment modality offered to children will depend on the operability of the current tumour, the larger proportions of the tumour that are solid and cystic, and whether primary radiotherapy was employed in treatment. Radical secondary surgery is associated with a reduced success rate in terms of gross total resection, and also an increase in mortality (Wisoff 2001). However, excellent long-term control of tumour can be achieved with external beam irradiation for children who have not previously received this treatment modality (Weiss et al. 1989). As discussed above, the role of chemotherapy may merit consideration by international cooperative groups for this rare tumour at relapse. Another study has also indicated the importance of young age at diagnosis, the presence of severe hydrocephalus and large tumour size for the risk of tumour recurrence (De Vile et al. 1996c).

Prognosis and late effects of treatment

The 10- and 20-year progression-free survival rates for craniopharyngioma have been reported to be in the range of 60–80% (Rajan et al. 1993, Habrand et al. 1999), and the 10-year overall survival rate also approximates to these figures. Therefore, any treatment-related morbidity will carry significant implications for these children.

The growth and endocrine sequelae of treatment for craniopharyngioma have been well characterized for children. Following surgery for this condition, multiple endocrinopathies are almost universal, such that 75% of children have panhypopituitarism at follow-up (De Vile et al. 1996b). In particular, replacement therapy with growth hormone, thyroid hormone, hydrocortisone and antidiuretic hormone are required in the majority of cases. The severity of endocrinological outcome relates to risk factors such as hypothalamic manifestations at presentation, tumour size greater than 3.5 cm and hypothalamic injury during radical resection (Habrand et al. 1999). However, one of the most significant morbidities to affect children with craniopharyngioma following treatment is that of obesity. Nearly one-half of children develop severe obesity following operation, which relates to tumour factors such as hydrocephalus and tumour size, and also familial obesity (Muller et al. 2001). Moreover, the extent of hypothalamic damage following surgery for craniopharyngioma related to hypothalamic damage as assessed by cranial MRI. Patients with increasing evidence of damage to the hypothalamus were found to be more at risk of excessive weight gain in the postoperative period (De Vile et al. 1996a).

Improvement in visual function following therapy has been reported for visual field loss, strabismus and reduced visual acuity in most published series (Habrand et al. 1999). However, craniopharyngioma is associated with significant permanent visual dysfunction in children. In particular, age younger than 6 years at presentation in association with visual symptoms before treatment has been correlated with a significantly poorer visual outcome than that for older children and adults (Abrams and Repka 1997).

The cognitive and neuropsychological sequelae for children following treatment for craniopharyngioma have been reported in a limited number of cases. Carpentieri et al. (2001) described specific memory problems, in both the language and visuospatial domains, in children following surgery for craniopharyngioma. In addition, children treated with surgery alone have been reported to experience a clinically significant loss of full scale IQ compared to children receiving combined-modality treatment with surgery and radiotherapy (Merchant et al. 2002). Moreover, children with craniopharyngioma have commonly been found to exhibit disorders of behaviour (Anderson et al. 1997).

Neuropsychological deficits may seriously impact upon the quality of life for survivors of craniopharyngioma. In the series of Habrand et al. (1999), one-third of children were reported to have psychological disorders and poor school performance following treatment.

Similarly, in the report of Vernet et al. (1999), 9 of 25 children who had received treatment for craniopharyngioma were described as having a poor outcome with severely delayed schooling or institutionalization as an adult. An indication of the overall morbidity can be found for 75 children treated at Great Ormond Street Hospital, London, where a review of morbidity focused on endocrine, visual, neurological, educational and hypothalamic sequelae. At assessment, performed at an average of 6.4 years following surgery, 76% of children had panhypopituitarism and 13% had panhypopituitarism and impaired thirst. Approximately one-half of children had severely impaired vision affecting at least one eye, 40% had a motor disorder, and 56% had hypothalamic dysfunction as evidenced by obesity. In terms of education, only 37% of children had a normal IQ, with 27% having severe learning difficulties (De Vile et al. 1996c).

Future directions

The overall survival rates for children undergoing therapy for craniopharyngioma with radical surgery or with subtotal resection plus radiotherapy appear to be equivalent (Hayward 1999). However, further studies are needed to define the modality of treatment that is optimal in terms of the late sequelae of treatment experienced by children with this condition, as treatment-related sequelae will have an important bearing on their subsequent quality of life. For example, at the St Jude's Children's Research Hospital, Memphis, the Mean Heath Utility Index (a functional quality of life index) has been found to be higher for children receiving treatment with radiotherapy and surgery than for those receiving surgery alone (Merchant et al. 2002). Moreover, the burden of morbidity as described by De Vile et al. (1996c) was higher for children aged less than 5 years at presentation (30% of the series), for patients presenting with severe hydrocephalus and for those with intraoperative complications. The consequences of the development and therapy of craniopharyngioma in children may influence their life expectancy, as an association between premature mortality and causes of hypopituitarism such as craniopharyngioma has been described for adults (Tomlinson et al. 2001). Therefore, strategies of therapy that include staged surgical procedures (Hayward 1999), chemotherapy with existing cytotoxic agents or newer compounds such as interferon-alpha (Jakacki et al. 2000), and delaying definitive radiotherapy may be required to reduce the longer-term sequelae associated with the current treatment for craniopharyngioma. However, in the face of such a relatively rare tumour, it may be argued that a concentration of expertise in terms of the assessment, treatment and follow-up of these children would be warranted under the auspices of international collaborative studies.

REFERENCES

Abrams LS, Repka MX (1997) Visual outcome of craniopharyngioma in children. *J Pediatr Ophthalmol Strabismus* **34**: 223–228.
Anderson CA, Wilkening GN, Filley CM, Reardon MS, Kleinschmidt-DeMasters BK (1997) Neurobehavioural outcome in pediatric craniopharyngioma. *Pediatr Neurosurg* **26**: 255–260.
Blackburn TPD, Doughty D, Plowman PN (1999) Stereotactic intracavity therapy of recurrent cystic cranio-pharyngioma by instillation of 90yttrium. *Br J Neurosurg* **13**: 359–365.
Bremer AM, Nguyen TQ, Balsys R (1984) Therapeutic benefits of combination chemotherapy with vincristine, BCNU and procarbazine on recurrent cystic craniopharyngioma. A case report. *J Neurooncol* **2**: 47–51.

Bunin GR, Surawicz TS, Witman PA, Preston-Martin S, Davis F, Bruner JM (1998) The descriptive epidemiology of craniopharyngioma. *J Neurosurg* **89**: 547–551.

Carpentieri SC, Waber DP, Scott RM, Goumnervosa LC, Kieran MW, Cohen LE, Kim F, Billett AL, Tarbell NJ, Pomeroy SL (2001) Memory deficits among children with craniopharyngiomas. *Neurosurgery* **49**: 1053–1057.

Choux M, Lena G, Genitori L (1991) Le craniophayyngiome de l'enfant. *Neurochirurgie* **37**: 1–174.

De Vile CJ, Grant DB, Hayward RD, Kendall BE, Neville BGR, Stanhope R (1996a) Obesity in childhood craniopharyngioma: relation to post-operative hypothalamic damage shown by magnetic resonance imaging. *J Clin Endocrin Metabol* **81**: 2734–2737.

De Vile CJ, Grant DB, Hayward RD, Stanhope R (1996b) Growth and endocrine sequelae of craniopharyngioma. *Arch Dis Child* **75**: 108–114.

De Vile CJ, Grant DB, Kendall BE, Neville BG, Stanhope R, Watkins KE, Hayward RD (1996c) Management of childhood craniopharyngioma: can the morbidity of radical surgery be predicted. *J Neurosurg* **85**: 73–81.

Fisher PG, Jenab J, Gopldthwaite PT, Tihan T, Wharam MD, Foer DR, Burger PC (1998) Outcomes and failure patterns in childhood craniopharyngioma. *Child's Nerv Syst* **14**: 558–563.

Habrand J-L, Ganry O, Couanet D, Rouxel V, Levy-Piedbios C, Pierre-Kahn A, Kalifa C (1999) The role of radiation therapy in the management of craniopharyngioma: a 25 year experience and review of the literature. *Int J Radiat Oncol Biol Phys* **44**: 255–263.

Hayward R (1999) The present and future management of childhood craniopharyngioma. *Child's Nerv Syst* **15**: 764–769.

Jakacki RI, Cohen BH, Jamison C, Mathews VP, Arenson E, Longee DC, Hilden J, Cornelius A, Needle M, Heilman D, Boaz JC, Luerssen TG (2000) Phase II evaluation of interferon-alpha-2a for progressive or recurrent craniopharyngiomas. *J Neurosurg* **92**: 255–260.

Kennedy HB, Smith RJ (1975) Eye signs in craniopharyngioma. *Br J Ophthalmol* 59: 689–695.

Lippens RJJ, Rotteveel JJ, Otten BJ, Merx H (1998) Chemotherapy with adriamycin (doxorubicin) and CCNU (lomustine) in four children with recurrent craniopharyngioma. *Eur J Paediatr Neurol* **2**: 263–268.

Merchant TE, Kiehna EN, Sanfod RA, Mulhern RK, Thompson SJ, Wilson MW, Lustig RH, Kun LE (2002) Craniopharyngioma : the St Jude Research Hospital experience 1984–2001. *Int J Radiat Oncol Phys* **53**: 533–542.

Mottolese C, Stan H, Hermier M, Berlier P, Convert J, Frappaz D, Lapras C (2001) Intracystic chemotherapy with bleomycin in the treatment of craniopharyngiomas. *Child's Nerv Syst* **17**: 724–730.

Muller HL, Bueb K, Bartels U, Roth C, Harz K, Graf N, Korinthenber R, Bettendorf M, Kuhl J, Gutjahr P, Sorensen N, Calaminus G (2001) Obesity after childhood craniopharyngioma – German multicenter study on pre-operative risk factors and quality of life. *Klin Pädiatr* **213**: 244–249.

Plowman PN, Wraith C, Royle N, Grossman AB (1999) Stereotactic radiosurgery. IX. Craniopharyngioma: durable complete imaging responses and indications for treatment. *Br J Neurosurg* **13**: 352–358.

Rajan B, Ashley S, Gorman C, Jose CC, Horwich A, Bloom HJG, Marsh H, Brada M (1993) Craniopharyngioma – long-term results following limited surgery and radiotherapy. *Radiother Oncol* **26**: 1–10.

Sung DI, Chang CH, Harisiadis L, Carmel PW (1981) Treatment results of craniopharyngiomas. *Cancer* **47**: 847–852.

Tomlinson JW, Holden N, Hills RK, Wheatley K, Clayton RN, Bates AS, Sheppard MC, Stewart PM (2001) Association between premature mortality and hypopituitarism : West Midlands Prospective Hypopituitary Study Group. *Lancet* **357**: 425–431.

Vernet O, Montes JL, Farmer J-P, Blundell JE, Bertrand G, Freeman CR (1999) Long term results of multi-modality treatment of craniopharyngioma in children. *J Clin Neurosci* **6**: 199–203.

Weiner HL, Wisoff JH, Rosenberg ME, Kupersmith MJ, Cohen H, Zagzag D, Shiminski-Maher T, Flamm ES, Epstein FJ, Miller DC (1994) Craniopharyngiomas: A clinicopathological analysis of factors predictive of recurrence and functional outcome. *Neurosurgery* **35**: 1001–1011.

Weiss M, Sutton L, Marcial V, Fowble B, Packer R, Zimmerman R, Schut L, Bruce D, D'Angio G (1989) The role of radiation therapy in the management of childhood craniopharyngioma. *Int J Radiat Oncol Biol Phys* **17**: 1313–1321.

Wisoff JH (2001) Craniopharyngioma. In: Keating RF, Goodrich JT, Packer RJ, eds. *Tumors of the Pediatric Central Nervous System*. New York: Thieme, pp 276–291.

Yasargil MG, Curcic M, Kis M, Siegenthaler G, Teddy PJ, Roth P (1990) Total removal of craniopharyngiomas. Approaches and long-term results in 144 patients. *J Neurosurg* **73**: 3–11.

17
MIXED NEURONAL TUMOURS

Eddy Estlin

Mixed neuronal tumours are relatively rare CNS tumours that may occur in childhood, and characteristically present in children at the end of their first decade of life with a preceding history of drug-resistant epilepsy. The two main tumour types, dysembryoplastic neuroepithelial tumour (DNET) and ganglioglioma, carry an excellent prognosis and have an indolent clinical course.

Dysembryoplastic neuroepithelial tumour

DNETs were first described as a clinical entity by Daumas-Duport et al. (1988). Although the World Health Organization has classified DNET as a neuronal and mixed neuronal tumour, some authors consider it to represent a malformative or hamartomatous lesion (Schneider and Insinga 2001). The true incidence of this tumour is unknown, but DNETs represent approximately 1% of CNS tumours in the childhood population. However, DNETs are more frequently found following surgery for temporal lobe tumours in association with intractable epilepsy, where this diagnosis is made histologically in 5–15% of cases (Schneider and Insinga 2001). There is no obvious causal association for this tumour, although DNETs have been reported in association with neurofibromatosis type 1 (Schneider and Insinga 2001).

The histological features of DNETs are heterogenous (Honavar et al. 1999), but classically comprise a specific ganglioneuronal element with small blue oligodendroglial-like cells and neurons in a mucinous background. The tumours are characteristically nodular and there is adjacent cortical dysplasia (Schneider and Insinga 2001). DNETs typically present with a long-standing history of a refractory seizure disorder, typically partial complex seizures, which have an onset at approximately 10 years of age. Symptoms associated with raised intracranial pressure or visual field deficit are rare, and there are normally no abnormalities to be found on neurological examination (Daumas-Duport et al. 1988).

DNETs typically involve the temporal lobe in approximately 60% of patients, the frontal lobe in 31% of cases and the parietal and/or occipital lobes in the remainder (Daumas-Duport et al. 1988).

DNETs demonstrate some characteristic findings with radiological imaging. On CT they are sharply demarcated and moderately hypodense tumours which may be calcified and enhance minimally with contrast. On MRI (Fig. 17.1), they show low signal intensity on T1-weighted scans and increased intensity on T2-weighted scans, and demonstrate little gadolinium enhancement (Schneider and Insinga 2001).

The treatment of choice for DNETs remains surgical resection, and gross total resection rates of 50–70% (Daumas-Duport et al. 1988, 1999). However, even subtotal resection is

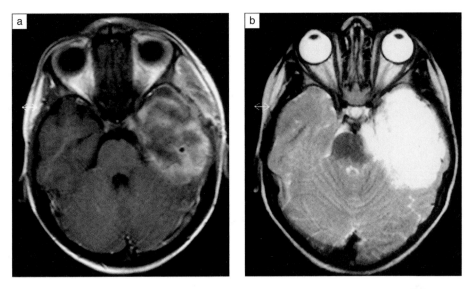

Fig. 17.1. (a) T_1-weighted axial MRI shows a well-defined, multilobulated mass within the left temporal lobe, which is markedly expanded. The mass shows heterogenous enhancement following administration of gadolinium. (b) T_2-weighted axial MRI demonstrates the characteristic high signal intensity of a DNET.

often valuable in terms of long-term control of intractable epilepsy (Schneider and Insinga 2001), and residual tumours are characteristically stable on postoperative surveillance imaging (Daumas-Duport et al. 1999). Therefore, the prognosis for children diagnosed with DNT is excellent, and malignant transformation is an extremely rare event in this tumour (Hammond et al. 2000).

Gangliogliomas

Gangliogliomas are rare CNS neoplasms, accounting for 1–4% of primary CNS tumours in children (Johnson et al. 1997). In the paediatric age group, the mean age at diagnosis is 9.5 years, and there have been no associations made between factors such as sex or ethnicity and the incidence of this tumour (Schneider and Insinga 2001). As with DNETs, gangliogliomas most commonly present with seizures, experienced on average 2 years before diagnosis of the tumour. Gangliogliomas are most often found in the temporal lobes (38%), with other sites in the parietal (30%) and frontal lobes (18%) (Johnson et al. 1997). Overall, approximately 90% of gangliogliomas are supratentorial and 10% are infratentorial in location (Schneider and Insinga 2001).

The pathological features of ganglioglioma are characterized by mature, well-differentiated ganglion cells, glial stroma, lack of perineuronal clustering of glial cells and GFAP positivity (Schneider and Insinga 2001). The imaging appearances of gangliogliomas are similar to those of DNETs. The tumours may show cystic areas, calcification and variable enhancement on CT, while MRI (Fig. 17.2) may demonstrate variable signal on T_1-weighted

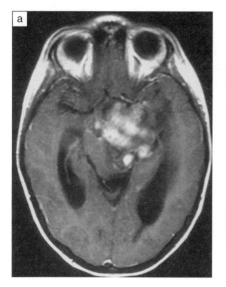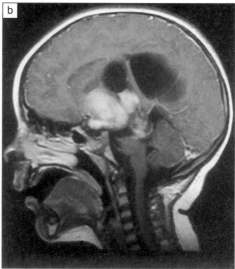

Fig. 17.2. T_1-weighted axial (a) and sagittal (b) post-gadolinium MRI showing large, part solid enhancing, part cystic mass in the suprasellar cistern and extending into the hypothalamus, right basal ganglia and thalamus. There is also compression of the left cerebral peduncle, and the left lateral ventricle is compressed.

scans, increased signal on T_2-weighted scans, and variable enhancement with gadolinium (Schneider and Insinga 2001).

The natural history of ganglioglioma appears to be relatively benign, and is characterized by slow growth of the glial element of the tumour. Treatment of choice is gross total excision of the tumour if possible. In terms of long-term prognosis, the location of the tumour appears to be the most important prognostic factor. Hemispheric tumours carry the most favourable prognosis, with a 5-year survival rate of over 90%, compared with 5-year survival rates of 84% and 73% for spinal cord and brainstem tumours, respectively (Schneider and Insinga 2001). For the purposes of adjuvant therapy, gangliogliomas are usually treated according to institutional or national guidelines for the treatment of low-grade gliomas. Therefore, recurrent tumours, or those growing and threatening function following subtotal resection, will be initially treated with chemotherapy in young children and radiotherapy in older children. Rapid regrowth of gangliogliomas has been described as indicative of anaplastic transformation of the glial elements of the tumour and portends a poor prognosis (Schneider and Insinga 2001).

A further variant of ganglioglioma, described as desmoplastic infantile ganglioglioma, in which the ganglioglioma is associated with a desmoplastic matrix, occurs primarily in infancy (Duffner et al. 1994). Desmoplastic infantile gangliogliomas are usually very large, supratentorial cystic masses that present in children less than 1 year of age (Fig. 17.3). Despite their massive size and pathologically malignant appearance, they tend to run a relatively benign clinical course, and a good prognosis can be expected if a gross total resection can

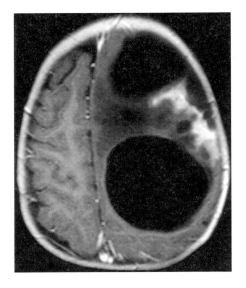

Fig. 17.3. T_1-weighted axial post-gadolinium MRI showing a very large, multicystic intrinsic mass in the left frontoparietal region with surrounding oedema and enhancing solid components on its superolateral aspect. There is associated mass effect with compression of the body of the left lateral ventricle, effacement of the ipsilateral cortical sulci and midline shift.

be achieved surgically. However, the role of adjuvant therapy is controversial (Duffner et al. 1994).

Conclusions

Although rare, DNETs and gangliogliomas are important as a cause of intractable epilepsy in children. These tumours are characterized by an indolent, but not necessarily benign clinical course, and gross total resection remains the treatment of choice for these tumours. When these tumours are associated with seizures, 60–90% of children may be rendered seizure-free by surgery (Johnson et al. 1997, Aronica et al. 2001). In particular, younger age at surgery, gross total resection, shorter duration of pre-existing epilepsy, absence of generalized seizures and absence of epileptiform discharge in the postoperative EEG predict a better postoperative seizure outcome (Aronica et al. 2001). In view of the relative rarity of these tumours, international cooperative studies would be required to formally assess the role of adjuvant radiotherapy and chemotherapy, which are probably more indicated for ganglioglioma than DNET.

REFERENCES

Aronica E, Leenstra S, van Veelen CW, van Rijen PC, Hulsebox TJ, Tersmette AC, Yankaya B, Troost D (2001) Glioneuronal tumours and medically intractable epilepsy: a clinical study with long term follow up of seizure outcome after surgery. *Epilepsy Res* **43**: 179–191.
Daumas-Duport C, Scheithauer BW, Chodkiewicz JP, Laws ER, Vedrenne C (1988) Dysembryoplastic neuroepithelial tumor: a surgically curable tumor of young patinets with intractable partial seizures. Report of thirty-nine cases. *Neurosurgery* **23**: 545–556.
Daumas-Duport C, Varlet P, Bacha S, Beuvon F, Cervera-Pierot P, Chodkiewicz JP (1999) Dysembryoplastic neuroepithelial tumors: non-specific histological forms – a study of 40 cases. *J Neurooncol* **41**: 267–280.
Duffner PK, Burger PC, Sanford RA, Krischer JP, Elterman R, Aronin PA, Pullen J, Horowitz ME, Parent A (1994) Desmoplastic infantile ganglioglioma: an approach to therapy. *Neurosurgery* **34**: 583–589.

Hammond RR, Duggal N, Woulfe JM, Girvin JP (2000) Malignant transformation of a dysembryoplastic neuroepithelial tumour. A case report. *J Neurosurg* **92**: 722–725.

Honavar M, Janota I, Polkey CE (1999) Histological heterogeneity of dysembryoplastic neuroepithelial tumour: identification and differential diagnosis in a series of 74 cases. *Histopathology* **34**: 242–256.

Johnson JH, Hariharan S, Berman J, Sutton LN, Rorke LB, Molloy P, Philips PC (1997) Clinical outcome of pediatric gangliogliomas: ninety-nine cases over 20 years. *Pediatr Neurosurg* **27**: 203–207.

Schneider SJ, Insinga SA (2001) Miscellaneous brain tumours. In: Keating RF, Goodrich JT, Packer RJ, eds. *Tumors of the Pediatric Central Nervous System*. New York: Thieme, pp. 398–412.

18
SPINAL CORD TUMOURS IN CHILDREN

Douglas J Hyder, Peter B Dirks, Ute Bartels and Eric Bouffet

Among CNS tumours, intramedullary spinal cord tumours (IMSCTs) require special consideration. Although histologically similar to tumours in the brain, spinal cord tumours have a different prognosis, and the literature suggesting optimal management is frequently limited. This chapter will be confined to IMSCTs. Metastatic tumours and extradural tumours that impinge on the spinal cord or upon spinal roots or plexuses will not be addressed. Spinal cord tumour epidemiology, presentation and evaluation, individual tumour types, and long-term sequelae will be discussed.

Intradural spinal cord tumours are rare in children, accounting for 1–9% of all childhood malignancies (Hardison et al. 1987, Stiller and Nectoux 1994, Constantini and Epstein 1996, Allen et al. 1998). IMSCTs occur in boys slightly more frequently than in girls, with a ratio of approximately 1.4 to 1. Although the most common age of presentation is between 7 and 10 years, IMSCTs have been reported in the neonatal and infant periods. IMSCTs can occur anywhere along the vertebral axis or in multiple locations (Goh et al. 1997).

The most common types of spinal cord tumours in children are fibrillary astrocytoma, ganglioglioma and ependymoma, but numerous other pathologies have been described including high-grade astrocytoma, myxopapillary ependymoma, other mixed glial–neuronal tumours and haemangioblastoma (Miller 2000). Each of these tumours poses therapeutic challenges when considering the relative benefits and risks of surgery, radiation therapy and chemotherapy.

As with other CNS tumours, two factors are important when considering outcome: (1) tumour control, as measured by progression free survival and overall survival, and (2) neurological function, as measured by the presence or absence of neurological deficits, and the extent to which these deficits impair quality of life. Unfortunately, the best possible outcome in many circumstances may be a compromise between maximizing tumour control and minimizing neurological sequelae.

Presenting symptoms and radiology

The diagnosis of an IMSCT is usually difficult. Children may present with back pain, scoliosis, walking difficulties, headaches, weakness, numbness, incoordination, or bowel or bladder dysfunction (DeSousa et al. 1979, Rossitch et al. 1990, Goh et al. 1997). Rarely, children may present with symptoms of increased intracranial pressure secondary to hydrocephalus (Caviness et al. 1998). Frequently, initial referral is made to an orthopaedist for management of back pain or a suspected muscle or joint disorder, and only upon the failure of an initial management plan or progression of symptoms is a tumour suspected.

The most common symptoms of a spinal cord tumour are pain, gait disturbances, bladder or bowel dysfunction, scoliosis and torticollis (DeSousa et al. 1979).

MRI is the imaging modality of choice in the diagnosis and management of spinal cord tumours. When a spinal cord tumour is suspected, the entire spine should be imaged to check for metastases. A brain MRI should also be performed, and this may identify a primary brain tumour or CNS dissemination. MRI localizes the tumour and characterizes any solid and cystic components, blood vessels, and syrinxes. MRI resolution may not be sufficient to characterize very small lesions. It is frequently difficult to delineate exactly where a tumour ends and where peritumoural oedema begins. Since intramedullary tumours impinge upon both ascending and descending spinal cord tracts, degenerative changes may be difficult to distinguish from tumour on MRI.

General principles of surgery for IMCST

Generally, MRI interpretation will not provide a definitive diagnosis, so a surgical biopsy may be necessary. Depending on the type of tumour, a surgical resection may outweigh the potential risks of the procedure. Advances in imaging and in microsurgical technique have made IMSCTs amenable to surgical resection. Surgical resection is the mainstay of therapy for spinal cord astrocytomas and ependymomas. Following a careful review of neuroimaging studies, a posterior approach via a laminotomy or laminectomy is performed. A laminotomy involves removal of contiguous laminae en bloc (if more than two segments are required) using a high-speed surgical saw with replacement at the end of the procedure. This technique may reduce the chance for progressive kyphosis associated with laminectomy for IMSCTs, especially in the cervical region. Intraoperative somatosensory and motor evoked potentials are used to monitor cord function during the operation.

Following dural exposure, intraoperative ultrasound is used to localize the solid tumour within the cord and can identify associated tumour cysts or a spinal cord syrinx, which is often found rostral or caudal to the tumour. Ultrasound confirms adequate bony removal and directs where the midline dural opening will occur. Under the operating microscope, a midline dorsal myelotomy is then made. The midline is determined using the dorsal root entry zones bilaterally as a guide, as the cord can be rotated. The myelotomy is made either over the maximal bulk of the tumour or into a rostral or caudal syrinx. Entry into a syrinx cavity first will aid greatly in developing a plane of dissection between tumour and normal cord. After myelotomy, there is usually 1–2 mm thickness of cord tissue over the tumour that is dissected using small surgical spatulas aided by bipolar coagulation. Once the tumour is found, the myelotomy is extended over the rostral–caudal extent of the tumour.

Management of specific tumour types

ASTROCYTOMA

Astrocytoma is the most common spinal cord tumour in children, accounting for up to 40% of tumours in some series. Most of these astrocytomas have low-grade, fibrillary histology. Fibrillary astrocytomas account for 25–30% of all spinal cord tumours in children; pilocytic astrocytomas are uncommon. Anaplastic astrocytomas account for about 9% of all spinal cord tumours in children; glioblastoma multiforme is rare (Miller 2000).

The most common age at presentation is 7–8 years, although tumours may be seen at any age. Astrocytomas occur anywhere from the cervicomedullary junction to the filum terminale. They are found most frequently in the thoracic cord, primarily because of the relative size of this area (Goh et al. 1997).

MRI usually reveals an iso- to slightly hypointense signal on T_1 weighting, hyperintense on T_2. Cysts are commonly seen associated with the tumour. Astrocytomas may not enhance, but when they do enhance, it is generally less intense and more eccentric than is seen with ependymomas (Houten and Cooper 2000).

In the past, holocord tumours were believed to be quite common; however, this was based on myelograms and CT myelograms (Epstein and Epstein 1982, Vles et al. 1990). With MRI, holocord tumours are unusual. Most spinal cord astrocytomas span a few vertebral segments, but cord swelling, cysts, syrinx and other non-neoplastic cord changes may be present in many more segments.

Prognosis is influenced by duration of symptoms and tumour grade. Acute symptom presentation suggests a more aggressive tumour, and these children may have a worse prognosis. Chronic symptoms, sometimes spanning years, implies a more indolent tumour and perhaps a better chance at successful tumour control. In the series reported by Bouffet et al. (1998), children with a history of symptoms of less than two months duration had a 34% survival rate; children with a longer duration of symptoms had a 90% survival. In the same series, children with low-grade tumours had a 76% survival whereas those with anaplastic astrocytomas had a 32% survival with a median follow-up of 4 years.

The initial treatment of spinal cord low-grade astrocytoma is surgery. At the time of surgery, an astrocytoma is usually firm and grey in colour. Astrocytomas do not usually have a good plane of cleavage between the tumour and surrounding spinal cord, making circumferential dissection difficult. The tumour removal occurs from the inside to the outside, first internally debulking the tumour and gradually working toward the tumour–cord interface. An ultrasonic surgical aspirator is used that allows delivery of the tumour tissue without manipulation of the surrounding spinal cord. In the end, under high-power magnification, the tumour is shaved down until small pieces of tumour are gently removed adjacent to normal cord. It can be difficult to know exactly where the tumour–cord interface is, so the surgeon proceeds until this distinction is left uncertain.

One of the largest series of spinal cord astrocytoma, reported by Constantini et al. (2000), included 164 patients aged less than 21 years. A gross total resection could be achieved in 77% and a subtotal resection in 20%. When compared to preoperative and 3 month postoperative functional grades, 60% of patients stayed the same, 16% improved and 24% worsened. Of the patients who worsened, 13 did so by more than one functional grade.

For low-grade astrocytoma, it is unclear whether adjuvant therapy is necessary. Radiation therapy is conventionally performed at many centres, but this is largely based on the adult experience, and there are no reports of a controlled trial looking at outcome either with or without adjuvant radiation therapy for spinal cord astrocytoma in children. Some series report good survival with surgery alone or that survival is not improved by postoperative radiation therapy, even when the tumour is incompletely resected (Constantini et al. 2000). Reports on the use of chemotherapy for low-grade astrocytomas of the spine are uncommon. Fort

291

et al. (1998) reported 5 children aged 11 to 27 months who received a combination of intravenous carboplatin and vincristine: 1 patient had a complete response, 2 patients had minimal responses, and 2 had progressive disease. At a mean follow-up of 22 months, all were alive, 3 with no further therapy and 2 with additional surgery at the time of progression. Hassall et al. (2001) reported three children with progressive low-grade tumours treated with carboplatin that resulted in one complete response, one partial response and one patient with stable disease. Doireau et al. (1999) reported 8 children who received multi-agent chemotherapy according to the baby SFOP protocol: at a mean follow-up of 3 years from the beginning of chemotherapy, 7 were alive, 4 with complete remission.

Higher-grade astrocytomas have a much worse prognosis. The tumours may be disseminated at diagnosis, and a complete surgical resection is difficult or impossible. High-grade spinal astrocytomas are generally treated with adjuvant radiation therapy and chemotherapy based on their poor prognosis. Despite aggressive treatments, progression-free survival remains poor (Merchant et al. 1999). Even when radical excision is accomplished, prognosis is poor. In the series reported by Cohen et al. (1989), 19 patients with high-grade astrocytomas underwent radical excision. Eighteen of these patients received adjuvant radiation therapy and 10 received chemotherapy. Four of the 19 patients were still alive at the time of the report, with a median survival of 6 months. Allen et al. (1998) reported the use of '8 in 1' chemotherapy in 13 children with high-grade spinal cord astrocytoma, 9 of whom also received radiation therapy. Seven patients developed tumour recurrence, with over half relapsing at the primary site, often with leptomeningeal metastases. Seven of the 13 patients were alive at the follow-up review, with a median follow-up of 59 months.

MIXED GLIOMAS

Mixed neuronal glial tumours, most commonly gangliogliomas, account for about 10–40% of spinal cord tumours in children, depending on the series (see review by Miller and McCutcheon 2000). These tumours are generally managed as low-grade astrocytomas with surgical resection and the consideration of adjuvant radiation therapy depending on institutional practice (Merchant et al. 2000).

EPENDYMOMA

Ependymoma is the third most common type of spinal cord tumour in children and accounts for about 15% of patients (Miller 2000). Ependymomas are usually tumours of the posterior fossa, with a smaller percentage in the supratentorial brain. While brain ependymoma tends to be more common in infants and young children, spinal cord ependymoma is more common in older children and adults.

MRI is the most informative diagnostic imaging modality; however, ependymomas and astrocytomas may be indistinguishable on routine scans. Ependymoma is more likely when the tumour is located in the center of the spinal cord or the tumour margins are distinct. Gadolinium enhancement tends to be homogenous or cap-like in appearance with a higher signal at both tumour poles (Fine et al. 1995).

Complete surgical removal of the ependymoma is considered by many to be the treatment of choice (Brotchi et al. 1992, Lonjon et al. 1998). At surgery, an ependymoma is relatively discrete. It is usually soft and reddish-purple in color. Typically, there is a good plane between the tumour surface and the spinal cord. Tumour is removed using a technique similar to that used for astrocytoma. The tumour is debulked internally initially and gradually the cleavage plane between tumour and cord is dissected. Ependymomas are more likely to be completely removed than are astrocytomas.

Lonjon et al. (1998) reported 20 children with intramedullary spinal cord ependymomas who underwent complete resection and were not treated with radiation, 14 had a complete resection, 6 a subtotal resection. Eighteen patients survived at 10-year follow-up. Three patients had a recurrence, 2 at the primary site and 1 at a distant site. Following surgery, 8 patients clinically improved, 10 were unchanged, and 2 deteriorated. Centres that routinely use radiation also report good long-term results (Merchant et al. 2000, O'Sullivan et al. 1994). However, no randomized controlled trial to determine whether radiation therapy is indicated following complete resection of spinal cord ependymoma in children has yet been done.

Adjuvant therapy for incompletely resected ependymoma or when anaplastic features are present is usually radiation for children older than 3 years at diagnosis (Shaw et al. 1987, Merchant et al. 2000). Whole brain and spine radiation is currently not in favour since most relapses are local and the risk of neuroaxis dissemination is believed to be low (McLaughlin et al. 1998). Chemotherapy may be the preferred adjuvant therapy when a spinal cord ependymoma is diagnosed in a child less than 3 years of age, with the hope of either delaying or avoiding radiation.

MYXOPAPILLARY EPENDYMOMA (MPE)

MPE is a variant of ependymoma, histologically characterized by the pseudopapillary architecture, arborizing vasulature and mucin production (Chan et al. 1984). It is a relatively common spinal intradural neoplasm in adults and is diagnosed most frequently during the fourth decade of life. It is rare in children and usually presents following a prolonged period (usually 12 months) of unexplained chronic back pain and musculoskeletal complaints (Gagliardi et al. 1993, Nagrib and O'Fallon 1997). MPE is almost always seen in the conus medullaris and filum terminale, although it may occur elsewhere in the CNS. MPEs show hyperintense signal on T_2-weighted MRI. Most tumours have clear margins and exhibit uniform contrast enhancement. MPE is usually considered a benign tumour, although relapses and metastatic disease have been reported (Nagib and O'Fallon 1997).

Total resection of this tumour is the treatment of choice. However, when total resection is not possible due to tumour infiltration of the root nerves, a partial resection followed by postoperative radiation therapy may be considered, although this is primarily based on experience with adults. Metastatic MPE has been successfully treated with craniospinal radiation (Chinn et al. 2000). Recently, one patient who had tumour recurrence following partial resection and involved field radiation received a combination of oral etoposide and tamoxifen on an experimental protocol and had a partial response with residual tumour stabilization for 19 months following chemotherapy initiation (Madden et al. 2001).

HAEMANGIOBLASTOMA

Although relatively common in the adult population, haemangioblastomas are quite rare in children, accounting for less than 5% of all spinal cord tumours (Miller and McCutcheon 2000). About 35% of adults with haemangioblastoma have von Hippel–Lindau syndrome (VHL), an autosomal dominant condition that maps to chromosome 3p25–26. In addition to CNS haemangioblastoma, VHL may be associated with renal and pancreatic cysts, epidydimal cystadenoma, retinal angioma, pheochromocytoma and renal cell carcinoma (Miller and McCutcheon 2000). VHL protein suppresses vascular endothelial growth factor (VEGF) expression, but it is not known if this plays a causal role in the development of haemangioblastoma (Leung and Ohh 2002). In children, haemangioblastoma does not appear to be exclusively seen with VHL, although the aetiology remains unclear (Fisher et al. 2002).

Haemangioblastoma is most common in the posterior fossa (80%), with the remainder in the spine. When one haemangioblastoma is diagnosed, a thorough evaluation of the CNS should be undertaken.

On MRI, haemangioblastomas have characteristic findings including enlargement of the spinal cord with associated cysts or syrinx, and with a seemingly disproportional amount of oedema and venous congestion. The tumour is isointense on T_1, enhances with gadolinium, and has high signal intensity on T_2. Serpigious flow voids may be present, but angiography will more clearly demonstrate the vascular nature of the tumour and the characteristically large draining veins (Lowe 2000).

Treatment of spinal haemangioblastoma is surgical resection when feasible, and the potential benefits are judged less than the risks. Haemangioblastomas are very discrete and can be completely resected using microsurgical techniques. As with other highly vascular lesions, preoperative embolization may be a consideration, but there is always concern regarding the risks of this procedure. In circumstances where multiple hemangioblastomas are present in the same patient, only the symptomatic tumour is surgically addressed. The remaining tumours are followed with serial imaging, and resection is usually considered at symptom progression when the tumour increases in size and symptoms are imminent (Miller and McCutcheon 2000).

Conclusion

Spinal cord tumours are rare in children, making their management difficult because there is often little empirical evidence to support clinical practices. The prognosis for tumour control and for neurological function is dependent upon several factors including: tumour histology, location, size, duration and type of symptoms, and surgical resectability.

The most important factor when predicting functional recovery (if there is to be any) is the time to recovery: the longer the interval between neurological improvements, the more pessimistic one becomes for any meaningful recovery. While physical and occupational therapy, satisfactory skin care, management of bowel and bladder continence, and attention to joint stability and flexibility may have some impact on neurological recovery, the ability of these interventions to positively influence neurological recovery is modest since they primarily set the stage for potential central and peripheral nervous system recovery. While stem cell therapies are now more commonly discussed, their feasibility for improving or reversing spinal cord damage is only in the developmental stage.

REFERENCES

Allen JC, Aviner S, Yates AJ, Boyett JM, Cherlow JM, Turski PA, Epstein F, Finlay JL (1998) Treatment of high-grade spinal cord astrocytoma of childhood with "8 in 1" chemotherapy and radiotherapy: a pilot study of CCG-945. *J Neurosurg* **88**: 215–220.

Bouffet E, Pierre Kahn A, Marchal JC, Jouvet A, Kalifa C, Choux M, Dhellemmes P, Guerin J, Tremoulet M, Mottolese C (1998) Prognostic factors in pediatric spinal cord astrocytoma. *Cancer* **83**: 2391–2398.

Brotchi J, Noterman J, Baleriaux D. (1992) Surgery of intramedullary spinal cord tumours. *Acta Neurochir* **116**: 176–178.

Caviness JA, Tucker MH, Pia SK, Tam DA (1998) Hydrocephalus as a possible early symptom in a child with a spinal cord tumor. *Pediatr Neurol* **18**: 169–171.

Chan HS, Becker LE, Hoffman HJ, Humphreys RP, Hendrick EB, Fitz CR, Chuang SH (1984) Myxopapillary ependymoma of the filum terminale and cauda equine in childhood: report of seven cases and review of the literature. *Neurosurgery* **14**: 204–211.

Chinn DM, Donaldson SS, Dahl GV, Wilson JD, Huhn SL, Fisher PG (2000) Management of children with metastatic spinal myxopapillary ependymoma using craniospinal irradiation. *Med Ped Oncol* **35**: 443–445.

Cohen AR, Wishoff JH, Allen JC, Epstein FJ (1989) Malignant astrocytomas of the spinal cord. *J Neurosurg* **70**: 50–54.

Constantini S, Epstein FJ (1996) Intraspinal tumors in infants and children. In: Youmans JR, ed. *Neurological Surgery*. Philadelphia: WB Saunders, pp. 3123–3133.

Constantini S, Miller DC, Allen JC, Rorke LB, Freed D, Epstein FJ (2000) Radical excision of intramedullary spinal cord tumors: surgical morbidity and long-term follow-up evaluation in 164 children and young adults. *J Neurosurg* **93**: 183–193.

DeSousa AL, Kalsbeck JE, Mealey J, Campbell RL, Hockey A (1979) Intraspinal tumors in children. *J Neurosurg* **51**: 437–445.

Doireau V, Grill J, Zerah M, Lellouch-Tubiana A, Couanet D, Chastagner P, Marchal JC, Grignon Y, Chouffai Z, Kalifa C (1999) Chemotherapy for unresectable and recurrent intramedullary glial tumours in children. Brain Tumours Subcommittee of the French Society of Paediatric Oncology (SFOP). *Br J Cancer* **81**: 835–840.

Epstein FJ, Epstein N (1982) Surgical treatment of spinal cord astrocytomas of childhood. *J Neurosurg* **57**: 685–689.

Fine MJ, Kricheff II, Freed D, Epstein FJ (1995) Spinal cord ependymomas: MR imaging features. *Radiology* **197**: 655–658.

Fisher PG, Tontiplaphol A, Pearlman EM, Duffner PK, Hyder DJ, Stolle CA, Vortmeyer AO, Zhuang Z (2002) Childhood cerebellar hemangioblastoma does not predict germline or somatic mutations in the von Hippel–Lindau tumor suppressor gene. *Ann Neurol* **2**: 257–260.

Fort DW, Packer RJ, Kirckpatrick GB, Kuttesch JF, Ater JL (1998) Carboplatin and vincristine for pediatric spinal cord astrocytoma (8th International Neuro-Oncology Symposium Abstract). *Child's Nerv Syst* **14**: 484.

Gagliardi FM, Cervoni L, Domenicucci M, Celli P, Salvati M (1993) Ependymomas of the filum terminale in childhood: report of four cases and review of the literature. *Child's Nerv Syst* **9**: 3–6.

Goh KY, Velasquez L, Epstein FJ (1997) Pediatric intramedullary spinal cord tumors: is surgery alone enough? *Pediatric Neurosurg* **27**: 34–39.

Hardison HH, Packer RJ, Rorke LB, Schut L, Sutton LN, Bruce DA (1987) Outcome of children with primary intramedullary spinal cord tumors. *Child's Nerv Syst* **3**: 89–92.

Hassall TE, Mitchell AE, Ashley DM (2001) Carboplatin chemotherapy for progressive intramedullary spinal cord low-grade gliomas in children: three case studies and a review of the literature. *Neuro-oncol* **3**: 251–257.

Houten JK, Cooper PR (2000) Spinal cord astrocytomas: presentation, management and outcome. *J Neurooncol* **47**: 219–224.

Leung SK, Ohh M (2002) Playing Tag with HIF: The VHL Story. *J Biomed Biotechnol* **2**: 131–135.

Lonjon M, Goh KY, Epstein FJ (1998) Intramedullary spinal cord ependymomas in children: treatment, results and follow-up. *Pediatr Neurosurg* **29**: 178–183.

Lowe GM (2000) Magnetic resonance imaging of intramedullary spinal cord tumors. *J Neurooncol* **47**: 195–210.

Madden JR, Fenton LZ, Weil M, Winston KR, Partington M, Foreman NK (2001) Experience with tamoxifen/etoposide in the treatment of a child with myxopapillary ependymoma. *Med Ped Oncol* **37**: 67–69.

McLaughlin MP, Marcus RB, Buatti JM, McCollough WM, Mickle JP, Kedar A, Maria BL, Million RR (1998) Ependymoma: results, prognostic factors and treatment recommendations. *Int J Radiat Oncol Biol Phys* **40**: 845–850.

Merchant TE, Nguyen D, Thompson SJ, Reardon DA, Kun LE, Sanford RA (1999) High-grade pediatric spinal cord tumors. *Pediatr Neurosurg* **30**: 1–5.

Merchant TE, Kiehna EN, Thompson SJ, Heideman RL, Sanford RA, Kun LE (2000) Pediatric low-grade and ependymal spinal cord tumors. *Pediatr Neurosurg* **32**: 30–36.

Miller DC (2000) Surgical pathology of intramedullary spinal cord neoplasms. *J Neurooncol* **47**: 189–194.

Miller DJ, McCutcheon IE (2000) Hemangioblastoma and other uncommon intramedullary tumors. *J Neurooncol* **47**: 253–270.

Nagib MG, O'Fallon MT (1997) Myxopapillary ependymoma of the conus medullaris and filum terminale in the pediatric age group. *Pediatr Neurosurg* **26**: 2–7.

O'Sullivan C, Jenkins RD, Doherty MA, Hoffman HJ, Greenberg ML (1994) Spinal cord tumors in children: long term results of combined surgical and radiation treatment. *J Neurosurg* **81**: 507–512.

Rossitch E, Ziedman SM, Burger PC, Curnes JT, Harsh C, Anscher M, Oakes WJ (1990) Clinical and pathological analysis of spinal cord astrocytomas in children. *Neurosurgery* **27**: 193–196.

Shaw EG, Evans RG, Scheithauer BW, Ilstrup DM, Earle JD (1987) Postoperative radiotherapy of intracranial ependymoma in pediatric and adult patients. *Int J Radiat Oncol Biol Phys* **10**: 1457–1462.

Stiller CA, Nectoux J (1994) International incidence of childhood brain and spinal tumors. *Int J Epidemiol* **23**: 458–464.

Vles JS, Grubben CP, van Ooy A, Weil EH (1990) Holocord astrocytomas in childhood. *Clin Neurol Neurosurg* **92**: 361–364.

19
METASTATIC DISEASE AFFECTING THE CNS

Stephen Lowis

Leukaemia

CNS involvement with acute leukaemia, defined as more than 5 unequivocal leukaemia cells per cubic millimetre of CSF, occurs in fewer than 5% of patients with acute lymphoblastic leukaemia (ALL) at diagnosis, although in the 1960s, when increased haematological remissions began to be seen, the CNS was the main site of relapse (Bleyer and Poplack 1985, Kreuger et al. 1991, Reiter et al. 1994). The incidence of CNS relapse has been greatly reduced by CNS-directed therapy, but remains an important sanctuary site, particularly for T-lineage leukaemias and those presenting in infancy (Chessells et al. 1994). CNS involvement may be asymptomatic, and identified by lumbar puncture as part of standard initial assessment, or may be associated with symptoms or signs suggestive of local brain or meningeal involvement. Unexplained hydrocephalus or symptoms of raised intracranial pressure are the most frequently encountered symptoms (Hardisty and Norman 1967), but behavioural change, weight gain, visual symptoms and isolated cranial nerve palsies are all reported features of newly diagnosed or recurrent leukaemia. A young child presenting with a lower motor VII nerve palsy should not be assumed to have an idiosyncratic cause (Bell's palsy), and steps should be taken to exclude malignancy, including ALL. Patients may also present with signs of meningeal irritation, with focal neurological signs, or with acute intracranial haemorrhage, particularly in association with high-count leukaemia and an associated coagulopathy. Rarely, CNS recurrence may be seen in the spine and lead to compression (Kataoka et al. 1995).

CNS involvement confers a somewhat worse prognosis for the patient with these conditions, but current treatment strategies still offer 5 year overall survival, which is comparable to other patients, provided appropriate CNS-directed therapy is administered. Craniospinal radiotherapy is necessary for patients with known CNS leukaemia, whereas this can usually be avoided in the absence of overt disease. The current UK protocol requires a dose of 24 Gy to the craniospinal axis, in 15 fractions, given to patients who are older than 2 years at diagnosis.

Solid tumours

The development of brain metastases in adult patients with solid malignancy is relatively common, arising in 20–30% of patients. Metastases arise most commonly from melanoma, and lung, breast, renal or colonic carcinoma (Le Chevalier et al. 1985). In up to a quarter of such patients, the metastatic disease will be a presenting feature of the patient's illness.

TABLE 19.1
Reported tumour types in brain metastases from three series

	Vannucci + Graus (combined)*	Bouffet**
Ewing's sarcoma	2/27	3/54
Neuroblastoma	2/114	3/160
Wilms' tumour	4/31	1/78
Soft tissue sarcoma	6/66	1/53
Osteogenic sarcoma	6/50	3/66
Germ cell tumour	4/8	0/27
Other	7/60	1/48
Total	31/356	12/486
Frequency	8.7%	2.5%

*Vannucci and Baten (1974), Graus et al. (1983).
**Bouffet et al. (1997a).

Brain metastasis arising from solid malignancies is less common, with incidences of 6.0% and 9.8% in two series (Vannucci and Baten 1974, Graus et al. 1983). These reports came from post-mortem examination of patients who had died from malignant solid tumours, most commonly osteogenic sarcoma, Ewing's sarcoma, soft tissue sarcoma and neuroblastoma, but also Wilms' tumour, germ cell tumour, retinoblastoma and melanoma. Perhaps more relevant is the series of Bouffet et al. (1997a) of patients presenting with CNS involvement and investigated before death, where 12 patients from a total population of 486 patients with solid organ malignancy showed brain metastasis, an incidence of 2.5%. These data are summarized in Table 19.1. The majority of these patients presented with clinical features suggestive of CNS disease, but 2 had no symptoms. Nine patients had metastatic disease at presentation, and 11 had already received intensive multi-agent chemotherapy (including 6 with high-dose chemotherapy and autologous stem cell reconstitution). The median time from diagnosis to presentation of brain metastases was 15 months. All except one patient died soon after presentation (median 3 months), despite intervention. One patient with retinoblastoma responded to chemotherapy, and went on to receive high-dose chemotherapy and local radiotherapy, and was alive at the time of publication.

The prognosis for patients with brain metastasis is therefore extremely poor, and management is often supportive. However, this is not the case universally, and a series of six patients with Wilms' tumour showed successful treatment in three, which is comparable to the outcome of patients with relapsed disease at other sites (Lowis et al. 1998).

Spinal metastatic disease
The development of metastatic disease affecting the spinal cord also appears to be significantly less common in children than in adults, and the pattern of involvement is different. Typically, adults will develop bony extradural disease. Compressive cord symptoms develop because of either bony vertebral collapse or expansion of involved bone. Plain spinal X-ray has a high (90%) likelihood of identifying an abnormality leading to diagnosis (Portenoy et al. 1989). In children, however, metastatic disease often involves intradural spread or

298

direct extension through an intervertebral foramen, with no bony involvement. The diagnostic yield from plain spinal radiographs is therefore less than for adult patients, with abnormalities visible in only 30–50% of cases (Lewis et al. 1986). The frequency of spinal cord disease is also less than in adult patients, being 2.7% in the series of Lewis et al. (1986) and Bouffet et al. (1997). The majority of these cases were in patients with known solid tumour malignancy, and a median delay from initial diagnosis to spinal recurrence of between 13 and 21 months (absolute range 2 to 84 months) has been reported (Baten and Vannucci 1977, Lewis et al. 1986, Bouffet et al. 1997). In a significant number of patients, cord compression is the presenting feature of malignancy. Significant diagnostic delay is a feature of such patients.

The most common area for spinal cord compression to occur is in the thoracic spine, with cervical compression the least common. The most common symptoms are back pain (17/24 patients in the series of Lewis), weakness affecting one or more limbs (14/24), and loss of sphincter control and sensory loss (approximately half of all patients). Three distinct patterns of presentation can be identified, depending on whether the cord, conus medullaris or cauda equina is affected (Lewis et al. 1986), and it is worthwhile describing these.

In patients with compression of the cord itself, there is moderate or severe flaccid weakness. Deep tendon reflexes are reduced, plantars extensor. Sphincter control is usually preserved.

In patients with a lesion affecting the conus medullaris, there is loss of power, but relatively normal tone. Reflexes are variably affected, plantars extensor, and sensory loss is variable, often affecting the perineal region or posterior thigh.

A lesion involving the cauda equina will typically cause relatively mild loss of power, ipsilateral loss of deep tendon reflexes, flexor plantars and a dermotomal pattern of sensory loss. Approximately half of such patients will have loss of sphincter control.

When symptoms and signs of disease are clear cut there should be little difficulty in making a diagnosis and investigating appropriately. Whole spine MRI is indicated for any patient with suspected cord compression. Other investigations are rarely necessary.

Treatment of spinal cord compression is discussed in Chapter 9. Initial treatment will usually be with high-dose dexamethasone, although the value of this is uncertain. For a patient presenting with newly diagnosed disease, surgical decompression may be indicated, but in the context of recurrent metastatic disease, extensive decompressive laminectomy is less likely to be of benefit. The large majority of such patients will die of their disease within a short space of time (median 2 months in Bouffet's series), and therefore an approach that limits overall morbidity in the short term is often preferred (Bouffet et al. 1997). Radiotherapy is most often an appropriate alternative, and is particularly effective in relief of pain. Recovery of mobility in patients who have lost their ability to walk, and of continence where this has been lost, is seen in approximately 50% of patients.

Summary
Metastatic disease affecting the brain should be considered in patients with advanced malignant disease, particularly where there is recurrent tumour. Whilst the overall prognosis for many such patients is poor, the patient must be assessed as an individual. Isolated metastasis may be amenable to active, aggressive treatment.

It is clear that, although uncommon, metastatic disease affecting the spine is likely to cause significant morbidity in a group of patients approaching the end of life. Any symptoms that may suggest cord compression in a patient with known malignancy must be taken as strong indications for whole spine MRI, and active intervention considered as soon as possible in order to avoid unnecessary morbidity.

REFERENCES

Baten M, Vannucci RC (1977) Intraspinal metastatic disease in childhood cancer. *J Pediatr* **90**: 207–212.
Bleyer WA, Poplack DG (1985) Prophylaxis and treatment of leukemia in the central nervous system and other sanctuaries. *Semin Oncol* **12**: 131–148.
Bouffet E, Doumi N, Thiesse P, Mottolese C, Jouvet A, Lacroze M, Carrie C, Frappaz D, Brunat-Mentigny M (1997a) Brain metastases in children with solid tumors. *Cancer* **79**: 403–410.
Bouffet E, Marec-Berard P, Thiesse P, Carrie C, Risk T, Jouvet A, Brunat-Mentigny M, Mottolese C (1997b) Spinal cord compression by secondary epi- and intradural metastases in childhood. *Child's Nerv Syst* **13**: 383–387.
Chessells JM, Eden OB, Bailey CC, Lilleyman JS, Richards SM (1994) Acute lymphoblastic leukaemia in infancy: experience in MRC UKALL trials. Report from the Medical Research Council Working Party on Childhood Leukaemia. *Leukemia* **8**: 1275–1279.
Graus F, Walker RW, Allen JC (1983) Brain metastases in children. *J Pediatr* **103**: 558–561.
Hardisty RM, Norman PM (1967) Meningeal leukaemia. *Arch Dis Child* **42**: 441–447.
Kataoka A, Shimizu K, Matsumoto T, Shintaku N, Okuno T, Takahashi Y, Akaishi K (1995) Epidural spinal cord compression as an initial symptom in childhood acute lymphoblastic leukemia: rapid decompression by local irradiation and systemic chemotherapy. *Pediatr Hematol Oncol* **12**: 179–184.
Kreuger A, Garwicz S, Hertz H, Jonmundsson G, Lanning M, Lie SO, Moe PJ, Salmi TT, Schroder H, Siimes MA, et al. (1991) Central nervous system disease in childhood acute lymphoblastic leukemia: prognostic factors and results of treatment. *Pediatr Hematol Oncol* **8**: 291–299.
Le Chevalier T, Smith FP, Caille P, Constans JP, Rouesse JG (1985) Sites of primary malignancies in patients presenting with cerebral metastases. A review of 120 cases. *Cancer* **56**: 880–882.
Lewis DW, Packer RJ, Raney B, Rak IW, Belasco J, Lange B (1986) Incidence, presentation, and outcome of spinal cord disease in children with systemic cancer. *Pediatrics* **78**: 438–443.
Lowis SP, Foot A, Gerrard MP, Charles A, Imeson J, Middleton H, Coakham H, Bouffet E (1998) Central nervous system metastasis in Wilms' tumor: a review of three consecutive United Kingdom trials. *Cancer* **83**: 2023–2029.
Portenoy RK, Galer BS, Salamon O, Freilich M, Finkel JE, Milstein D, Thaler HT, Berger M, Lipton RB (1989) Identification of epidural neoplasm. Radiography and bone scintigraphy in the symptomatic and asymptomatic spine. *Cancer* **64**: 2207–2213.
Reiter A, Schrappe M, Ludwig WD, Hiddemann W, Sauter S, Henze G, Zimmermann M, Lampert F, Havers W, Niethammer D, et al. (1994) Chemotherapy in 998 unselected childhood acute lymphoblastic leukemia patients. Results and conclusions of the multicenter trial ALL-BFM 86. *Blood* **84**: 3122–3133.
Vannucci RC, Baten M (1974) Cerebral metastatic disease in childhood. *Neurology* **24**: 981–985.

SECTION THREE

LATE EFFECTS,
REHABILITATION
AND
PALLIATIVE CARE

20
LATE EFFECTS OF CNS TUMOURS

Adam Glaser and Gary Butler

Survival from childhood cancer represents a success story for modern medicine. However, up to 50% of all survivors are thought to be at risk of developing a disability with resultant impairment in quality of life (Meadows and Hobbie 1986). This figure is likely to be an underestimate for survivors of CNS tumours, although accurate estimates of the comprehensive burden of morbidity experienced by this group have not been made.

This chapter will outline the late effects for which survivors of CNS tumours are at risk, as well as identifying strategies to document late effects in a standardized and systematic manner. Specific areas of concern will be explored under the categorization of the components of health, e.g. physical, mental, social and autonomous sequelae.

Aetiology

Brain damage following cancer treatments is recognized (Bleyer 1998). Late sequelae of CNS tumours on the developing brain may result from either the tumour itself or therapeutic modalities used for its treatment: primary brain and spinal tumours have the potential to cause direct tumoral effects and raised intracranial pressure with significant local and global structural morbidity. Radiation-induced morbidity may have dramatic consequences, developing many years after therapy has been completed. Leukoencephalopathy may result, as well as being caused by chemotherapy (Ball et al. 1992). Drug-induced late effects may involve multiple organs depending upon the agents used. Chemotherapy dose intensification and high-dose regimes continue to be introduced for the management of CNS tumours, and these may have far-reaching consequences. Renal, hepatic, cardiac and pulmonary impairment, along with second malignancies and infertility may all be experienced after cytotoxic drug exposure. Potential late effects will depend upon the chemotherapeutic agents administered. Long-term surveillance strategies to identify these will need to be tailored to the specific treatment regime (Kissen and Wallace 1995).

Following completion of therapy, children frequently experience great difficulties in returning to a normal life. Reintegration into society and maintenance of as normal a lifestyle as possible are two of the primary aims of children's cancer services (SIOP 1995). Consequently, the concepts of *quality of life* and *health-related quality of life* must be considered when evaluating the late effects associated with survival from CNS tumours.

Quality of life

Determination of morbidity following survival from life-threatening conditions is essential. Detection of emerging problems will allow attempts to be made to ameliorate them and to enable provision of support services to enhance function and reintegration within society. Equally, future treatment strategies can be refined to reduce negative late sequelae, through the identification of the consequences of survival for individuals treated in a specified manner for a specific tumour.

The 'cost of cure' is not restricted to the individual but impacts on society in general. Increasing numbers of survivors with disability and health problems make previously unencountered demands on their carers and healthcare providers. Systematic monitoring of the morbidity burden is required if an appropriate infrastructure to support these needs is to be provided. Government agencies have identified 'outcomes' as an important part of the wider health agenda (Calman 1996). The majority of major clinical trial sponsors (including the Medical Research Council and National Cancer Institute) insist that new trials consider inbuilt quality of life assessments if they are to be supported (Nayfield et al. 1992, Medical Research Council 1996).

Despite its widespread use and recognition of its importance as an outcome measure, little concensus exists regarding the definition of 'quality of life' (*Lancet* 1991). The World Health Organization has provided the following definition: "Quality of life is defined as an individual's perception of their position in life in the context of the culture and value systems in which they live and in relation to their goals, expectations, standards and concerns. It is a broad ranging concept affected in a complex way by the person's physical health, psychological state, level of independence, social relationships, and their relationships to salient features of their environment" (WHOQUOL Group 1993).

Complex issues of *growth* (an increase in size), *development* (the acquisition of new skills) and *dependence on others* must all be considered when evaluating quality of life in children (Glaser and Walker 1995). The American Cancer Society has acknowledged these issues in their definition of 'quality of life' in children: "Quality of life is multidimensional. It includes, but is not limited to, the social, physical and emotional functioning of the child and adolescent, and when indicated, his/her family. Measurement of quality of life must be from the perspective of the child, adolescent and family, and it must be sensitive to the changes that occur through development" (Bradlyn et al. 1996).

Health and health-related quality of life

While monitoring for late effects of CNS tumours, it is reasonable to focus on health-related quality of life, thereby excluding factors such as spirituality, finance and income, freedom and quality of environment. This restriction is justified as the goal of health care is to maximize the health component of quality of life. Health equates to "a state of complete physical, mental and social well-being and not merely the absence of disease or infirmity" (WHO 1947); subsequently the term "autonomy" has been added to this definition (WHO 1987).

Childhood illness often manifests itself as inappropriate physical, emotional or intellectual development rather than as specific clinical symptoms or signs (Starfield et al. 1993). Hence, child health can be defined as "the ability to participate fully in developmentally appropriate activities and requires physical, psychological and social energy" (Pantel and Lewis 1987).

Physical sequelae

NEUROENDOCRINE DYSFUNCTION

Although current treatment regimens for childhood brain tumours have resulted in increased survival, the frequency of long-term side-effects is therefore greater, and persistent and progressive dysfunction is seen in the endocrine system. The effects are multifactorial and are dependent on the timing, dosage and combination of treatments given (surgery, radiotherapy and chemotherapy). For central tumours involving the hypothalamo-pituitary axis, it is not surprising that either they will present with endocrine symptoms and signs, or endocrine dysfunction will arise from the direct effects of surgery and radiotherapy. However, it is also apparent from several studies that radiotherapy directed to tumours distant from the hypothalamo-pituitary axis will have endocrine side-effects resulting from spread outside the radiation field. These tend to occur in a dose-dependent relationship. This dysfunction may not be apparent initially and may evolve over time. It is also clear that the younger the child at the time of treatment, the more severe the eventual endocrine deficit will become.

EFFECTS ON SPECIFIC ENDOCRINE AXES

Growth and growth hormone (GH) secretion

It is clear from many studies that the most radiosensitive pituitary cell type is the gonadotroph and that abnormalities of GH secretory dynamics are common after as little as 10 Gy, whereas doses of more than 30 Gy directly or indirectly to the hypothalamus/pituitary are likely to cause a permanent loss of GH secretion. This may become apparent shortly after the course of radiotherapy is finished, but GH deficiency may evolve more slowly, depending on the age, dose and fractionation of the radiation regimen (Ogilvy-Stuart and Shalet 1995a, Schmiegelow et al. 2000). Reductions in GH secretion are directly correlated to the height velocity, so regular monitoring of a child's growth from diagnosis is advisable in order to detect faltering at the earliest opportunity. The earlier the diagnosis of GH deficiency is made, the earlier GH replacement can begin and consequently the total loss of height can be minimized, and many GH-treated children can now attain normal adult stature.

Knowledge of the normal rates of growth at each age is essential, alongside pubertal staging, in managing a child following cranial radiotherapy. Both true precocious puberty and an earlier then expected onset of puberty with an accelerated transit time through puberty are common following cranial radiation, and growth failure can paradoxically be masked by a blunted precocious pubertal growth spurt masquerading as an apparently normal height velocity (Ogilvy-Stuart and Shalet 1995a, Bozzola et al. 2001).

Radiotherapy may also limit growth by direct effects on the skeleton. Craniospinal irradiation causes impairment of spinal growth and consequently a reduced adult height and obvious body disproportion, often causing a disordered body image in the adolescent. The younger the age at irradiation, the worse this disproportion becomes (Clayton and Shalet 1991).

Chemotherapy is frequently given as an adjunct to radiotherapy and may have an added effect on growth impairment (Ogilvy-Stuart and Shalet 1995b). Standard chemotherapeutic agents as well as glucocorticoids have also been demonstrated in vitro to have a growth suppressive effect (Crofton et al. 1998).

305

Thyroid axis

Central hypothyroidism is less common than GH deficiency and may evolve more slowly, rather similar to the situation in idiopathic hypopituitarism. Although this may suggest that the pituitary thyrotroph cells are relatively radioresistant, this is not true for the thyroid gland itself. The gland may receive a small dose of radiation as scatter from a cranial beam, or may suffer damage from the radiation beam directly during spinal radiotherapy (Ogilvy-Stuart et al. 1991, Schmiegelow et al. 2003). In the latter case, hypothyroidism is inevitable and needs to be screened for as a matter of routine. Patients should have their thyroid function checked at least annually from the end of treatment. The level of thyroxine (T4, free or total) should be carefully monitored, as a rise in thyroid stimulating hormone may not be apparent due to hypothalamo-pituitary damage. Checking pretreatment thyroxine levels at first diagnosis is most helpful here as a permanent downward drift in T4 can be watched for and replacement started before thyroxine levels become subnormal and the patient clinically hypothyroid. In the absence of pre-treatment thyroxine levels, treatment should aim to pitch T4 levels in the upper-normal range, ignoring TSH completely.

Occasionally the need for acute surgery (such as a tumour recurrence or a blocked CSF drainage shunt) may precipitate a hypothyroid crisis manifested by slow or absent recovery from a general anaesthetic. In this situation, once the diagnosis is confirmed and adrenal support given if required, treatment should begin with triiodothyronine (T3) as well as T4. The T3 can be discontinued once a clinical improvement is seen and T3 levels are normal. If hypothyroidism is found at first diagnosis and surgery is urgent, then thyroid replacement should begin with both T3 and T4 simultaneously.

Adrenal axis

The extent of the effect of cranial irradiation on the hypothalamo-pituitary–adrenal axis is debated. Whereas in adult patients it is the third most commonly affected axis, in children this may be as low as 10% or as high as 60%, with dysfunction beginning soon after high-dose irradiation finishes (Fujiwara et al. 1995, Spoudeas et al. 2000). Symptoms are non-specific, mainly tiredness, lethargy, a tendency to fall asleep easily, and a loss of stamina and concentration. The defect appears to be central, affecting ACTH responsiveness. Pituitary–adrenal function is rarely completely absent, but the cortisol stress response is frequently reduced. Therefore patients who require cortisol replacement with hydrocortisone need to mimic this response by doubling their replacement doses during acute illnesses and trauma. In grave situations the hydrocortisone should be given intravenously. At present there is no evidence to suggest that this axis is affected by chemotherapy alone or in combination with radiotherapy for brain tumours. Mineralocorticoid secretion is not ACTH dependent so is not affected by any treatment regimens.

Puberty and fertility axis

The second most commonly affected hormone by cranial irradiation is GnRH. Pituitary FSH and LH release is very sensitive to subtle variations in the pulsatile secretion of GnRH. The variability in the dynamics of this hormone system is what is responsible for the onset and progression of puberty, spermatogenesis and the menstrual cycle. Whereas doses greater than 50 Gy may causes loss of GnRH secretion, doses commonly used for brain tumours (25–50 Gy) can cause paradoxical effects on this axis (Ogilvy-Stuart and Shalet 1993, 1995a). Precocious puberty is frequently seen. A reduction in the age at starting puberty is inversely related to the dose of radiation received. This is thought to be a direct central effect but hypothalamic damage is associated with obesity (Lustig et al. 1999) and the consequent increase in insulin and the adipocyte hormone leptin may also contribute to the occurrence of early puberty.

Signs of sexual development should be checked for regularly in young children as an early onset and a rapid progression through the process of puberty can occur. The result of this is a significant diminution in adult stature from the loss of childhood growing time and a blunted adolescent growth spurt. Even if growth hormone is replaced, it is necessary to intervene by blocking FSH and LH secretion with one of the long-acting GnRH analogues. Once treatment is discontinued, one can see paradoxical GnRH insufficiency with failure to progress in puberty after high-dose irradiation, and this requires sex hormone replacement with testosterone or oestradiol.

Secondary infertility is rare and relatively easy to treat with exogenous gonadotrophins if no gonadotoxic chemotherapy has been given. However, alkylating agents are frequently used as an adjunct to radiotherapy in brain tumour regimens and are likely to have a direct effect on the oocyte in the female and the germinal epithelium in the male causing significant impairment (Clayton et al. 1988, 1989). In males, this can be predicted by raised gonado-trophins (especially FSH) alongside low inhibin B (Thomson et al. 2002) during and after puberty and reduced testicular volume in postpubertal males. The most reliable investigation is semen analysis. In the female, primary or secondary amenorrhoea, reduced ovarian size on ultrasound, low oestradiol and raised gonadotrophins are suggestive but not absolutely predictive of impaired fertility, since as in the male, late recovery is sometimes possible. Rarely the ovary may be damaged if it falls within the radiation field. The ovary is a very mobile organ and oophoropexy can be performed with success to move the ovary away from the radiation field.

Second malignancies

After recurrence of primary malignancy, second neoplasms are the commonest cause of death in long-term survivors (5 years and over from completion of therapy) of childhood and adolescent cancer (Mertens et al. 2001. Neglia et al. 2001). The risk depends upon the original diagnosis, presence of genetic predisposition syndromes and therapeutic modalities administered.

Neurofibromatosis with mutation of the NF1 gene is associated with astrocytomas, dermal and plexiform neurofibromas, as well as acute myeloid leukaemia, rhabdomyosarcoma and phaeochromocytoma (Pollack and Mulvihill 1997, Listernick et al. 1999).

Li–Fraumeni syndrome due to a p53 gene germline mutation is associated with intracranial (low- and high-grade gliomata, primitive neuroectodermal and choroid plexus tumours) and extracranial neoplasms (adrenocortical carcinoma, breast cancer, sarcomas, leukaemia) (Malkin et al. 1990).

Medulloblastoma occurs in 3% of individuals with *Gorlin syndrome*, which is associated with germline mutations of the PTCH sonic hedgehog receptor. Multiple skeletal anomalies and macrocephaly are found at birth. The risk of basal cell carcinoma is massively increased within cranial radiation fields (Kimonis et al. 1997). Medulloblastomas and gliomata occur in *Turcot syndrome*, a heterogeneous group of disorders associated with the occurrence of adenomatous polyposis (Hamilton et al. 1995). Turcot syndrome is discussed in greater detail in Chapter 2.

Chemotherapeutic agents may be carcinogenic. The epipodophyllotoxins, such as etoposide, increase the risk of acute non-lymphoblastic leukaemia. No significant cumulative effect has been found (Smith et al. 1999). Secondary leukaemia may occur following exposure to alkylating agents, with a mean latency period of 60–84 months and association with a myelodysplastic prodrome (Blayney et al. 1987).

Secondary solid tumours may result form radiation exposure. Skin cancers, thyroid carcinoma, soft-tissue sarcomas and secondary brain tumours (meningioma and glioma) may all arise within radiotherapy fields (Rosso et al. 1994. Neglia et al. 2001). Advice regarding sun exposure should be given to all survivors following radiation therapy.

Shunts

Brain tumours may result in hydrocephalus, requiring ventriculo-peritoneal shunt placement. It is essential that survivors and their health care providers remember that a shunt remains in situ. They may malfunction in three ways: infection, mechanical failure or functional failure with over- or under-draining (Chumas et al. 2001). Other shunt complications may include fracturing of the tubing or migration of part or all of the shunt (Drake and Saint-Rose 1995).

Bone and dental effects

Corticosteroids, frequently used to control symptoms of raised intracranial pressure, may lead to avascular necrosis, osteopenia and osteoporosis (Glaser et al. 1997a). Radiotherapy to the spine and prolonged periods of immobility may increase the risk of these complications (Tefft et al. 1976). Ovarian or testicular failure may increase the risk of osteopenic changes. Abnormalities may be diagnosed with plain radiographs, although assessment of bone mineral density with DEXA scans is more sensitive (Leiper 1998). Symptomatic treatment is indicated.

Scoliosis may develop many years after spinal surgery, involving laminectomy or spinal radiotherapy (Mehlman et al. 1999).

Dental complications follow cranial radiotherapy. Delayed or arrested dental development may be seen after low doses of cranial irradiation (~1.8 Gy). Higher radiation exposure increases the risks of malocclusion and dental caries (Dens et al. 1995). The younger the age at which radiation is administered, the more marked the effects are (Kaste et al. 1997). Regular dental review and good levels of dental hygiene should be recommended to all following cranial radiotherapy (Holtta et al. 2002).

Neurocognitive and behavioural sequelae

Tumour location, patient age at treatment and the administered therapies may all influence the severity of late cognitive deficits. Brainstem and hypothalamic tumours, or those extending into the fourth ventricle, have been associated with more severe deficits in IQ than those in other locations (Danoff et al. 1982, Hirsh et al. 1979).

The nature of brain damage that occurs after some cancer therapies is recognized. Cranial radiotherapy for leukaemia is known to cause impaired school performance ratings and reductions in IQ of up to 20 points (along with poor growth and disordered pubertal development). These effects are more severe in younger children, with those under 7 years being most susceptible (Ellenberg et al. 1987, Radcliffe et al. 1992, Anderson et al. 1994). In the case of primary brain and spinal tumours, the radiotherapy doses are frequently much greater than for leukaemia treatment. The use of focused doses of cranial radiation, given at the limits of brain tissue tolerance, enhances the risks and severity of these effects. Local damage resulting from the tumour itself and neurosurgery may serve to compound these established mechanisms of injury.

Late cognitive effects of chemotherapy are less well defined. Methotrexate may lead to leukoencephalopathy with resultant chronic dementia (Allen et al. 1980). However, the cognitive effects of high-dose methotrexate are being evaluated as part of ongoing leukaemia trials (Medical Research Council Working Party on Leukaemia 1997).

Deficits in IQ in long-term survivors of CNS tumours over 10 years from completion of therapy have been documented. In one study, following surgical resection and radiation for medulloblastoma, average IQ was 78, whilst an age- and sex-matched cohort of children with posterior fossa astrocytomas treated with surgery alone (IQ 99) had no significant differences from a control group (IQ 104) (Spiegler et al. 1998). The same study demonstrated that functional deficits were not confined to the irradiated medulloblastoma patients. Following surgery alone, the astrocytoma survivors perceived they had cognitive and mobility problems as assessed by the Health Utilities Index (Barr et al. 1994). Utility score for the controls was 0.97, for posterior fossa astrocytoma survivors 0.89, and for medulloblastoma survivors 0.84 (1.00 equates to perfect health, 0.00 to death).

Behavioural and adjustment problems are commonly reported after CNS tumours, with one-quarter of survivors requiring special educational courses (Slavc et al. 1994). Survivors of cancers with severe late effects are known to experience poor self-esteem and to be less confident about themselves, while feeling less in control of their lives (Glaser et al. 1997b, Greenberg et al. 1989). In keeping with this is the finding that following cancer, children may be less sociable, more isolated and withdrawn (Larcombe et al. 1990, Eiser 1991).

Social sequelae and autonomy

Survivors of childhood CNS tumours have repeatedly been found to have economic sequelae of cancer extending beyond the first decade after treatment (Hays et al. 1992). Therefore, it is essential that attention is paid to issues surrounding their education, employment and ability to function as adults within society. However, despite significant problems having been identified, a significant number do cope well and achieve similar lifestyle goals to their siblings (Evans and Radford 1995).

EDUCATION
A study of survivors of CNS tumours in school has demonstrated impaired cognition,

emotion and self-esteem. However, they attended school willingly and interacted well with their peer-groups (Glaser et al. 1997b). Normal school behaviour has been found by other studies (Gregory et al. 1994). This may in part reflect the increasing use of education intervention programmes (utilizing teams of liaison nurses, teachers and social workers) to support active reintegration within the classroom (Baysinger et al. 1993).

The reduced health status of this group of individuals identifies them as having 'special educational need' under the UK Education Acts 1981 and 1993, requiring intensive physical and psychosocial support during and after treatment (Glaser et al. 1997b).

Following treatment for CNS tumours, individuals are equally as likely as their siblings and peers to complete secondary or high school education. However, many fewer complete university or higher education courses (Charlton et al. 1991, Hays et al. 1992).

EMPLOYMENT
Studies of survivors of childhood CNS tumours in the USA and Europe have found that they are less likely to be employed than either the general population or survivors of non-CNS tumours (Hays et al. 1992, Pastore et al. 2001). Discrimination in the work place and lower incomes were reported. Survivors of all forms of childhood malignancies experience difficulties in gaining recruitment to the armed forces (Dolgin et al. 1999).

ACTIVITIES OF DAILY LIVING
Many survivors of childhood CNS tumours achieve independent living and normal adult life goals. However, others are left with significant difficulties. Marriage rates are lower and divorce rates higher in studies of this cohort of cancer survivors (Hays et al. 1992).

LIFE INSURANCE
Difficulties in obtaining life insurance are reported by adult survivors of childhood cancer (Green et al. 1991). Individuals have also experienced difficulties in obtaining mortgages, although there are few published data.

Clinical trials
Attempts to assess the impact of therapy on the health status of survivors of CNS tumours have not revealed a clearly definable picture. Results are frequently neither reproducible nor consistent. Up to 80% of survivors have been shown to have some cognitive deficit (Gamis and Nesbit 1991, Glauser and Packer 1991), whilst the developmental trajectory for the majority of late sequelae is not established.

In view of the complex potential array of late effects of CNS tumours in childhood and the increasingly aggressive therapies being adopted, it is essential that comprehensive assessment of outcome is performed.

Systematic and standardized approaches to the longitudinal evaluation of these individuals are increasingly being taken within the context of international clinical trials. Frameworks for comprehensive assessment are being developed (Glaser et al. 1999). These should include descriptions of not just physical outcome parameters but also the mental, social and health-related quality of life domains as described in this chapter. Longitudinal data will be invaluable in clarifying late sequelae associated with survivorship from CNS tumours and may enable effects of tumour and individual therapeutic interventions to be teased out. Additionally, comprehensive evaluation of these issues may enhance our ability to intervene to maximize individual survivors' health-related quality of life and functioning within society.

REFERENCES

Allen JC, Rosen G, Mehta BM, Horten B (1980) Leukoencephalopathy following high-dose iv methotrexate chemotherapy with leucovorin rescue. *Cancer Treat Rep* **64**: 1261–1273.

Anderson V, Smibert E, Ekert H, Godber T (1994) Intellectual, educational, and behavioural sequelae after cranial irradiation and chemotherapy. *Arch Dis Child* **70**: 476–483.

Ball WS, Prenger EC, Ballard ET (1992) Neurotoxicity of radio/chemotherapy in children: pathologic and MR correlation. *AJNR* **13**: 761–776.

Barr RD, Pai MKR, Weitzman S, Feeny D, Furlong W, Rosenbaum P, Torrance GW (1994) A multi-attribute approach to health status measurement and clinical management – illustrated by an application to brain tumours in children. *Int J Oncol* **4**: 639–948.

Baysinger M, Heiney SP, Creed JM, Ettinger RS (1993) A trajectory approach for education of the child/adolescent with cancer. *J Ped Oncol Nurs* **10**: 133–138.

Blayney DW, Longo DL, Young RC, Greene MH, Hubbard SM, Postal MG, Duffey PL, DeVita VT (1987) Decreasing risk of leukemia with prolonged follow-up after chemotherapy and radiotherapy for Hodgkin's disease. *N Engl J Med* **316**: 710–714.

Bleyer WA (1998) Chemotherapy interactions in the central nervous system. *Med Pediatr Oncol*, Suppl 1: 10–16.

Bozzola M, Albanese A, Butler GE, Cherubini V, Cicognani A, Caruso-Nicoletti M, Crowne E, De Sanctis V, Di Battista E, Hokken-Koelega AC, Severi F, Wonke B, Cavallo L; International Workshop on Management of Puberty for Optimum Auxological Results (2001) Unresolved problems in optimal therapy of pubertal disorders in oncological and bone marrow transplanted patients. *J Pediatr Endocrinol Metab* **14** Suppl 2: 997–1002.

Bradlyn AS, Ritchey AK, Harris CV, Moore IM, O'Brien RT, Parsons SK, Patterson K, Pollock BH (1996) Quality of life research in pediatric oncology. Research methods and barriers. *Cancer* **78**: 1333–1339.

Calman KC (1996) Departmental news from the chief medical officer. *Health Trends* **28**: 1–2.

Charlton A, Larcombe IJ, Meller ST, Morris Jones PH, Mott MG, Potton MW, Tranmer MD, Walker JJ (1991) Absence from school related to cancer and other chronic conditions. *Arch Dis Child* **66**: 1217–1222.

Chumas P, Tyagi A, Livingston J (2001) Hydrocephalus – what's new? *Arch Dis Child Fetal Neonatal Ed* **85**: F149–F154.

Clayton PE, Shalet SM (1991) The evolution of spinal growth after irradiation. *Clin Oncol* **3**: 220–222.

Clayton PE, Shalet SM, Price DA, Campbell RH (1988) Testicular damage after chemotherapy for childhood brain tumors. *J Pediatr* **112**: 922–926.

Clayton PE, Shalet SM, Price DA, Jones PH (1989) Ovarian function following chemotherapy for childhood brain tumours. *Med Pediatr Oncol* **17**: 92–96.

Crofton PM, Ahmed SF, Wade JC, Stephen R, Elmlinger MW, Ranke MB, Kelnar CJ, Wallace WH (1998) Effects of intensive chemotherapy on bone and collagen turnover and the growth hormone axis in children with acute lymphoblastic leukemia. *J Clin Endocrinol Metab* **83**: 3121–3129.

Danoff BF, Cowchock FS, Marquette C, Mulgrew L, Kramer S (1982) Assessment of the long-term effects of primary radiation therapy for brain tumors in children. *Cancer* **49**: 1580–1586.

Dens F, Boute P, Otten J, Vinckier F, Declerck D (1995) Dental caries, gingival health, and oral hygiene of long term survivors of paediatric malignant diseases. *Arch Dis Child* **72**: 129–132.

Dolgin MJ, Somer E, Buchvald E, Zaizov R (1999) Quality of life in adult survivors of childhood cancer. *Soc Work Health Care* **28**: 31–43.

Drake JM, Saint-Rose C (1995) *The Shunt Book*. New York: Blackwell Scientific.

Eiser C (1991) Cognitive deficits in children treated for leukaemia. *Arch Dis Child* **66**: 164–168.

Ellenberg L, McComb JG, Siegel SE, Stowe S (1987) Factors affecting intellectual outcome in pediatric brain tumor patients. *Neurosurgery* **21**: 638–644.

Evans SE, Radford M (1995) Current lifestyle of young adults treated for cancer in childhood. *Arch Dis Child* **72**: 423–426.

311

Fujiwara I, Igarashi Y, Ogawa E (1995) A comparison of pituitary–adrenal responses to corticotropin-releasing hormone, hypoglycaemia and metyrapone in children with brain tumours and growth hormone deficiency. *Eur J Pediatr* **154**: 717–22.

Gamis AS, Nesbit ME (1991) Neuropsychologic (cognitive) disabilities in long-term survivors of childhood cancer. *Pediatrician* **18**: 11–19.

Glaser A, Walker D (1995) Quality of life. *Lancet* **346**: 444.

Glaser AW, Buxton N, Walker D (1997a) Corticosteroids in the management of central nervous system tumours. Kids Neuro-Oncology Workshop (KNOWS). *Arch Dis Child* **76**: 76–78.

Glaser AW, Abdul Rashid NF, U CL, Walker DA (1997b) School behaviour and health status after central nervous system tumours in childhood. *Br J Cancer* **76**: 643–650.

Glaser AW, Kennedy C, Punt J, Walker DA (1999) Standardized quantitative assessment of brain tumor survivors within clinical trials in childhood. *Int J Cancer*, Suppl 12: 77–82.

Glauser TA, Packer RJ (1991) Cognitive deficits in long-term survivors of childhood brain tumours. *Child's Nerv Syst* **7**: 2–12.

Green DM, Zevon MA, Hall B (1991) Achievement of life goals by adult survivors of modern treatment for childhood cancer. *Cancer* **67**: 206–213.

Greenberg HS, Kazak AE, Meadows AT (1989) Psychologic functioning in 8–16 year old cancer survivors. *J Pediatr* **114**: 488–493.

Gregory K, Parker L, Craft AW (1994) Returning to primary school after treatment for cancer. *Pediatr Hematol Oncol* **11**: 105–109.

Hamilton SR, Liu B, Parsons RE, Papadopoulos N, Jen J, Powell SM, Krush AJ, Berk T, Cohen Z, Tetu B, et al. (1995) The molecular basis of Turcot's syndrome. *N Engl J Med* **332**: 839–847.

Hays DM, Landsverk J, Sallan SE, Hewett KD, Patenaude AF, Schoonover D, Zilber SL, Ruccione K, Siegel SE (1992) Educational, occupational, and insurance status of childhood cancer survivors in their fourth and fifth decades of life. *J Clin Oncol* **10**: 1397–1406.

Hirsch JF, Renier D, Czernichow P, Benveniste L, Pierre-Kahn A (1979) Medulloblastoma in childhood. Survival and functional results. *Acta Neurochir* **48**: 1–15.

Holtta P, Alaluusua S, Saarinen-Pihkala UM, Wolf J, Nystrom M, Hovi L (2002) Long-term adverse effects on dentition in children with poor-risk neuroblastoma treated with high-dose chemotherapy and autologous stem cell transplantation with or without total body irradiation. *Bone Marrow Transplant* **29**: 121–127.

Kaste SC, Hopkins KP, Jones D, Crom D, Greenwalk CA, Santana VM (1997) Dental abnormalities in children treated for acute lymphoblastic leukemia. *Leukemia* **11**: 792–796.

Kimonis VE, Goldstein AM, Pastakia B, Yang ML, Kase R, DiGiovanna JJ, Bale AE, Bale SJ (1997) Clinical manifestations in 105 persons with nevoid basal cell carcinoma syndrome. *Am J Med Genet* **69**: 299–308.

Kissen GDN, Wallace WHB (1995) *The United Kingdom Children's Cancer Study Group Late Effects Group: Long Term Follow Up Therapy Based Guidelines*. Milton Keynes: Pharma Endocrine Care.

Lancet (1991) Quality of life. *Lancet* **338**: 350–351 (editorial).

Larcombe IJ, Walker J, Charlton A, Meller S, Morris Jones P, Mott MG (1990) Impact of childhood cancer on return to normal schooling. *BMJ* **74**: 219–223.

Leiper AD (1998) Osteoporosis in survivors of childhood malignancy. *Eur J Cancer* **34**: 770–772.

Listernick R, Charrow J, Guttmann DH (1999) Intracranial gliomas in neurofibromatosis type 1. *Am J Med Genet* **89**: 38–44.

Lustig RH, Rose SR, Burghen GA, Velasquez-Mieyer P, Broome DC, Smith K, Li H, Hudson MM, Heideman RL, Kun LE (1999) Hypothalamic obesity caused by cranial insult in children: altered glucose and insulin dynamics and reversal by a somatostatin agonist. *J Pediatr* **135**: 162–168.

Malkin D, Li FP, Strong LC, Fraumeni JF, Nelson CE, Kim DH, Kassel J, Gryka MA, Bischoff FZ, Tainsky MA, et al. (1990) Germ line p53 mutations in a familial syndrome of breast cancer, sarcomas, and other neoplasms. *Science* **250**: 1233–1238; erratum in *Science* 1993, **259**: 878.

Meadows AT, Hobbie WL (1986) The medical consequences of cure. *Cancer* **58**: 524–528.

Medical Research Council (1996) *The Assessment of MRC Trials 1996/1997*. London: MRC.

Medical Research Council Working Party on Leukaemia (1997) *UK National Lymphoblastic Leukaemia Trial ALL 97*. London: MRC.

Mehlman CT, Crawford AH, McMath JA (1999) Pediatric vertebral and spinal cord tumors: a retrospective study of musculoskeletal aspects of presentation, treatment, and complications. *Orthopedics* **22**: 49–55; discussion 55–56.

Mertens AC, Yasui Y, Neglia JP, Potter JD, Nesbit ME, Ruccione K, Smithson WA, Robison LL (2001) Late mortality experience in five-year survivors of childhood and adolescent cancer: the Childhood Cancer Survival Study. *J Clin Oncol* **19**: 3163–3172.

Nayfield SG, Ganz PA, Moinpour CM, Cella DF, Hailey BJ (1992) Report from a National Cancer Institute (USA) workshop on quality of life assessment in cancer clinical trials. *Qual Life Res* **1**: 203–210.

Neglia JP, Friedman DL, Yasui Y, Mertens AC, Hammond S, Stovall M, Donaldson SS, Meadows AT, Robison LL (2001) Second malignant neoplasms in five-year survivors of childhood cancer: childhood cancer survivor study. *J Natl Cancer Inst* **93**: 618–629.

Ogilvy-Stuart AL, Shalet SM (1993) Effect of radiotherapy on the human reproductive system. *Environ Health Perspect* **101**, Suppl 2: 109–116.

Ogilvy-Stuart AL, Shalet SM (1995a) Growth and puberty after growth hormone treatment after irradiation for brain tumours. *Arch Dis Child* **73**: 141–146.

Ogilvy-Stuart AL, Shalet SM (1995b) Effect of chemotherapy on growth. *Acta Paediatrica Suppl* **411**: 52–56.

Ogilvy-Stuart AL, Shalet SM, Gattamaneni HR (1991) Thyroid function after treatment of brain tumors in children. *J Pediatr* **119**: 733–737.

Pantel RH, Lewis CC (1987) Measuring the impact of medical care on children. *J Chronic Dis* **40** (Suppl.): 99S–108S.

Pastore G, Mosso ML, Magnani C, Luzzatto L, Bianchi M, Terracini B (2001) Physical impairment and social life goals among adult long-term survivors of childhood cancer: a population-based study from the childhood cancer registry of Piedmont, Italy. *Tumori* **87**: 372–378.

Pollack IF, Mulvihill JJ (1997) Neurofibromatosis 1 and 2. *Brain Pathol* **7**: 823–836.

Radcliffe J, Packer RJ, Atkins TE, Bunin GR, Schut L, Goldwein JW, Sutton LN (1992) Three- and four-year cognitive outcome in children with noncortical brain tumours treated with whole-brain radiotherapy. *Ann Neurol* **32**: 551–554.

Rosso P, Terracini B, Fears TR, Jankovic M, Fossati Bellani F, Arrighini A, Carli M, Cordero di Montezemolo L, Garre ML, Guazzelli C, et al. (1994) Second malignant tumours after elective end of therapy for a first cancer in childhood: a multicenter study in Italy. *Int J Cancer* **59**: 451–456.

Schmiegelow M, Lassen S, Poulsen HS, Feldt-Rasmussen U, Schmiegelow K, Hertz H, Muller J (2000) Cranial radiotherapy of childhood brain tumours: growth hormone deficiency and its relation to the biological effective dose of irradiation in a large population based study. *Clin Endocrinol* **53**: 191–197.

Schmiegelow M, Feldt-Rasmussen U, Rasmussen AK, Poulsen HS, Muller J (2003) A population-based study of thyroid function after radiotherapy and chemotherapy for a childhood brain tumor. *J Clin Endocrinol Metab* **88**: 136–140.

SIOP (1995) Guidelines for school/education. *Med Pediat Oncol* **25**: 429–430.

Slavc I, Salchegger C, Hauer C, Urban C, Oberbauer R, Pakisch B, Ebner F, Schwinger W, Mokry M, Ranner G, et al. (1994) Follow-up and quality of survival of 67 consecutive children with CNS tumors. *Child's Nerv Syst* **10**: 433–443.

Smith MA, Rubinstein L, Anderson JR, Arthur D, Catalano PJ, Freidlin B, Heyn R, Khayat A, Krailo M, Land VJ, Miser J, Shuster J, Vena D (1999) Secondary leukemia or myelodysplastic syndrome after treatment with epipodophyllotoxins. *J Clin Oncol* **17**: 569–577.

Spiegler B, Glaser A, Dennis M, Greenberg M (1998) Health-related quality of life following posterior fossa tumours. Paper presented at the 5th International Conference on Long-term Complications of Treatment of Children and Adolescents for Cancer, Niagara-on-the-Lake, Canada.

Spoudeas HA, Charmendari E, Brook CGD (2000) The effect of cranial irradiation for tumours distal to the pituitary on ACTH secretion. *Horm Res* **53**, Suppl 2: 549.

Starfield B, Bergner M, Ensminger M, Riley A, Ryan S, Green B, McGauhey P, Skinner A, Kim S (1993) Adolescent health status measurement: development of the Child Health and Illness Profile. *Pediatrics* **91**: 430–435.

Tefft M, Lattin PB, Jereb B, Cham W, Ghavimi G, Rosen G, Exelby P, Marcove R, Murphy ML, D'Angio GJ (1976) Acute and late effects on normal tissues following combined chemo- and radiotherapy for childhood rhabdomyosarcoma and Ewing's sarcoma. *Cancer* **37**: 1201–1217.

Testa MA, Simonson DC (1996) Assessment of quality-of-life outcomes. *N Engl J Med* **334**: 835–840.

Thomson AB, Campbell AJ, Irvine DC, Anderson RA, Kelnar CJ, Wallace WH (2002) Semen quality and spermatozoal DNA integrity in survivors of childhood cancer: a case control study. *Lancet* **360**: 361–367.

World Health Organization (1947) *Constitution of the World Health Organization*. Geneva: WHO.

WHOQUOL Group (1993) *Measuring Quality of Life: The Development of the World Health Organization Quality of Life Instrument*. Geneva: WHO.

21
AN OVERVIEW OF CEREBRAL FUNCTIONING AND ITS APPLICATION IN THE DEVELOPING BRAIN

Andrew Curran

This chapter aims to provide a readily understandable overview of the mechanisms of how basic functions, such as memory and the emotional content of thoughts, are now believed to work. The aim is to build a picture of brain functioning that allows the reader to place a tumour in any position in the brain and be able to have some idea of the impact that the tumour, surgical removal and radiotherapy will have on cognitive and emotional functions.

The first part outlines normal functioning of the brain, with particular reference to the key anatomical structures central to this functionality. Part two describes how structures in the developing brain gradually mature to integrate emotional perception into our memories. The penultimate section focuses on the effects of stress on the developing brain and reinforces the need for sensitive handling of children undergoing stressful experiences. The final section looks at the hemispheric lateralization of functionality.

In all fields of medicine, but especially in the care of children, the understanding of how the brain works, and especially the importance of emotional health in allowing the individual to achieve their maximal potential must, I believe, always be paramount in our thoughts.

The normal brain
THE REPTILIAN BRAIN
The control of sophisticated structures, such as the bodies of multicellular living organisms, requires coordination and control beyond that seen in simpler organisms. A unified 'master control system' to govern these activities in lesser systems is provided by the spinal cord, brainstem and corpus striatum (Fig. 21.1), the so-called reptilian brain, in higher organisms. MacLean (1990) has described this as the first step towards the "triune brain", the ultimate expression of which is seen in modern man.

Compared to the complexity of a modern human brain the reptilian brain is an unsophisticated and simple structure that is poor at responding to novel situations. The corpus striatum can store a small number of behavioural responses related to self-preservation and survival of the species, i.e. it is a neural repository for genetically determined forms of behaviour as well as learned behaviours. Interestingly there are strong parallels to these behaviours in all animals and these behaviours are also stored in the corpus striatum despite the existence of other phylogenetically younger and more complex higher structures. In

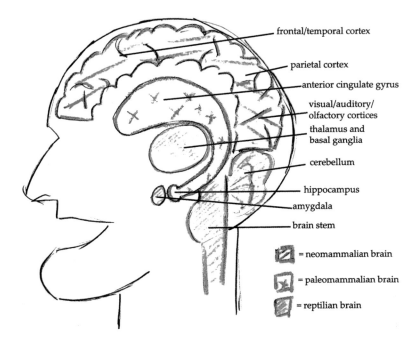

frontal/temporal cortex

parietal cortex

anterior cingulate gyrus

visual/auditory/
olfactory cortices

thalamus and
basal ganglia

cerebellum

hippocampus

amygdala

brain stem

= neomammalian brain

= paleomammalian brain

= reptilian brain

Fig. 21.1. Schematic representation of the brain showing the three main parts of the triune brain.

humans, the reptilian brain "appears to be a slave to precedent" (MacLean 1970) and is responsible for obsessive–compulsive behaviours, stereotyped behaviours, a predisposition to imitation in social situations and an inability to learn to cope with new situations, and may also contribute to superstitions and obeisance to precedent in ceremonial rituals, religious convictions and political persuasions.

The corpus striatum and related structures express themselves through the brainstem and spinal cord. These act as a signal pathway to and from higher centres in the brain and contain: (1) motor effector structures, and (2) the main tracts of the activating systems such as the reticular activating system. These structures have various functions. The motor effector nuclei are concerned primarily with large postural movement such as axial correction during walking. The activating systems (of which five have been described) are responsible for the level of arousal of the brain as a whole.

THE PALEOMAMMALIAN BRAIN

The next major level of complexity of the brain is the paleomammalian brain (Fig. 21.1), which involves essentially the addition of the limbic system and a larger mass of cortex to the reptilian brain. The paleomammalian brain allows much more sophisticated behaviours as a direct result of the hugely increased number of neurones that are now available to the animal. It is a common denominator in all mammals and is centrally involved in emotional experience and behaviour, allowing feelings to guide self-preservation and survival of the species. The possession of a paleomammalian brain is associated with the desire to care for and nurture the young (MacLean 1982, 1985).

The two oldest components of the paleomammalian brain are closely related to the olfactory apparatus and are the amygdala (which is concerned with feeding, fighting and self-preservation) and the septal nuclei (which are concerned with genital and procreational functions) (MacLean 1977, Holden 1979). The third subdivision bypasses the olfactory apparatus on its way to link up with what corresponds to the frontal cortex. It becomes progressively larger in higher primates and is concerned with empathy, compassion, and a 'far-seeing concern' for the species (MacLean 1977). It is felt that this subdivision reflects a change in emphasis from olfactory to visual influences in sociosexual behaviour (MacLean 1977).

The limbic and cortical structures control the corpus striatum, which is used increasingly in higher animals for processing information for behavioural and memory purposes while still retaining some of its own independent functionality.

THE NEOMAMMALIAN BRAIN

The last part of the triune brain is called the neomammalian brain (Fig. 21.1), and is characterized by a massive increase in the amount of cortex. It "provides a vast neural screen for the portrayal of symbolic language" (MacLean 1977). In the human it is represented by the huge bulk of the frontal cortex, the only part of the brain that can look inwards to the inside world (MacLean 1977). This evolutionary development made possible "the insight required for the foresight to plan for the needs of others as well as the self – to use our knowledge to alleviate suffering everywhere" (MacLean 1990). In its turn it acquired control over the previous structures and the resulting interrelating system evolved into the human brain as we know it today.

Patterns of learning

One of the main differences between the three different parts of the triune brain is the number of neurones that each contains. The more neurones available to a creature, the more sophisticated its behaviour can be, and this seems to be entirely based on the greater ability to store information that increased neuronal numbers confers. It seems that almost all behaviour is based on learning, and this in turn arises from patterns of neuronal firing in the brain, called templates or Hebbian assemblies (Damasio 1990, Bressler et al. 1993, Merzenich and Sameshima 1993, Vaadia and et al. 1995, Varela 1995, Kreiter and Singer 1996, Skrebitsky and Chepkova 1998, Rodriguez et al. 1999).

When an infant is exposed repeatedly to an emotionally important stimulus, such as the appearance and disappearance of her mother's face, there is, over time, the setting up and perpetuation of long-term potentiation (LTP) and depression (LTD) under the control of the limbic system. A pattern of spiny striatal neurones (a Hebbian assembly or template) becomes interconnected by both direct synapses with each other and through the agency of so-called tonically active neurones (TANs) (Hebb 1968, Merzenich and Sameshima 1993, Skrebitsky and Chepkova 1998, Bailey et al. 2000). This pattern of neurones will now preferentially fire whenever the child sees her mother's face. A final refinement to this summary is to say that the specificity of 'my mother's face' takes many months to develop. Initially the child will remember 'face', or perhaps just a small sub-category of face such as 'eyes'. The combination of repeated exposure to a specific face with its associated emotional import and the continuing maturation in both the anatomy and biochemistry of the infant's brain will lead to this initial generic memory being gradually refined until the child knows which 'face' is her mother's.

Neurochemical control of memory

This description of memory refers to the corpus striatum, the repository of 'non-declarative' memory, or memory that is not readily accessed by the conscious mind. The other main memory structure is the hippocampus which deals with 'declarative' memory, that which is readily available for conscious recall (Squire et al. 1993, Squire and Zola 1996). This is situated in the medial temporal lobes and is part of the limbic system (Fig. 21.1). The mechanisms of memory formation in the hippocampus rely on the establishment of long-term potentiation and long-term depression. These are triggered through the action of glutamate (Bliss and Collingridge 1993, Milner et al. 1998, Malenka and Nicoll 1999) and are sustained by the release of dopamine, which is primarily under the control of the limbic system.

To understand memory more fully, however, at least three other neurochemicals must be discussed. The first of these is the main inhibitory neurochemical in the brain, gamma-amino-butyric acid (GABA). This is also required for the formation of effective synapses (Silkis 2001). It exerts its effect through the sequence of reciprocal inhibition between striatal neurones that occurs through both GABAA and GABAB receptors (Shi and Rayport 1994, Silkis 2001) and so affects the efficacy of inhibitory connections (Silkis 1998).

The second neurochemical is acetylcholine, which is present in large amounts in the brain, especially in the frontal lobes, and may have the role of 'synapse control' (Girod et al. 2000, Girod and Role 2001, Jo and Role 2002). Through this proposed ability acetylcholine may also be part of the processes of forgetting previously learned data.

The final neurochemical involved in the process of learning is noradrenaline. Acting through both central brainstem arousal systems and the amygdala (see below), noradrenaline is responsible for adding 'energy' to memories. Changes in the concentration of noradrenaline, and of other neurochemicals such as acetylcholine and serotonin, in the brainstem activating systems (Fig. 21.1) cause a change in the state of arousal and hence wakefulness (Berlucchi 1997). The more activity in this system, the more aroused we are.

The brain also has systems to inhibit memory storage. GABA and endogenous opioids (such as enkephalins and substance P) both inhibit memory storage, as does a huge excess of noradrenaline (Izquierdo et al. 1980a,b, 1984; Brioni and McGaugh 1988; Brioni et al. 1989). The benzodiazepine group of drugs, which work on the GABAA receptor, are an example of an exogenous amnesiac (Izquierdo et al. 1990, 1991; Medina et al. 1992).

Structural aspects of memory

The description of memory processes may be divided into three main streams: (1) the corpus striatum, dealing with implicit memory with reference to the effect of the limbic system on this memory acquisition; (2) the amygdala, dealing with the emotional content of memory; (3) the hippocampus, dealing with explicit memory both short term and long term.

It is likely that memory processing is much more complex than described here, with significant interactions between the various systems and the involvement of other areas of the limbic system in a central way in memory processing and storage.

The amygdala and emotional content of memory

The amygdala (Fig. 21.1) is a phylogenetically primitive structure and is thought to be concerned first and foremost with fight and flight reactions, though this is probably an oversimplification (LeDoux 1998, 2000). The amygdala is also central to the emotional control of memory, regulating the strength of memories in relation to their emotional significance (McGaugh et al. 1996). It is connected to both the hippocampus and the corpus striatum (LeDoux 1993a,b): through these, and also through direct connections to cortex and to brainstem activating systems, the amygdala can modulate the storage of both conscious and unconscious memories (LeDoux 2000).

The connections to the hippocampus and striatum are glutamatergic (Krettek and Price 1977, Kita and Kitai 1990, Pitkanen et al. 2000), and their effect on memory is significantly affected by the level of emotional arousal present in the individual (Cahill and McGaugh 1996, McGaugh et al. 1996, Cahill 2000). One factor that affects this is the amount of stress the individual is feeling.

Stress has several effects on the amygdala and hence on memory. First, noradrenaline is released directly into the amygdala, increasing its activity (Cahill et al. 1994, McGaugh et al. 1996, van Stegeren et al. 1998). Second, the systemic release of adrenaline by the adrenal glands activates afferents to the amygdala from the vagus nerve, and also increases the level of excitation (van Stegeren et al. 1998, Clark et al. 1999, Cahill 2000). Third, the release of glucocorticoids from the adrenal glands has a direct effect on the amygdala to increase its level of excitation (Quirarte et al. 1997; Roozendaal 2000; Roozendaal et al. 2002a,b). These effects have a final common pathway through cholinergic interneurons that connect with the excitatory efferents from the amygdala to the hippocampus, caudate, substantia nigra, thalamus and frontal cortex (Packard and Cahill 2001), and stimulation of these enhances memory retention (Kesner and Wilburn 1974, McGaugh and Gold 1976). This enhancement can, however, become overdriven by excess stress: the effect of excessive stress on the amygdala results in a shift of memory storage from the explicit (conscious, cognitive) memory of the hippocampal system to the implicit (unconscious, cue–response) memory system of the caudate (Packard and Cahill 2001).

The hippocampus

The hippocampus is an essential component of the brain system, underlying the conscious recollection of past events (Squire 1992) and the processing of spatial, configural, contextual and/or relational information (O'Keefe and Nadel 1978, Eichenbaum 1992, Nadel 1992). The particular interest in the hippocampus is that it can encode and store memories that do not have an obvious emotional content, i.e. the storage of intellectual facts. However, it does receive outputs from the amygdala, and the limbic system can therefore exert some control over it (LeDoux 2000). Such memories are time-limited and will eventually become largely independent of the hippocampus, supported by the neocortex (Nadel and Bohbot 2001, Ryan et al. 2001).

Developmental aspects of memory

The age of an individual is critical to the patterns of memory storage they are capable of. Different areas of the limbic system mature at different times during infancy and this directly influences the learning patterns at different stages of development. This chronology of development can be clearly seen in the maturation of several limbic structures: the amygdala, the cingulate gyrus and the septate nuclei.

The *amygdala* dictates the early timing of socializing behaviours so the human infant will at first socialize indiscriminately (a need of the immature amygdala), then slowly develop stable and selective loving attachments and, at around 6 months to 1 year, express emotions such as anger, joy, and the fear of strangers (a function of the mature amygdala) (Joseph 1982, 1992).

The *cingulate gyrus* is closely associated with the amygdala and contributes to the establishment of infant-maternal attachment during the latter half of the first postnatal year, including the expression of maternal separation anxiety (MacLean 1990, Joseph 1992). As it (and the frontal lobes) continues to mature, up to (and beyond) the age of 3 years, the cingulate gyrus allows the expression of behaviours such as displaying emotions not felt by the infant, complex play, role playing and creative fantasy (Stroufe 1996).

The *septate nuclei* mature at the slowest rate, continuing well into adolescence (Joseph 1992, 1999). In the first year of life, they act to inhibit the over-zealous socializing driven by the amygdala (in conjunction with the cingulate gyrus and the orbital frontal lobes) and are felt to control the psychosocial development of the individual starting with the phallic stage of Freudian theory.

Environmental factors

Because of the slow rate of maturation of these structures, the medial amygdala and later the cingulate and septal nuclei are most vulnerable during the first 3 years of life when they are immature. There is now evidence to show that deprived or abnormal rearing conditions (i.e. where appropriate stimuli are absent or of poor quality) induce severe disturbance in all aspects of social and emotional functioning both behaviourally and at a neurochemical and anatomical level (Joseph and Gallagher 1980; Greer et al. 1982; Sesma et al. 1984; Carughi et al. 1989; Lachica et al. 1990; Joseph 1992, 1999). Normal development in the limbic and cortical systems requires "considerable social, emotional, perceptual, and cognitive stimulation during the first several months and years of life" (Joseph 1999). Insufficient or abnormal stimulation will lead to the abnormal growth or death of both neurones and neuronal connections within these structures.

The early years of development are also associated with a massive overgrowth of dendrites from neurones, the so-called 'mossy fibre' stage (Joseph 1982, Finlay and Slattery 1983, Rakic et al. 1986). Successful development requires that these be appropriately 'pruned' so that neural pathways can be fine tuned towards increasingly mature and efficient patterns. An abnormal rearing environment can not only significantly reduce the number of dendrites, but can also lead to the preservation of pathways that would otherwise have been discarded (Diamond et al. 1971, 1976; Bennett et al. 1974; Uylings et al. 1978; Greer et al. 1982; Carughi et al. 1989). These neuroanatomical effects can be seen in an inability of the forebrain to "discretely, purposefully, and selectively maintain control over behaviour", along with significant effects on all aspects of intellectual, perceptual, social and emotional development (Joseph 1999).

Specific patterns of abnormal behaviour have been identified with anatomical structures. For example, bilateral septate nuclei damage or destruction leads to an irrepressible drive for social contact and also to explosive violence (a behaviour especially associated with humans who have suffered maternal deprivation during development) (Corman et al. 1967; Jonason and Enloe 1971, Jonason et al. 1973, Meyer et al. 1973, 1978). Destruction of the amygdala abolishes the desire for social contact and emotional functioning is virtually extinguished (Dicks et al. 1968, Kling et al. 1970; Kling and Cornell 1971, Lilly et al. 1983, Ramamurthi 1988). This loss of emotional functioning includes the ability to interpret social nuances including facial expression and body language.

The role of stress
Children undergoing investigation and treatment are likely to be experiencing stress, which can often be chronic. An environment that contains excessive stress, either continuously or intermittently, produces damage to the hippocampi, the amygdala and the septal nuclei. This occurs by two separate routes, related to (1) catecholamine, and (2) enkephalin/corticosteroid activity.

THE ROLE OF CATECHOLAMINES
Catecholamines do not pass the blood–brain barrier in any quantity (McGaugh et al. 1996). Any effect that they have on neurones is therefore either from their effect on peripheral receptors via vagus nerve innervation of the nucleus of the solitary tract to release noradrenaline within the amygdala (Schreurs et al. 1986) or through the release from other routes of noradrenaline directly into the amygdala (Liang et al. 1990, 1995; McGaugh et al. 1996).

Noradrenaline exerts a stimulating effect on neuronal growth, significantly influences neuronal maturation, and promotes neural plasticity and synaptic development during early development (Bear and Singer 1986, Rosenblum et al. 1994, Joseph 1999). It therefore enhances memory at low doses through its effect on β-adrenergic receptors. This mechanism is thought to be active during the encoding and storage of aversive events but seems to be active in any emotionally arousing circumstance (Joseph 1999). Catecholamines are also neuroprotective (Joseph 1998; Sapolsky 1996, 2000), but high doses can impair memory (through their effect on β-adrenergic receptors) (Joseph 1999). In chronic stress, reserves of noradrenaline become depleted with subsequent loss of their neuroprotective and memory enhancing effects.

THE ROLE OF ENKEPHALINS AND CORTICOSTEROIDS
Enkephalins and corticosteroids are released during stress and can actively damage the

hippocampi and amygdala (Sapolsky et al. 1990; Starkman et al. 1992, 1999; Uno et al. 1994; Sheline 1996; Sheline et al. 1998, 1999). This damage interferes not only with emotional responsiveness but also with the ability to remember faces, people, objects and locations – all essential in the formation of emotional attachments.

Stress, especially chronic or severe intermittent stress, therefore carries with it the ability to profoundly influence the growth and development of the immature brain. Whilst it is likely that some of these effects can be reversed over time, others may not be, especially if the child remains in an environment where the stresses are still present and active.

Lateralization of function within the cerebral hemispheres

The hemispheres contain some functions that are not lateralized, for example vision, hearing, and the motor and sensory cortex. Each cortex controls these functions for the contralateral side of the body, but these cortical areas do roughly mirror each other, both in structure and function. Superimposed on this symmetry however are the hemispheric specializations. The left hemisphere (usually the dominant hemisphere even in left-handed individuals) deals with linguistic, analytic and sequential processing, and the right deals with nonverbal, holistic and parallel processing (Benowitz et al. 1983, Berlucchi et al. 1997). Why hemispheric specialization occurred is not known. It can be hypothesized that speed of processing might have dictated a function residing in one hemisphere rather than both – communication between two functionally similar areas of cortex in opposite hemispheres might slow down a behaviour that needs to occur quickly.

Lateralization should be thought of in terms of complementary hemispheric specialization (Heilman and Gilmore 1998): even in visual and auditory cortices where both hemispheres carry equal functionality, specific items of information are stored preferentially in one side or the other. Information presented to one hemisphere and learned by that hemisphere has been shown not to be available to the other hemisphere when the main connection between the two hemispheres, the corpus callosum, is divided (Gazzaniga 1998, Spence et al. 2001, Corballis et al. 2002). The two hemispheres can, however, process information simultaneously and independently (Zaidel 2001). Anatomically the corpus callosum is subdivided into sections each of which carries specific information between the two hemispheres. The posterior section carries visual information and, moving anteriorly, auditory and tactile information. The anterior corpus callosum is involved in higher order transfer of semantic information. For correct interpretation of a stimulus by both hemispheres, therefore, information transfer must involve both the posterior corpus callosum, to carry the stimulus itself, and the anterior corpus callosum, to carry semantic information about the stimulus.

THE LEFT HEMISPHERE

One of the most important specialized functions of the left hemisphere is language, for which the specialized area resides on the superior border of the temporal lobe and includes Wernicke's area. This region, which has shown to be larger on the left than the right, is termed the planum temporale and underlies the sylvian fissure near Wernicke's area. PET and fMRI studies suggest that this area may be responsible for phonological decoding and auditory comprehension (Zaidel 2001). The lateral posterior nucleus of the thalamus also tends to be larger on the left (Gazzaniga et al. 2002).

Language is best thought of as comprising grammar (the rules of language) and the lexicon (the dictionary). The lexicon is present in both hemispheres, but a larger part seems to reside in the left (Gazzaniga 1970, Zaidel 1991). Grammar resides almost entirely in the left hemisphere, which is also responsible for speech production (Gazzaniga 2000).

Higher order cognition and problem-solving also reside in the left hemisphere (LeDoux et al. 1977, Gazzaniga 2000), i.e. the left hemisphere is specialized for intelligent behaviour. This is shown in its function in hypothesis formation. Whilst the right hemisphere approaches a task in the simplest possible manner, the left hemisphere tries to make order out of chaos (Gazzaniga 2000). The left hemisphere is also the interpreter of events, even those generated in the right hemisphere (Gazzaniga 2000). Positive and negative moods generated in the right hemisphere drive the left hemisphere to interpret the present circumstance in a positive or negative way respectively.

Attention is divided between the two hemispheres (Zaidel 2001). The left hemisphere specializes in spatial compatibility and divided attention tasks. For motor skills, the left hemisphere is specialized for action.

THE RIGHT HEMISPHERE

The right hemisphere has a better ability to see the 'whole picture' or totality of a problem or stimulus set rather than to do a step-by-step analysis (Lamm and Gordon 1984). Stimuli that preferentially activate the right hemisphere are those that are unfamiliar (Kimura 1963), spatial (Kimura 1969), and nonverbal (Milner 1968). Attention is divided between the two hemispheres. The right hemisphere specializes in sustained attention and the orienting of visuospatial attention, and has a greater specialization for facial recognition and for perception of smell than the left.

CONCLUDING REMARKS ABOUT LATERALIZATION

Cerebral lateralization has fascinated neuroscience since the late 1900s, and recent work has led to a greater understanding of how it might work. The left hemisphere deals with higher order functions, while the right deals predominantly with emotions, though in many ways it is very 'concrete' in its processes. An example of this is that when a patient with a 'split-brain' (i.e. a divided corpus callosum) is asked to decide whether a series of stimuli appeared in a study set or not, the right hemisphere is able to identify correctly items that have been seen previously and to reject new items. The left hemisphere, however, tends to falsely recognize new items when they are similar to previously presented items, presumably because they fit into the schema it has constructed (Phelps and Gazzaniga 1992, Metcalfe et al. 1995). This 'concreteness' is because the right hemisphere does not engage in interpretative processes, maintaining instead an accurate record of events (Gazzaniga 2000). It is interesting to note that gender differences in lateralization of emotional memory have recently been demonstrated, with females being much more likely to activate the left amygdala after an emotionally arousing memory task, while males activated the right (Cahill et al. 2001). The two hemispheres therefore complement each other, allowing elaborative processing to occur without sacrificing veracity (Gazzaniga 2000).

When thinking about the likely deficits that might occur because of the anatomical position of a tumour, it is important to remember that the outcome for that individual can only be guessed at. Nothing can replace careful neuropsychological assessment to accurately delineate the actual deficits that the individual has.

Treatment of brain tumours and neurological injury

Cognitive deficit after brain tumour treatment is common and may worsen over time as the developing brain is unable to 'bring online' areas that have been irreversibly damaged by treatment early in life. Full scale IQ has been shown to be significantly decreased in children treated with cranial irradiation (Ilveskoski et al. 1996, Fossen et al. 1998, Grill et al. 1999), and this effect is dependent on both the dose (Grill et al. 1999) and age of the child, where children younger than 3 years have a more marked reduction in full scale IQ than those over 3 years (Johnson et al. 1994). There is also evidence that the effects of cranial irradiation continue over time, so that intellectual deterioration continues to progress even years after the treatment dose was received (Hoppe-Hirsch et al. 1995).

Children with intracranial tumours also show evidence of impairments across a wide range of cognitive functions including visual attention and memory, verbal fluency, perceptual abilities, performance (nonverbal), attention and memory, and social problem solving (Butler et al. 1994, Garcia-Perez et al. 1994, Lewis et al. 2000). It is obvious that any one of these deficits can have a significant impact on academic performance and on normal day-to-day living, and children may have several of these problems concurrently after treatment for an intracerebral tumour. The magnitude of the effect of these problems is such that 58% of children in one study showed poor academic performance after treatment for an intracranial tumour (Yang et al. 1997).

The elements of treatment that cause this significant reduction in intellectual abilities are poorly understood but include cranial irradiation and chemotherapy, tumour site and histopathological type, quality of surgery and perioperative complications, pituitary hormone status, and the presence or absence of ventricular-peritoneal shunting (Brookshire et al. 1990; Glauser and Packer 1991; Dennis et al. 1992; Hoppe-Hirsch et al. 1993, 1995; Johnson et al. 1994; Kao et al. 1994; Levisohn et al. 2000).

Neurological outcome of paediatric brain tumours

Intracranial imaging (see Chapter 3) produces detailed images of the anatomical brain but tells us very little about the function of the brain and nothing about microscopic damage to neuronal structures. It is how these structures function after treatment that dictates the lifelong outcome for the child.

In terms of gross functional outcome, approximately 50% of children have at least one significant problem (Ilveskoski et al. 1996;Slavc et al. 1994). The commonest physical problems among survivors attending special schools are limb paralysis, affecting approximately 20%, and epilepsy (10–30%) (Ilveskoski et al. 1996). These physical disabilities alone represent a significant need for thoughtful, whole-person orientated, multidisciplinary rehabilitation, even without the cognitive and behavioural deficits common after treatment

TABLE 21.1
**Appropriate members of a multidisciplinary rehabilitation
team for neuro-oncology patients**

Oncologist
Paediatric neurologist or community paediatrician with an
   interest in rehabilitation
Neuropsychologist
Nursing staff (both hospital and community) with an interest
   in rehabilitation
Physiotherapist
Occupational therapist
Speech and language therapist
Specialist teacher(s) and play therapists

for intracerebral tumours. Such a rehabilitation team should therefore ideally consist of groups of professionals able to address such variable needs (Table 21.1).

When considering rehabilitation needs, it should be remembered that recovery from brain injury contains at least three stages: (1) the initial period when overt deficits are present; (2) a period following recovery from overt deficits within which covert deficits can be reinstated by a pharmacological challenge; and (3) a period following recovery from both overt and covert deficits. Covert deficits can persist long after the recovery of overt deficits.

In the paediatric population it must also be remembered that many of the functions of the developing brain are specifically directed at acquiring new information and interpreting incoming stimuli (Ewing-Cobbs et al. 1989). Disruption or damage to these centres during development will therefore have an impact on the child's ability to acquire new and higher functions by impeding the normal processing of new information. As a result, injury to the developing brain could affect the ability to retain what has already been learned as well as the ability to process new information in the future (Adelson and Kochanek 1998).

With time, the focus of rehabilitation moves from the immediate physical and emotional needs of the child and his or her family to wider issues involving education and the broader arena of psychosocial interactions (Sherwin and O'Shanick 2000). The core philosophy behind rehabilitation in all ages must therefore be the facilitation of an individual's attempts to reclaim their life as they recover from brain injury. In children and adolescents, the driving need is to help the child resume a normal developmental trajectory. This cannot be achieved by too narrow a focus on specific issues, but rather requires a broad view encompassing both the specific issues and the longer term needs for increasingly sophisticated understanding of the individual and the environment in which they have to function. One of the main criticisms levelled at the literature on rehabilitation is its tendency to adopt a narrow, over-focused view on specific aspects of care (Sherwin and O'Shanick 2000), i.e. decreased awareness, cognitive impairment, family therapy, school re-entry, etc. Whilst these needs must be met, it is the detailed understanding of how the specific problems they represent interfere with the child's ability to function in and adapt to their environment that determines how accurately interventions can be put in place that will genuinely improve their reintegration.

As development is a continuum, a child's needs after brain injury must be identified by their developmental age rather then by chronological age (Sherwin and O'Shanick 2000). The assessment of developmental age must be based on the cognitive, physical, emotional and behavioural difficulties that the child experiences at that time.

It is not possible in this chapter to explore all the various aspects of rehabilitation in detail, but the following points must always be borne in mind (Sherwin and O'Shanick 2000):

- the needs of the child and family will often be constantly changing as the rehabilitation process proceeds; this is related to the stages of recovery of the healing brain and the requirements this places on the child's environment to adopt a dynamic stance to the child's changing needs
- the grief that the family is suffering
- the understanding that the damage caused by treatment is often irreversible, though the effects of it, such as difficult behaviours are often not
- children with a brain tumour may have the majority of their life ahead of them, but even if this is not the case, optimizing the child and family's quality of life at any point in time is of central importance
- families both are members of a culture, and are themselves a culture; they will have their own expression of social mores and communication, and will achieve a better understanding of the issues surrounding their child if these are recognized, accepted and, where possible, used in caring for the family (Leaf 1993, DePompei and Williams 1994).

Conclusion

Placing a tumour and the effects of its treatment on an anatomical map of brain function is important, but only a small part of the picture.

From the moment the child is admitted, there is a risk of conflict between the experts who know about brain tumours, and the family experts who know about their family member who has experienced the brain injury. The treatment of intracerebral tumours results in complex and life-changing damage. The entire experience of diagnosis, treatment and long-term survival carry with them the potential to distort normal brain development, and it must therefore be central to our practice to care for each patient and their family in an holistic and sympathetic way: to view each one as a human who has a disease, as opposed to a disease that happens to have a human attached. The process of rehabilitation must be built into all aspects of care, and the process of holistic care should start as soon as the child is admitted. It is central to the management of these children therefore that care does not stop with the eradication of disease but continues for as long as is necessary to ensure that they are given the fullest possible chance to reach the potentials that are left to them following treatment.

REFERENCES

Adelson PD, Kochanek PM (1998) Head injury in children. *J Child Neurol* **13**: 2–15.
Bailey CH, Giustetto M, Huang YY, Hawkins RD, Kandel ER (2000) Is heterosynaptic modulation essential for stabilizing Hebbian plasticity and memory? *Nat Rev Neurosci* **1**: 11–20.
Bear MF, Singer W (1986) Modulation of visual cortical plasticity by acetylcholine and noradrenaline. *Nature* **320**: 172–176.

Bennett EL, Rosenzweig MR, Diamond MC, Morimoto H, Hebert M (1974) Effects of successive environments on brain measures. *Physiol Behav* **12**: 621–631.

Benowitz LI, Bear DM, Rosenthal R, Mesulam MM, Zaidel E, Sperry RW (1983) Hemispheric specialization in nonverbal communication. *Cortex* **19**: 5–11.

Berlucchi G (1997) One or many arousal systems? Reflections on some of Giuseppe Moruzzi's foresights and insights about the intrinsic regulation of brain activity. *Arch Ital Biol* **135**: 5–14.

Berlucchi G, Aglioti S, Tassinari G (1997) Rightward attentional bias and left hemisphere dominance in a cue–target light detection task in a callosotomy patient. *Neuropsychologia* **35**: 941–952.

Berman SM, Mandelkern MA, Phan H, Zaidel E (2003) Complementary hemispheric specialization for word and accent detection. *Neuroimage* **19**: 319–331.

Bliss TVP, Collingridge GL (1993) A synaptic model of memory – long-term potentiation in the hippocampus. *Nature* **361**: 31–39.

Bressler SL, Coppola R, Nakamura R (1993) Episodic multiregional cortical coherence at multiple frequencies during visual task performance. *Nature* **366**: 153–156.

Brioni JD, McGaugh JL (1988) Post-training administration of GABAergic antagonists enhances retention of aversively motivated tasks. *Psychopharmacology* **96**: 505–510.

Brioni JD, Nagahara AH, McGaugh JL (1989) Involvement of the amygdala GABAergic system in the modulation of memory storage. *Brain Res* **487**: 105–112.

Brookshire B, Copeland DR, Moore BD, Ater J (1990) Pretreatment neuropsychological status and associated factors in children with primary brain tumors. *Neurosurgery* **27**: 887–891.

Butler RW, Hill JM, Steinherz PG, Meyers PA, Finlay JL (1994) Neuropsychologic effects of cranial irradiation, intrathecal methotrexate, and systemic methotrexate in childhood cancer. *J Clin Oncol* **12**: 2621–2629.

Cahill L (2000) Neurobiological mechanisms of emotionally influenced, long-term memory. *Prog Brain Res* **126**: 29–37.

Cahill L, McGaugh JL (1996) The neurobiology of memory for emotional events: adrenergic activation and the amygdala. *Proc West Pharmacol Soc* **39**: 81–84.

Cahill L, Prins B, Weber M, McGaugh JL (1994) Beta-adrenergic activation and memory for emotional events. *Nature* **371**: 702–704.

Cahill L, Haier RJ, White NS, Fallon J, Kilpatrick L, Lawrence C, Potkin SG, Alkire MT (2001) Sex-related difference in amygdala activity during emotionally influenced memory storage. *Neurobiol Learn Mem* **75**: 1–9.

Carughi A, Carpenter KJ, Diamond MC (1989) Effect of environmental enrichment during nutritional rehabilitation on body growth, blood parameters and cerebral cortical development of rats. *J Nutr* **119**: 2005–2016.

Clark KB, Naritoku DK, Smith DC, Browning RA, Jensen RA (1999) Enhanced recognition memory following vagus nerve stimulation in human subjects. *Nat Neurosci* **2**: 94–98.

Corballis PM, Funnell MG, Gazzaniga MS (2002) Hemispheric asymmetries for simple visual judgments in the split brain. *Neuropsychologia* **40**: 401–410.

Corman CD, Meyer PM, Meyer DR (1967) Open-field activity and exploration in rats with septal and amygdaloid lesions. *Brain Res* **5**: 469–476.

Damasio AR (1990) Synchronous activation in multiple cortical regions: a mechanism for recall. *Neuroscience* **2**: 287–297.

Dennis M, Spiegler BJ, Obonsawin MC, Maria BL, Cowell C, Hoffman HJ, Hendrick EB, Humphreys RP, Bailey JD, Ehrlich RM (1992) Brain tumors in children and adolescents—III. Effects of radiation and hormone status on intelligence and on working, associative and serial-order memory. *Neuropsychologia* **30**: 257–275.

DePompei R, Williams J (1994) Working with families after TBI: a family-centered approach. *Top Lang Disord* **15**: 68–81.

Diamond MC, Johnson RE, Ingham C (1971) Brain plasticity induced by environment and pregnancy. *Int J Neurosci* **2**: 171–178.

Diamond MC, Ingham CA, Johnson RE, Bennett EL, Rosenzweig MR (1976) Effects of environment on morphology of rat cerebral cortex and hippocampus. *J Neurobiol* **7**: 75–85.

Dicks D, Myers RE, Kling A (1968) Uncus and amygdala lesions: effects on social behavior in the free-ranging rhesus monkey. *Science* **165**: 69–71.

Eichenbaum H (1992) The hippocampal system and declarative memory in animals. *J Cogn Neurosci* **4**: 217–231.

Ewing-Cobbs L, Miner ME, Fletcher JM, Levin HS (1989) Intellectual, motor, and language sequelae following closed head injury in infants and preschoolers. *J Pediatr Psychol* **14**: 531–547.

Finlay BL, Slattery M (1983) Local differences in the amount of early cell death in neocortex predict adult local specializations. *Science* **219**: 1349–1351.

Fossen A, Abrahamsen TG, Storm-Mathisen I (1998) Psychological outcome in children treated for brain tumor. *Pediatr Hematol Oncol* **15**: 479–488.

Garcia-Perez A, Sierrasesumaga L, Narbona-Garcia J, Calvo-Manuel F, Aguirre-Ventallo M (1994) Neuropsychological evaluation of children with intracranial tumors: impact of treatment modalities. *Med Pediatr Oncol* **23**: 116–123.

Gazzaniga MS (1970) *The Bisected Brain*. New York: Appleton-Century-Crofts.

Gazzaniga MS (1998) The split brain revisited. *Sci Am* **279**: 50–55.

Gazzaniga MS (2000) Cerebral specialization and interhemispheric communication: does the corpus callosum enable the human condition? *Brain* **123**: 1293–1326.

Gazzaniga MS, Ivry RB, Mangun GR (2002) *Cognitive Neuroscience: The Biology of the Mind, 2nd edn*. New York: WW Norton.

Girod R, Role LW (2001) Long-lasting enhancement of glutamatergic synaptic transmission by acetylcholine contrasts with response adaptation after exposure to low-level nicotine. *J Neurosci* **21**: 5182–5190.

Girod R, Barazangi N, McGehee D, Role LW (2000) Facilitation of glutamatergic neurotransmission by presynaptic nicotinic acetylcholine receptors. *Neuropharmacology* **39**: 2715–2725.

Glauser TA, Packer RJ (1991) Cognitive deficits in long-term survivors of childhood brain tumors. *Child's Nerv Syst* **7**: 2–12.

Greer ER, Diamond MC, Tang JM (1982) Environmental enrichment in Brattleboro rats: brain morphology. *Ann NY Acad Sci* **394**: 749–752.

Grill J, Renaux VK, Bulteau C, Viguier D, Levy-Piebois C, Sainte-Rose C, Dellatolas G, Raquin MA, Jambaque I, Kalifa C (1999) Long-term intellectual outcome in children with posterior fossa tumors according to radiation doses and volumes. *Int J Radiat Oncol Biol Phys* **45**: 137–145.

Hebb DO (1968) Concerning imagery. *Psychol Rev* **75**: 466–477.

Heilman KM, Gilmore RL (1998) Cortical influences in emotion. *J Clin Neurophysiol* **15**: 409–423.

Holden C (1979) Paul MacLean and the triune brain. *Science* **204**: 1066–1068.

Hoppe-Hirsch E, Hirsch JF, Lellouch-Tubiana A, Pierre-Kahn A, Sainte-Rose C, Renier D (1993) Malignant hemispheric tumors in childhood. *Child's Nerv Syst* **9**: 131–135.

Hoppe-Hirsch E, Brunet L, Laroussinie F, Cinalli G, Pierre-Kahn A, Renier D, Sainte-Rose C, Hirsch JF (1995) Intellectual outcome in children with malignant tumors of the posterior fossa: influence of the field of irradiation and quality of surgery. *Child's Nerv Syst* **11**: 340–345.

Ilveskoski I, Pihko H, Wiklund T, Lamminranta S, Perkkio M, Makipernaa A, Salmi TT, Lanning M, Saarinen UM (1996) Neuropsychologic late effects in children with malignant brain tumors treated with surgery, radiotherapy and "8 in 1" chemotherapy. *Neuropediatrics* **27**: 124–129.

Izquierdo I, Dias RD, Souza DO, Carrasco MA, Elisabetsky E, Perry ML (1980a) The role of opioid peptides in memory and learning. *Behav Brain Res* **1**: 451–468.

Izquierdo I, Souza DO, Carrasco MA, Dias RD, Perry ML, Eisinger S, Elisabetsky E, Vendite DA (1980b) Beta-endorphin causes retrograde amnesia and is released from the rat brain by various forms of training and stimulation. *Psychopharmacology* **70**: 173–177.

Izquierdo I, Souza DO, Dias RD, Perry ML, Carrasco MA, Volkmer N, Netto CA (1984) Effect of various behavioral training and testing procedures on brain beta-endorphin-like immunoreactivity and the possible role of beta-endorphin in behavioral regulation. *Psychoneuroendocrinology* **9**: 381–389.

Izquierdo I, Da Cunha C, Huang CH, Walz R, Wolfman C, Medina JH (1990) Post-training down-regulation of memory consolidation by a GABA-A mechanism in the amygdala modulated by endogenous benzodiazepines. *Behav Neurol Biol* **54**: 105–109.

Izquierdo I, Medina JH, Da Cunha C, Wolfman C, Jerusalinsky D, Ferreira MB (1991) Memory modulation by brain benzodiazepines. *Braz J Med Biol Res* **24**: 865–881.

Jo YH, Role LW (2002) Cholinergic modulation of purinergic and GABAergic co-transmission at in vitro hypothalamic synapses. *J Neurophysiol* **88**: 2501–2508.

Johnson DL, McCabe MA, Nicholson HS, Joseph AL, Getson PR, Byrne J, Brasseux C, Packer RJ, Reaman G (1994) Quality of long-term survival in young children with medulloblastoma. *J Neurosurg* **80**: 1004–1010.

Jonason KR, Enloe LJ (1971) Alterations in social behavior following septal and amygdaloid lesions in the rat. *J Comp Physiol Psychol* **75**: 286–301.

Jonason KR, Enloe LJ, Contrucci J, Meyer PM (1973) Effects of simultaneous and successive septal and amygdaloid lesions on social behavior of the rat. *J Comp Physiol Psychol* **83**: 54–61.

Joseph R (1982) The neuropsychology of development hemispheric laterality, limbic language, and the origin of thought. *J Clin Psychol* **38**: 4–33.

Joseph R (1992) The limbic system: emotion, laterality, and unconscious mind. *Psychoanal Rev* **79**: 405–456.

Joseph R (1998) Traumatic amnesia, repression, and hippocampus injury due to emotional stress, corticosteroids and enkephalins. *Child Psychiatry Hum Dev* **29**: 169–185.

Joseph R (1999) Environmental influences on neural plasticity, the limbic system, emotional development and attachment: a review. *Child Psychiatry Hum Dev* **29**: 189–208.

Joseph R, Gallagher RE (1980) Gender and early environmental influences on activity, overresponsiveness, and exploration. *Dev Psychobiol* **13**: 527–544.

Kao GD, Goldwein JW, Schultz DJ, Radcliffe J, Sutton L, Lange B (1994) The impact of perioperative factors on subsequent intelligence quotient deficits in children treated for medulloblastoma/posterior fossa primitive neuroectodermal tumors. *Cancer* **74**: 965–971.

Kesner RP, Wilburn MW (1974) A review of electrical stimulation of the brain in context of learning and retention. *Behav Biol* **10**: 259–293.

Kimura D (1963) Right temporal lobe damage: perception of unfamiliar stimuli after damage. *Arch Neurol* **8**: 264–271.

Kimura D (1969) Spatial localization in left and right visual fields. *Can J Psychol* **23**: 445–458.

Kita H, Kitai ST (1990) Amygdaloid projections to the frontal cortex and the striatum in the rat. *J Comp Neurol* **298**: 40–49.

Kling A, Cornell R (1971) Amygdalectomy and social behavior in the caged stump-tailed macaque (*Macaca speciosa*). *Folia Primatol* **14**: 190–208.

Kling A, Lancaster J, Benitone J (1970) Amygdalectomy in the free-ranging vervet (*Cercopithecus aethiops*). *J Psychiatr Res* **7**: 191–199.

Kreiter AK, Singer W (1996) Stimulus dependent synchronisation of neuronal responses in the visual cortex of the awake macaque monkey. *J Neurosci* **16**: 2381–2396.

Krettek JE, Price JL (1977) Projections from the amygdaloid complex to the cerebral cortex and thalamus in the rat and cat. *J Comp Neurol* **172**: 687–722.

Lachica EA, Crooks MW, Casagrande VA (1990) Effects of monocular deprivation on the morphology of retino-geniculate axon arbors in a primate. *J Comp Neurol* **296**: 303–323.

Lamm O, Gordon HW (1984) Right hemisphere superiority in processing new symbols for arithmetic operators. *Acta Psychol* **57**: 29–45.

Leaf LE (1993) Traumatic brain injury: affecting family recovery. *Brain Inj* **7**: 543–546.

LeDoux J (1998) Fear and the brain: where have we been, and where are we going? *Biol Psychiatry* **44**: 1229–1238.

LeDoux JE (1993a) Emotional memory systems in the brain. *Behav Brain Res* **58**: 69–79.

LeDoux JE (1993b) Emotional memory: in search of systems and synapses. *Ann NY Acad Sci* **702**: 149–157.

LeDoux JE (2000) Emotion circuits in the brain. *Annu Rev Neurosci* **23**: 155–184.

LeDoux JE, Risse GL, Springer SP, Wilson DH, Gazzaniga MS (1977) Cognition and commissurotomy. *Brain* **100**: 87–104.

Levisohn L, Cronin-Golomb A, Schmahmann JD (2000) Neuropsychological consequences of cerebellar tumour resection in children: cerebellar cognitive affective syndrome in a paediatric population. *Brain* **123**: 1041–1050.

Lewis JK, Morris MK, Morris RD, Krawiecki N, Foster MA (2000) Social problem solving in children with acquired brain injuries. *J Head Trauma Rehabil* **15**: 930–942.

Liang KC, Chen LL, Huang TE (1995) The role of amygdala norepinephrine in memory formation: involvement in the memory enhancing effect of peripheral epinephrine. *Chin J Physiol* **38**: 81–91.

Liang KC, McGaugh JL, Yao HY (1990) Involvement of amygdala pathways in the influence of post-training intra-amygdala norepinephrine and peripheral epinephrine on memory storage. *Brain Res* **508**: 225–233.

Lilly R, Cummings JL, Benson DF, Frankel M (1983) The human Kluver–Bucy syndrome. *Neurology* **33**: 1141–1145.

MacLean PD (1970) The triune brain, emotion, and scientific bias. In: Schmitt FO, ed. *The Neurosciences. Second Study Program*. New York: Rockefeller University Press, pp. 336–349.

MacLean PD (1977) The triune brain in conflict. *Psychother Psychosom* **28**: 207–220.

MacLean PD (1982) On the origin and progressive evolution of the triune brain. In: Armstrong E, Falk D, eds. *Primate Brain Evolution*. New York: Plenum Press, pp. 291–316.

MacLean PD (1985) Brain evolution relating to family, play, and the separation call. *Arch Gen Psychiatry* **42**: 405–417.

MacLean PD (1990) *The Triune Brain in Evolution*. New York: Plenum Press.

Malenka RC, Nicoll RA (1999) Long-term potentiation – a decade of progress? *Science* **285**: 1870–1874.

McGaugh JL, Gold PE (1976) Chapter title? In: Rosenzweig MR, Bennett EL, eds. *Neural Mechanisms of Learning and Memory*. Cambridge, MA: MIT Press, pp. 549–560.

McGaugh JL, Cahill L, Roozendaal B (1996) Involvement of the amygdala in memory storage: interaction with other brain systems. *Proc Natl Acad Sci USA* **93**: 13508–13514.

Medina JH, Pena C, Piva M, Wolfman C, de Stein ML, Wasowski C, Da Cunha C, Izquierdo I, Paladini AC (1992) Benzodiazepines in the brain. Their origin and possible biological roles. *Mol Neurobiol* **6**: 377–386.

Merzenich MM, Sameshima K (1993) Cortical plasticity and memory. *Curr Opin Neurobiol* **3**: 187–196.

Metcalfe J, Funnell M, Gazzaniga MS (1995) Right-hemisphere memory superiority: studies of a split-brain patient. *Psychol Sci* **6**: 157–164.

Meyer DR, Ruth RA, Lavond DG (1978) The septal social cohesiveness effect: its robustness and main determinants. *Physiol Behav* **21**: 1027–1029.

Meyer PM, Dalby DA, Glendenning KK, Lauber SM, Meyer DR (1973) Behavior of cats with lesions of the septal forebrain or anterior sigmoid neocortex. *J Comp Physiol Psychol* **85**: 491–501.

Milner B (1968) Visual recognition and recall after right temporal lobe excision in man. *Neuropsychologia* **6**: 191–209.

Milner B, Squire LR, Kandel ER (1998) Cognitive neuroscience and the study of memory. *Neuron* **20**: 445–468.

Nadel L (1992) Multiple memory systems: what and why. *J Cogn Neurosci* **4**: 179–188.

Nadel L, Bohbot V (2001) Consolidation of memory. *Hippocampus* **11**: 56–60.

O'Keefe J, Nadel L (1978) *The Hippocampus as a Cognitive Map*. Oxford: Clarendon Press.

Packard MG, Cahill L (2001) Affective modulation of multiple memory systems. *Curr Opin Neurobiol* **11**: 752–756.

Phelps EA, Gazzaniga MS (1992) Hemispheric differences in mnemonic processing: the effects of left hemisphere interpretation. *Neuropsychologia* **30**: 293–297.

Pitkanen A, Pikkarainen M, Nurminen N, Ylinen A (2000) Reciprocal connections between the amygdala and the hippocampal formation, perirhinal cortex, and postrhinal cortex in rat. A review. *Ann NY Acad Sci* **911**: 369–391.

Pollmann S, Zaidel E, von Cramon DY (2003) The neural basis of the bilateral distribution advantage. *Exp Brain Res* **153**: 322–333.

Quirarte GL, Roozendaal B, McGaugh JL (1997) Glucocorticoid enhancement of memory storage involves noradrenergic activation in the basolateral amygdala. *Proc Natl Acad Sci USA* **94**: 14048–14053.

Rakic P, Bourgeois JP, Eckenhoff MF, Zecevic N, Goldman-Rakic PS (1986) Concurrent overproduction of synapses in diverse regions of the primate cerebral cortex. *Science* **232**: 232–235.

Ramamurthi B (1988) Stereotactic operation in behaviour disorders. Amygdalotomy and hypothalamotomy. *Acta Neurochir Suppl* **44**: 152–157.

Rodriguez E, George N, Lachaux J-P, Martinerie J, Renault B, Varela FJ (1999) Perceptions shadow: long-distance synchronization of human brain activity. *Nature* **397**: 430–433.

Roozendaal B (2000) 1999 Curt P. Richter award. Glucocorticoids and the regulation of memory consolidation. *Psychoneuroendocrinology* **25**: 213–238.

Roozendaal B, Brunson KL, Holloway BL, McGaugh JL, Baram TZ (2002a) Involvement of stress-released corticotropin-releasing hormone in the basolateral amygdala in regulating memory consolidation. *Proc Natl Acad Sci USA* **99**: 13908–13913.

Roozendaal B, Quirarte GL, McGaugh JL (2002b) Glucocorticoids interact with the basolateral amygdala beta-adrenoceptor—cAMP/cAMP/PKA system in influencing memory consolidation. *Eur J Neurosci* **15**: 553–560.

Rosenblum LA, Coplan JD, Friedman S, Bassoff T, Gorman JM, Andrews MW (1994) Adverse early experiences affect noradrenergic and serotonergic functioning in adult primates. *Biol Psychiatry* **35**: 221–227.

Ryan L, Nadel L, Keil K, Putnam K, Schnyer D, Trouard T, Moscovitch M (2001) Hippocampal complex and retrieval of recent and very remote autobiographical memories: evidence from functional magnetic resonance imaging in neurologically intact people. *Hippocampus* **11**: 707–714.

Sapolsky RM (1996) Why stress is bad for your brain. *Science* **273**: 749–750.

329

Sapolsky RM (2000) Stress hormones: good and bad. *Neurobiol Dis* **7**: 540–542.

Sapolsky RM, Uno H, Rebert CS, Finch CE (1990) Hippocampal damage associated with prolonged glucocorticoid exposure in primates. *J Neurosci* **10**: 2897–2902.

Schreurs J, Seelig T, Schulman H (1986) Beta 2-adrenergic receptors on peripheral nerves. *J Neurochem* **46**: 294–296.

Sesma MA, Irvin GE, Kuyk TK, Norton TT, Casagrande VA (1984) Effects of monocular deprivation on the lateral geniculate nucleus in a primate. *Proc Natl Acad Sci USA* **81**: 2255–2259.

Sheline YI (1996) Hippocampal atrophy in major depression: a result of depression-induced neurotoxicity? *Mol Psychiatry* **1**: 298–299.

Sheline YI, Gado MH, Price JL (1998) Amygdala core nuclei volumes are decreased in recurrent major depression. *Neuroreport* **9**: 2023–2028.

Sheline YI, Sanghavi M, Mintun MA, Gado MH (1999) Depression duration but not age predicts hippocampal volume loss in medically healthy women with recurrent major depression. *J Neurosci* **19**: 5034–5043.

Sherwin ED, O'Shanick GJ (2000) The trauma of paediatric and adolescent brain injury: issues and implications for rehabilitation specialists. *Brain Inj* **14**: 267–284.

Shi WX, Rayport S (1994) GABA synapses formed in vitro by local axon collaterals of nucleus accumbens neurons. *J Neurosci* **14**: 4548–4560.

Silkis I (2001) The cortico-basal ganglia-thalamocortical circuit with synaptic plasticity. II. Mechanism of synergistic modulation of thalamic activity via the direct and indirect pathways through the basal ganglia. *Biosystems* **59**: 7–14.

Silkis IG (1998) The unitary modification rules for neural networks with excitatory and inhibitory synaptic plasticity. *Biosystems* **48**: 205–213.

Skrebitsky VG, Chepkova AN (1998) Hebbian synapses in cortical and hippocampal pathways. *Rev Neurosci* **9**: 243–264.

Slavc I, Salchegger C, Hauer C, Urban C, Oberbauer R, Pakisch B, Ebner F, Schwinger W, Mokry M, Ranner G, et al. (1994) Follow-up and quality of survival of 67 consecutive children with CNS tumors. *Child's Nerv Syst* **10**: 433–443.

Spence C, Kingstone A, Shore DI, Gazzaniga MS (2001) Representation of visuotactile space in the split brain. *Psychol Sci* **12**: 90–93.

Squire LR (1992) Declarative and nondeclarative memory: multiple brain systems supporting learning and memory. *J Cogn Neurosci* **4**: 232–243.

Squire LR, Zola SM (1996) Structure and function of declarative and nondeclarative memory systems. *Proc Natl Acad Sci USA* **93**: 13515–13522.

Squire LR, Knowlton B, Musen G (1993) The structure and organization of memory. *Annu Rev Psychol* **44**: 453–495.

Starkman MN, Gebarski SS, Berent S, Schteingart DE (1992) Hippocampal formation volume, memory dysfunction, and cortisol levels in patients with Cushing's syndrome. *Biol Psychiatry* **32**: 756–765.

Starkman MN, Giordani B, Gebarski SS, Berent S, Schork MA, Schteingart DE (1999) Decrease in cortisol reverses human hippocampal atrophy following treatment of Cushing's disease. *Biol Psychiatry* **46**: 1595–1602.

Stroufe LA (1996) *Emotional Development*. New York: Cambridge University Press.

Uno H, Eisele S, Sakai A, Shelton S, Baker E, DeJesus O, Holden J (1994) Neurotoxicity of glucocorticoids in the primate brain. *Horm Behav* **28**: 336–348.

Uylings HB, Kuypers K, Diamond MC, Veltman WA (1978) Effects of differential environments on plasticity of dendrites of cortical pyramidal neurons in adult rats. *Exp Neurol* **62**: 658–677.

Vaadia E, Haalman I, Abeles M, Bergman H, Prut Y, Slovin H, Aertsen A (1995) Dynamics of neuronal interaction in the monkey cortex in relation to behavioural events. *Nature* **373**: 515–518.

van Stegeren AH, Everaerd W, Cahill L, McGaugh JL, Gooren LJ (1998) Memory for emotional events: differential effects of centrally versus peripherally acting beta-blocking agents. *Psychopharmacology* **138**: 305–310.

Varela FJ (1995) Resonant cell assemblies: a new approach to cognitive function and neuronal synchrony. *Biol Res* **28**: 81–95.

Yang TF, Wong TT, Cheng LY, Chang TK, Hsu TC, Chen SJ, Chuang TY (1997) Neuropsychological sequelae after treatment for medulloblastoma in childhood—the Taiwan experience. *Child's Nerv Syst* **13**: 77–80.

Zaidel E (1991) Language function in the two hemispheres following complete cerebral commissurotomy and hemispherectomy. In: Boller F, Grafman J, eds. *Handbook of Neuropsychology, 4th edn*. Amsterdam: Elsevier, pp. 115–150.

22
PALLIATIVE CARE

Erica Mackie

> *"a time to be born and a time to die,*
> *a time to weep and a time to laugh,*
> *a time to mourn and a time to dance"*
> *Ecclesiastes* **3**: 2–4

The undoubted challenge for childhood CNS tumours remains the introduction of novel therapeutic methods aimed at improving current survival figures (Wolff and Egeler 1999). Although significant progress has been made in our understanding of the biology for many of these tumours, parallel improvements in clinical outcomes have not yet been achieved (Reddy 2001). Indeed, the anaplastic astrocytomas, and in particular the diffuse high-grade pontine gliomas, often present without the hope of cure with currently available therapy (Shiminski-Maher 1996, Cohen et al. 2001, Farmer et al. 2001). Low survival rates continue to present a clinical dilemma for children under the age of 2, with only limited progress achieved in the last three decades (Stiller and Bunch 1992).

CNS tumours are unique in the challenges that arise for families during palliative care. It is well recognized that a long pre-diagnostic period exists for many of these children, engendering an underlying sense of insecurity before active treatment has even commenced. Presenting symptoms can be subtle and nonspecific, such as changes in behaviour and intermittent headaches (Gordon et al. 1995, Edgeworth et al. 1996). This enhances the uncertainty with which these families live, during both active therapy and the palliative phase.

Following diagnosis, the outcome and prognosis can remain uncertain. Treatment is offered to many children without the promise of 'cure', but with the hope of living alongside the tumour. This may be relatively optimistic for children with a low-grade glioma or cranio-pharyngioma, but less so for those with a brainstem tumour or an unresectable astrocytoma. Consequently, children and families can be living with the threat of a life-limiting disease prior to the time of tumour progression.

Palliative care
The report from the Joint Working Party of the Association for Children with Life-Threatening or Terminal Conditions and their Families (ACT) and the Royal College of Paediatrics and Child Health (RCPCH) defined palliative care for children and young people with life-limiting conditions as "an active and total approach to care, embracing physical, emotional, social and spiritual elements. It focuses on enhancement of quality of life for the child and support for the family and includes the management of distressing symptoms, provision of respite

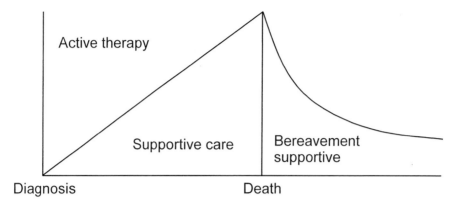

Fig. 22.1. Relationship between active and palliative care.

and care through death and bereavement" (ACT/RCPCH 1997). This clearly defines the areas of holistic care required for a child with a brain tumour. Importantly it emphasizes support for the whole family, which includes not only the primary caregivers (usually the parents), but also siblings and other members of the extended family, including grandparents. A further collaborative document from ACT, the National Council for Hospice and Specialist Palliative Care Services and the Scottish Partnership Agency for Palliative and Cancer Care reiterates the importance of holistic care for young people aged 13–24 years with a life-limiting condition (ACT/NCHSPCVS/SPAPCC 2001).

As for all children with cancer, treatment usually commences with the optimism of cure. The transition between curative and palliative care can be gradual, and importantly, as illustrated in Figure 22.1, active involvement with the family continues after the death of the child.

Many years after the death of a child, a family may find it helpful to revisit their child's illness, review the scans and raise questions that were perhaps too painful to face earlier. Siblings who were initially too young to remember many details may wish to visit the ward where their brother/sister was treated and have the opportunity to address their own anxieties.

Decision making

"a time to search and a time to die"

Ecclesiastes **3**: 6

The smooth transition to the palliative phase of an illness is dependent on good communication between the health professionals, the family and the child. Some families find it easier to accept that no further active therapy is available, whereas others will want to pursue experimental avenues. Research has identified that parents of children with cancer have difficulty in distinguishing between research and treatment and consequently can feel that they are not in control of the choices available (Broome et al. 2001, Deatrick et al. 2002). End-of-life decisions were found to be more challenging for parents than decisions based around other areas of treatment (Hinds et al. 1997).

Throughout all these discussions, it is essential to listen sensitively to the wishes of the child, providing them with appropriate information with regard to the progress of their illness, together with a full explanation about the treatment options. When a child is deemed competent, they should be able to take part fully in the decision making process, and a decision to refuse a certain treatment choice should be respected. Although a child is legally not able to dissent from a decision until the age of 18, both the UN Convention on the Rights of the Child (1991) and the UK Children's Act 1989 emphasize the importance of considering a child's views in relation to any decision affecting the child's future.

With little clarity and much controversy regarding the optimum therapeutic choice for many CNS tumours, it is not surprising that families sometimes find it difficult to accept that the only realistic therapy offers little hope of cure. Time spent discussing 'internet discoveries' and novel agents with the family can provide a background on which to develop a dialogue about the 'best interests' of the child. A sympathetic second opinion can also be invaluable in helping a family comes to terms with the inevitable prognosis.

Symptoms care during palliation

"a time to tear and a time to mend"

Ecclesiastes **3**: 7

The clinical presentation and mode of progression will depend on the location of the tumour. Specific neurological deficits will identify the position, whereas generalized symptoms, such as headache, nausea, lethargy and irritability, may indicate only the presence of a space-occupying lesion, with or without associated raised intracranial pressure (ICP).

THE ROLE OF CORTICOSTEROIDS IN PALLIATIVE CARE

When the symptoms of progressive disease are confirmed, corticosteroids can be usefully prescribed. However, controversy surrounds the use of steroids in palliative care. In a recent single institution audit of steroid use for 47 children with brain tumours, 33 were given steroids at some point during the palliative period, of whom 14 experienced some symptomatic relief. Response was demonstrated in those with signs of raised ICP, but not in the group with ataxia, cranial nerve palsies and long tract signs. Significant sequelae were identified in 11 of the children, all of whom had received a prolonged course of steroids (Watterson et al. 2002).

There is currently no evidence base to inform this practice, although guidelines have been published outlining the use of steroids in the situation of raised ICP secondary to peritumoral oedema. Short pulses of dexamethasone ($10\,mg/m^2$/day for 3–5 days) were recommended, with symptomatic benefit often lasting for periods up to 4 weeks (Hardy et al. 2001).

Restricting the role of steroids is essential, with their use confined to those children who may achieve temporary relief, enabling them to attain short-term goals, such as a holiday or a family celebration. Immediate side-effects should be anticipated including oral candidiasis and gastrointestinal irritation (Glaser et al. 1997). These can be treated with oral nystatin or fluconazole and appropriate antacids, respectively. In addition, steroids have been reported to be associated with behavioural difficulties, emotional lability and night wakening (Satel 1990, Drigan et al. 1992, Soliday et al. 1999). Longer-term usage can cause unwanted weight gain, with a change in self-image, together with decreased mobility, compounded by possible proximal myopathy.

Corticosteroid therapy, however, has an important therapeutic role in preserving the neurological function and decreasing pain associated with spinal cord compression secondary to epidural metastases (Wolfe et al. 2002).

MANAGEMENT OF PAIN

Headache

Headache occurs classically as a consequence of raised ICP, where compression of structures remote to the tumour occurs. Infratentorial lesions are more likely to cause raised ICP, and are commonly associated with discomfort occurring in the nuchal region. Headaches also develop as a direct result of mechanical pressure, tissue destruction and tissue displacement by the tumour (Caracini and Martini 1997). Symptoms are heightened by the effect of oedema surrounding the tumour (Andersen et al. 1993, Caracini and Martini 1997). High-grade tumours are more likely to result in uncontrollable headaches, compared to those with slower growth, where compensatory changes in the cerebral vasculature and the cerebrospinal fluid volume may occur. If there is a sudden deterioration in the symptoms, a secondary haemorrhage or hydrocephalus must be considered.

Management follows the basic philosophy of symptom control in palliative care, whereby the aim is to achieve the minimal intervention required to produce symptom relief, with the goal of maintaining a good quality of life. Neurosurgical intervention may be appropriate to alleviate obstructive hydrocephalus, or occasionally, debulking of a tumour may result in a prolongation of useful life. Similarly, radiotherapy can also be given to produce temporary symptom relief, and this can be considered for the high-grade brainstem gliomas, where although the median survival may be prolonged, the majority will still have progressed 6–12 months after diagnosis (Reddy 2001).

Pain control can follow the WHO analgesic ladder, which recommends a stepwise use of medication, with opioids prescribed only when alternative, milder drugs have failed (WHO 1990) (Fig. 22.2). The reality is that headaches secondary to raised ICP will probably require the early use of strong analgesics, and it is essential that they be used with confidence and by the most effective route. A ceiling effect exists for both paracetamol and the mild opioids such as codeine, whereas morphine and diamorphine are not limited in this way (Royal College Of Paediatrics and Child Health 1997, Goldman 1998). Whatever the choice of analgesia, it should be prescribed regularly, avoiding the experience of breakthrough pain (McGrath 1997). The practice of reassessing pain routinely is also of paramount importance in providing optimum pain control (Stevens 1994, Hain 1997).

Corticosteroids have a place in the management of headache secondary to raised ICP, although they must be prescribed with the caution outlined previously. It is usually possible to avoid their use, if adequate analgesia, together with anti-emetics, is commenced as the pain re-emerges. If a child appears to be becoming dependent on steroids, it is worth considering a change to administering medication via a subcutaneous or intravenous infusion.

334

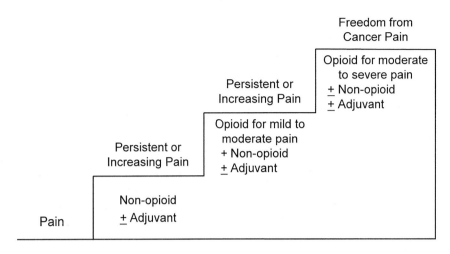

Fig. 22.2. The WHO 3-step analgesic ladder.

Neuropathic pain

This most commonly occurs following either infiltration or compression of the spinal cord or nerve roots secondary to a primary spinal cord tumour or leptomeningeal dissemination through the subarachnoid space (Kenner 1994). It can be a significant management challenge, most often presenting with waves of shooting pain, or severe burning pain. A background of altered sensation (dysaesthesia) can be experienced, and increased sensitivity to normal stimuli (allodynia) is also described. Similar principles of basic pain management apply, although conventional analgesics such as opioids are not always effective and it is essential to assess their therapeutic window with care (Twycross 1997).

Co-analgesics, including the tricyclic antidepressants (TCAs) can be used with some success, with evidence that their mechanism of action is independent from their anti-depressant activity. Amitriptyline is the most commonly used in children and is particularly successful for 'burning' pain (Royal College Of Paediatrics and Child Health 1997, Watson 2000). A nocturnal dose is usually recommended to avoid daytime sedation, allowing up to 4 days to evaluate the effect. Amitriptyline should be stopped if no response has been seen after 2 weeks at appropriate dosage.

Neuropathic symptoms are also responsive to anticonvulsant drugs (McQuay et al. 1995), in particular those that are stabbing in nature (Twycross 1997). There is some evidence that they are also useful in children experiencing continuous dyaesthesia. Carbamazepine is usually the first-line anticonvulsant drug prescribed, but there is evidence of successful use with several others, including sodium valproate and clonazapam. Clinical experience suggests that gabapentin has an important role to play in neuropathic pain, being both effective and with limited side-effects (Rosenberg et al. 1997, McGraw and Stacey 1998). As with the TCAs, the anticonvulsant dose needs to be increased gradually allowing up to 4 days to monitor the response. The combination of TCAs and anticonvulsants can also be a useful therapeutic manoeuvre.

In more resistant cases of neuropathic pain, it is worth considering nerve or intraspinal blocks, and early involvement of an experienced anaesthetist is important. Combinations of an anaesthetic agent such as bupivicaine, together with an opiate are useful in these cases (Collins et al. 1996). Data are also available in the paediatric population, demonstrating the potential use of a continuous infusion of ketamine, an n-methyl-d-aspartate (NMDA) antagonist, for refractory cases. Close monitoring for side-effects is essential, including hallucinations and dysphoria (Klepstead et al. 2001).

A useful strategy is to give children the opportunity to take some control of their pain. Transcutaneous electrical nerve stimulation (TENS) allows the patient to position and adjust both the timing and frequency of the electrical stimulation (Tulgar 1992). There is a variable outcome, but for limited periods it has been shown to help resistant pain. When a good response is observed, it can be possible to decrease the analgesic dosage.

The anxiety and fear that so often potentiates the experience of pain can be treated successfully with an anxiolytic, such as sublingual lorazepam. If this is shown to be effective in the acute situation, a regular small dose of an oral benzodiazepine or oral levomepromazine can be usefully prescribed. Both can also be administered successfully through a syringe driver if necessary. Equally, non-invasive distraction techniques play an essential role in the management of all pain, and advice from play therapists and teaching staff should be sought. Directed activity that fully absorbs the child will actually reduce the pain, by decreasing the neuronal responses evoked by tissue damage (McGrath 1997).

MUSCLE SPASMS

Involuntary muscle spasms are both distressing and often extremely painful. The most successful management is usually with a muscle relaxant, such as regular, low-dose diazepam (Goldman 1998). If the spasms are particularly refractory, an infusion of midazolam can be administered and is particularly useful during the terminal stage of the illness. Unacceptable drowsiness can occur, and then oral baclofen can be considered as an alternative therapy. Physiotherapy and gentle massage also have a useful role to play.

SEIZURES

Children with a CNS tumour, particularly one involving the cerebral hemispheres, may present with seizures and already be receiving regular anticonvulsant therapy at the time of tumour progression. In these cases, continued liaison with a paediatric neurologist can be extremely helpful. However, fits can be a new event in the terminal phase and it is important that families are forewarned about this possibility. Fear of the unknown, alongside anxiety about how to manage a new situation, can create further tension for the child and family. It is therefore essential to explain the nature of a fit, provide simple management strategies, and place the necessary medication in the child's home. Rectal diazepam is the simplest method for parents to manage an acute fit, although buccal midazolam (Scott et al. 1999) and sublingual clonazepam can also be useful. Diazepam and midazolam can also be administered through either a nasogastric tube or a gastrostomy.

Recurrent short-lived or focal seizures may not warrant active intervention during the terminal stages, and as with all symptoms, the balance between the benefit of additional therapy and the side-effects must be sensitively measured. Clearly, a child with a predicted life span of several months will benefit from regular anticonvulsant therapy.

Intractable fits as a child deteriorates can be treated with a subcutaneous infusion of midazolam or clonazepam. Both are sedative along with their anticonvulsant effect and are compatible with diamorphine and antiemetics such as cyclizine and levomepromazine.

ANXIETY AND AGITATION

The expression of anxiety in a child may reflect underlying fears related to symptoms of their progressive illness, or death. Enabling them to express and examine their feelings can help children regain control over both their emotions and future plans. When a child becomes more agitated, regular low-dose diazepam or levomepromazine can be useful. In a severe anxiety crisis or panic attack, sublingual lorazepam or antranasal midazolam have an important role (Cope et al. 2002). As a child approaches the terminal stages an infusion via a syringe driver of levomepromazine or midazolam can provide helpful sedation. All these therapies can be used in conjunction with adjunctive methods such as aromatherapy and massage (Wilkinson et al. 1999).

NAUSEA AND VOMITING

Although vomiting may be a direct result of raised ICP in a child with a brain tumour, it is essential to exclude other treatable causes, such as constipation, gastric irritation, side-effects of drugs or chemotherapy, and simple infections such as of the urinary tract. Corticosteroids, prescribed with caution, can resolve the nausea secondary to raised ICP and are also useful in the control of emesis secondary to chemotherapy. However, this effect is usually only temporary and alternative measures should be considered. Cyclizine is particularly useful in controlling the nausea and vomiting secondary to raised ICP and can be used as both an oral medication and an infusion, where it is compatible with an opioid. Levomepromazine, which has an important role as an anxiolytic and sedative, is also effective as an anti-emetic, confirming it as an essential drug in the symptomatic treatment for CNS tumours. Although anti-emetic drugs have specific sites of action, resistant vomiting often requires a combination of drugs. Ondansetron, a 5HT antagonist, available as both an oral and intravenous preparation, can be a useful addition to cyclizine and has been shown to be useful in palliation (Currow et al. 1997).

ARTIFICIAL NUTRITION AND HYDRATION

The role of artificial nutrition and hydration is dependent on the nature of the tumour and the stage of the disease process, and it is therefore important to regularly address the merits of these interventions in liaison with the family. Quality of life may be enhanced by nutritional supplementation in a child with a slowly progressive tumour, who although hungry, develops a bulbar palsy and is unable to swallow. Conversely, anorexia often accompanies the terminal stages of a child's illness, when artificial supplementation is unlikely to enhance life. However, some reversible causes should always be considered, such as nausea, sore mouth, constipation, depression, or the presentation of inappropriate or unappetising food (Miller-Thiel et al. 1993). Food is one area where parents feel they can maintain control

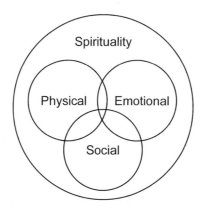

Fig. 22.3. The key elements of palliative care.

and it is likely that pursuing a good nutritional status will have been a priority during active therapy. If long-term assisted feeding becomes inevitable, a gastrostomy presents fewer complications than a nasogastric tube, and for the older child may help to preserve their self-esteem.

Families often express concern that their child will become distressed as a consequence of poor nutrition or dehydration, and clear explanations can help the family come to terms with this sensitive issue. There is no evidence base to suggest that dehydration is uncomfortable for children in the terminal stage and some observational data suggest that there is no association between fluid intake and thirst in the dying patient (Millard 1999). Indeed, the symptoms of cerebral oedema may be reduced and the indignity of incontinence helped by a decreased urine output. When a child demonstrates thirst, fluids can be administered via a nasogastric tube, but even in these cases, moistening the dry mouth with a sponge can often suffice. The ethical dilemma of balancing the benefits of intervention against the burdens is a continual challenge, with little research available to inform clinical decisions in this area. If there is doubt about the benefits/burden assessment in the palliative setting, the moral stance of non-treatment is preferable (Randall and Downie 1996). In all cases it is important that these decisions should involve the multidisciplinary team, including the child where possible, and parents.

Involuntary dribbling, with the risk of aspiration, is a potentially distressing and humiliating consequence for children unable to cough and swallow. Placing the unconscious child in the coma position is a simple measure to prevent aspiration, and a portable suction machine in the home can be helpful. Hyoscine hydrobromide has an important role to play in the reduction of secretions and is effective administered transdermally, using a patch that can be changed every 3 days. The subcutaneous route can also be used, either as a regular 6-hourly dose or as an infusion. Hyoscine hydrobromide also has a useful anti-emetic effect.

Supporting the child and family
Although good symptom control is an essential background on which to build other aspects

1. Every child shall be treated with dignity and respect and shall be afforded privacy whatever the child's physical or intellectual ability

2. Parents shall be acknowledged as the primary carers and shall be centrally involved as partners in all care and decisions involving their child

3. Every child shall be given the opportunity to participate in decisions affecting his or her care, according to age and understanding

4. Every family shall be given the opportunity of a consultation with a paediatric specialist who has particular knowledge of the child's condition

5. Information shall be provided for the parents, and for the child and siblings according to age and understanding. The needs of other relatives shall also be addressed

6. An honest and open approach shall be the basis of all communication which shall be sensitive and appropriate to age and understanding

7. The family home shall remain the centre of caring whenever possible. All other care shall be provided by paediatric trained staff in a child-centred environment

8. Every child shall have access to education. Efforts shall be made to enable the child to engage in other childhood activities

9. Every family shall be entitled to a named key-worker who will enable the family to build up and maintain an appropriate support system

10. Every family shall have access to flexible respite care in their own home and in a home-from-home setting for the whole family, with appropriate paediatric nursing and medical support

11. Every family shall have access to paediatric nursing support in the home when required

12. Every family shall have access to expert, sensitive advice in procuring practical aids and financial support

13. Every family shall have access to domestic help at times of stress at home

14. Bereavement support shall be offered to the whole family and be available for as long as is required

Fig. 22.4. Charter drawn up by the ACT (Association for Children with Life-Threatening or Terminal Conditions and their Families), outlining their recommendations for the holistic care of these children and their families.

of palliative care, it is imperative to integrate the management of physical difficulties with the emotional, social and spiritual elements of the child's care (Fig. 22.3).

Although spirituality is recognized as an important aspect of holistic care, it has been relatively neglected in the literature. Guidelines to assess spirituality have recently been described by the Children's International Project on Children's Palliative/Hospice Services (Davies et al. 2002). ACT has published a charter that summarizes the holistic care that all children and their families can expect to receive (Fig. 22.4).

Preparation for the terminal phase includes a discussion with regard to the place of death. Increasingly, families elect to look after their child at home (Chambers et al. 1989, Vickers and Carlisle 2000), and with forward planning between the general practitioner, community nurses, local hospice and other voluntary agencies, this can usually be facilitated. It is important that the child and parents feel that a choice is available and that they are supported in their decision. Since the opening of the first children's hospice, Helen House in 1982, a further 24 hospices have now been established throughout the UK. In the presence of a long palliative phase, together with the often distressing symptoms experienced by a child with a brain tumour, hospice care can be extremely helpful for periods of respite and, more rarely, the terminal event.

Effective communication, however, remains the key element in delivering good palliative care to these families. The journey travelled by each child has many potential paths, and although it is the health care professionals' responsibility to provide families with a map and guidebook, it is essential that the child and parents can choose to be actively involved in the decision-making process at each crossroad. Equally, it is essential that health professionals are supported in the service that they provide for these families, with appropriate resources available for both supervision and training.

REFERENCES

ACT/NCHSPCS/SPAPCC (2001) *Palliative Care for Young People Aged 13–24 Years*. Bristol: ACT.

ACT/RCPCH (1997) *A Guide to the Development of Children's Palliative Care Services*. Bristol: ACT.

Andersen C, Haselgrove JC, Doenstrup S, Astrup J, Gyldensted C (1993) Resorption of peritumoural oedema in cerebral gliomas during dexamethasone treatment evaluated by NMR relaxation time imaging. *Acta Neurochir* **122**: 218–224.

Broome ME, Richards DJ, Hall JM (2001) Children in research: the experience of ill children and adolescents. *J Fam Nurs* **7**: 214–218.

Caracini A, Martini (1997) Symptom management: neurological problems. In: Doyle D, Hanks G, MacDonald N, eds. *Oxford Textbook of Palliative Medicine, 2nd edn*. Oxford: Oxford University Press, pp. 727–728.

Chambers EJ, Oakhill A, Cornish JM, Curnick S (1989) Terminal care at home for children with cancer. *BMJ* **298**: 937–940.

Children's Act 1989. London: HMSO.

Cohen KJ, Broniscer A, Glod J (2001) Pediatric glial tumors. *Curr Treat Options Oncol* **2**: 529–536.

Collins JJ, Grier HE, Sethna NF, Wilder RT, Berde CB (1996) Regional anesthesia for pain associated with terminal pediatric malignancy. *Pain* **65**: 63–69.

Cope J, Bentley R, Jenney MEM, Hain R (2002) Use of intranasal/oral midazolam in paediatric palliative care. *Med Pediatr Oncol* **39**: 376 (abstract).

Currow DC, Coughlan M, Fardell B, Cooney NJ (1997) Use of ondansetron in palliative medicine. *J Pain Symptom Manage* **13**: 302–307.

Davies B, Brenner P, Orloff S, Sumner L, Worden W (2002) Addressing spirituality in pediatric hospice and palliative care. *J Palliat Care* **18**: 59–67.

Deatrick JA, Angst DB, Moore C (2002) Parents' views of their children's participation in phase 1 oncology clinical trials. *J Pediatr Oncol Nurs* **19**: 114–121.

Drigan R, Spirito A, Gelber RD (1992) Behavioral effects of corticosteroids in children with acute lympho-blastic leukemia. *Med Pediatr Oncol* **20**: 13–21.

Edgeworth J, Bullock P, Bailey A, Gallagher A, Crouchman M (1996) Why are brain tumours still being missed? *Arch Dis Child* **74**: 148–151.

Farmer JP, Montes JL, Freeman CR, Meagher-Villemure K, Bond MC, O'Gorman AM (2001) Brainstem gliomas. A 10-year institutional review. *Pediatr Neurosurg* **34**: 206–214.

Glaser AW, Buxton N, Walker D (1997) Corticosteroids in the management of central nervous system tumours. Kids Neuro-Oncology Workshop (KNOWS). *Arch Dis Child* **76**: 76–78.

Goldman A (1998) *Care of the Dying Child*. Oxford: Oxford University Press.

Gordon GS, Wallace SJ, Neal JW (1995) Intracranial tumours during the first two years of life: presenting features. *Arch Dis Child* **73**: 345–347.

Hain RDW (1997) Pain scales in children: a review. *Palliat Med* **11**: 341–350.

Hardy JR, Rees E, Ling J, Burman R, Feuer D, Broadley K, Stone P (2001) A prospective survey of the use of dexamethasone on a palliative care unit. *Palliat Med* **15**: 3–8.

Hinds PS, Oakes L, Furman W, Foppiano P, Olson MS, Quargnenti A, Gattuso J, Powell B, Srivastava DK, Jayawardene D, Sandlund JT, Strong C (1997) Decision making by parents and healthcare professionals when considering continued care for pediatric patients with cancer. *Oncol Nurs Forum* **24**: 1523–1528.

Kenner DJ (1994) Pain forum. Part 2. Neuropathic pain. *Aust Fam Physician* **23**: 1279–1283.

Klepstad P, Borchgrevink P, Hval B, Flaat S, Kaasa S (2001) Long-term treatment with ketamine in a 12-year-old girl with severe neuropathic pain caused by a cervical spinal tumor. *J Pediatr Hematol Oncol* **23**: 616–619.

McGrath PA (1997) Paediatric palliative care: pain control. In: Doyle D, Hanks G, MacDonald N, eds. *Oxford Textbook of Palliative Medicine, 2nd edn*. Oxford: Oxford University Press, pp. 1013–1028.

McGraw T, Stacey BR (1998) Gabapentin for treatment of neuropathic pain in a 12-year-old girl. *Clin J Pain* **14**: 354–356.

McQuay H, Carroll D, Jadad AR, Wiffen P, Moore A (1995) Anticonvulsant drugs for management of pain: a systematic review. *BMJ* **311**: 1047–1052.

Millard PH (1999) Ethical decisions at the end of life. *J R Coll Physicians Lond* **33**: 365–367.

Miller-Thiel J, Glover JJ, Beliveau E (1993) Caring for the dying child. *Hosp J* **9**: 55–72.

Randall F, Downie RS (1996) *Palliative Care Ethics: A Good Companion*. Oxford: Oxford University Press.

Reddy AT (2001) Advances in biology and treatment of childhood brain tumors. *Curr Neurol Neurosci Rep* **1**: 137–143.

Rosenberg JM, Harrell C, Ristic H, Werner RA, de Rosayro AM (1997) The effect of gabapentin on neuropathic pain. *Clin J Pain* **13**: 251–255.

Royal College Of Paediatrics and Child Health (1997) Management of long-term pain and pain during terminal care. In: *Prevention and Control of Pain in Children: a Manual for Health Care Professionals*. London: BMJ Publishing Group, pp. 1013–1028.

Satel SL (1990) Mental status changes in children receiving glucocorticoids; review of the literature. *Clin Pediatr* **29**: 383–388.

Scott RC, Besag FM, Neville BG (1999) Buccal midazolam and rectal diazepam for treatment of prolonged seizures in childhood and adolescence: a randomised trial. *Lancet* **353**: 623–626.

Shiminski-Maher T (1996) Brainstem tumors in childhood: preparing patients and families for long- and short-term care. *Pediatr Neurosurg* **24**: 267–271.

Soliday E, Grey S, Lande MB (1999) Behavioural effects of corticosteroids in steroid-sensitive nephrotic syndrome. *Pediatr* **104**: e51.

Stevens MM, Dalla Pozza L, Cavalletto B, Cooper MG, Kilham HA (1994) Pain and symptom control in paediatric palliative care. *Cancer Surv* **21**: 211–231.

Stiller CA, Bunch KJ (1992) Brain and spinal tumours in children aged under two years: incidence and survival in Britain, 1971–85. *Br J Cancer Suppl* **18**: S50–S53.

Tulgar M (1992) Advances in electrical nerve stimulation techniques to manage chronic pain: an overview. *Adv Ther* **9**: 366–372.

Twycross R (1997) *Introducing Palliative Care*. Oxford: Radcliffe Medical.

United Nations (1991) *Convention on the Rights of the Child*. London: HMSO.

Vickers JL, Carlisle C (2000) Choices and control: parental experiences in pediatric terminal home care. *J Pediatr Oncol Nurs* **17**: 12–21.

Watson CP (2000) The treatment of neuropathic pain: antidepressants and opioids. *Clin J Pain* **16** (Suppl 2): S49–S55.

Watterson G, Goldman A, Michalski A (2002) Corticosteroids in the palliative phase of paediatric brain tumours. *Arch Dis Child* **86**: A76 (abstract).

WHO (1990) *Cancer Pain Relief and Palliative Care in Children*. Geneva: World Health Organization.

Wilkinson S, Aldridge J, Salmon I, Cain E, Wilson B (1999) An evaluation of aromatherapy massage in palliative care. *Palliat Med* **13**: 409–417.

Wolfe J, Friebert S, Hilden J (2002) Caring for children with advanced cancer: integrating palliative care. *Pediatr Clin North Am* **49**: 1043–1062.

Wolff JEA, Egeler RM (1999) Investigational approaches to the treatment of brain tumors in children. *Med Pediatr Oncol* **32**: 135–138.

341

SECTION FOUR

SUMMARY

23
CONCLUSIONS AND FUTURE DIRECTIONS

Eddy Estlin and Stephen Lowis

The preceding sections have introduced the epidemiology, contemporary diagnosis, treatment and problems encountered in the longer term for children diagnosed with brain and spinal cord tumours.

In his chapter on epidemiology of paediatric brain tumours, Dr Burke has highlighted the varying and indeed apparently increasing incidence of this tumour type in western industrialized nations. The impact of genetic predisposition syndromes such as Li–Fraumeni syndrome and the neurofibromatoses has been summarized, recognizing that genetic influences are as yet identified only in the minority of patients with CNS malignancy. The importance of such syndromes for the affected individual lies in their impact on treatment, responsiveness of tumours to therapy, and their overall prognosis in the long term, and hence it is important to consider and recognize affected patients whenever possible.

With reference to the radiological investigation of children with CNS tumours, Dr Renowden has provided an exceptional collection of MR images, and a commentary that offers great insight into the process of diagnosis of CNS tumours. This chapter alone will prove a great aid to paediatric brain tumour management for many readers.

Drs Rorke and Biegel present a very comprehensive overview of the histological and cytogenetic characteristics for the large variety of CNS tumours that occur in children. In particular, the complimentary roles of histology, immunohistochemistry and cytogenetics for the diagnosis of paediatric CNS tumours are discussed, and these findings are related to tumour location and prognosis when possible.

In complement to this detailed description of histology and cytogenetics, Dr Gilbertson introduces the reader to the principles of molecular oncology and the application of this field to our understanding of the biology of, and rational selection of new therapeutic agents for, childhood CNS tumours. In the first section of his discussion, Dr Gilbertson outlines the advances in molecular biology techniques, with a description of global analyses of the genome, genomic losses and gains, gene expression assays and proteomics. The importance of these techniques in contemporary understanding of the tumour oncogenes and tumour suppressor genes that are being investigated for diseases such as primitive neuroectodermal tumour is highlighted. In addition, advances in preclinical disease models mean that it is now possible to produce mice with germline mutations that result in gain or loss of function, which holds great promise for studying tumorigenesis in the nervous system and potential for understanding the maintenance of tumour growth by stem-cell-like cancer cells. Finally, Dr Gilbertson relates molecular biology to contemporary disease management in the setting of childhood CNS tumours, and describes recent advances in the development of molecular targeted therapies such as drugs that target cell surface receptor kinases and inhibitors of angiogenesis.

When discussing the general principles of neurosurgery, Mr Ross and Mr Thorne provide an excellent overview of contemporary perioperative care and management of the common paediatric CNS tumours in their infratentorial and supratentorial locations. The discussion provides an insight into the technical difficulties to be overcome with these procedures, and a description of modern image-guided techniques of surgery, and their possible uses and limitations, is given. The recognition of the importance for completeness of surgical tumour resection and prognosis for many children's CNS tumours is discussed, along with the factors that limit this aim surgically. The authors conclude that neurosurgery will continue to play a pivotal role for the management of children with CNS tumours as advances in chemotherapy and radiotherapy are made.

For the radiotherapy of paediatric CNS tumours, Drs Estlin and Lowis describe the general principles of radiation physics and biology, and the role played by, and importance of, radiotherapy for the treatment of the common CNS tumours of childhood. The role of radiotherapy in the causation of the significant late effects of radiation for some children surviving CNS tumours is highlighted. Recent advances in radiotherapy scheduling and targeting may improve the efficacy of this modality and also reduce late effects such as neuropsychological deficits and ototoxicity.

Dr Estlin discusses the potential importance of the pharmacology of drugs in relation to the treatment of CNS tumours. The importance of the blood–brain barrier in limiting the access of most of the contemporary anticancer agents to tumour cells is highlighted. In addition, an overview of the lack of early clinical studies in determining the choice of treatment strategies that are employed in contemporary Phase III studies of diseases such as medulloblastoma is given. As a model of the potential importance of the knowledge of the interrelationship between drug effectiveness and the cellular determinants of chemosensitivity, the example of temozolomide/CCNU and the DNA repair enzyme AGT is discussed in terms of HGG therapy. Tumour AGTase levels have been shown to be an important determinant of response for adults receiving therapy with temozolomide for HGG, and similar studies are required in order to optimize our existing therapies for CNS tumours of childhood.

Dr Lowis discusses the management of acute complications appearing around the time of presentation of CNS tumours. Specifically, the issues relating to the drowsy or unconscious child are discussed, since the prompt recognition and treatment of the cause of an encephalopathy or confusional state will limit potentially severe morbidity. Similarly, the management of the patient with acute intrinsic and extrinsic cord compression is considered in the context of primary and metastatic malignant disease. Finally, the management of metabolic, electrolyte and fluid disturbance is discussed, since poor control of these in the perioperative period may also lead to significant morbidity.

In the second section of the book, specific paediatric tumours are considered. For low-grade glioma (LGG) and high-grade glioma (HGG), Drs Estlin and Lowis discuss the important principles of treatment, which have been defined in modern treatment protocols. Important questions remain unanswered, however. LGGs can follow an indolent course clinically, especially in the setting of neurofibromatosis type I. Total resection of a low-grade tumour is often curative, whereas even completely resected HGGs are almost always fatal. A low-grade tumour may be prevented from progressing by chemotherapy or radiotherapy, or a combination of these two treatment modalities, whereas the role of chemotherapy has yet to be fully defined for HGGs. Despite the high survival rate for LGG, improvements in disease control and survival are still needed for children who present with disease at a young age, and for those with disease that is inoperable.

Dr Bartels and his colleagues from the Pediatric Brain Tumour Program at the Hospital for Sick Children, Toronto, discuss the subject of paediatric ependymoma. A very comprehensive overview of the histology, cytogenetics and molecular oncology of this tumour type and the relationship of these to prognosis is presented. The vital importance of surgical resection for prognosis is discussed, along with consideration of factors such as infratentorial location of tumour that limit this aim for many children. The authors also highlight the lack of randomized clinical trials to support the use of radiotherapy that has become a standard postoperative treatment in many centres, and also the lack of clear phase II data to support the use of chemotherapy in this disease. Ongoing studies may help to clarify some of these areas in terms of techniques of radiotherapy, the role of chemotherapy to improve the success of second-look surgery and outcome, and the molecular characteristics of these tumours in relation to prognosis.

Diffuse intrinsic pontine glioma remains an essentially incurable condition for which new anti-tumour agents are needed. In the discussion of brainstem glioma, Drs Freeman and Farmer describe the clinicopathological characteristics of brainstem gliomas, those which are associated with a favourable prognosis, such as the dorsal exophytic tumour, and those for which prognosis has remained dismal for many years despite various trials of adjuvant treatment. The major controversy involved in the management of brainstem tumours is whether surgical biopsy or resection should be attempted, and a sensible approach to management of such patients is clearly described.

Primitive neuroectodermal tumour (PNET) is the most common primary malignant brain tumour of childhood, and one for which prognosis has generally improved greatly over the last two decades, albeit at the price of significant long-term morbidity. National and international collaboration has helped to define optimal strategies for treatment, and in particular has identified a role for adjuvant chemotherapy. Dr Lewis points out that the identification of risk factors beyond those traditionally used – age, site, completeness of resection, metastatic status – is progressing rapidly, and already, groups of children for whom significant reduction in therapy may be possible can be identified. The outcome for children with high-risk disease, particularly the very young and those with relapse, remains a challenge for which new strategies are being sought.

Drs Rogers and Saran have given an exceptionally clear overview of the management of germ cell tumours (GCTs). Primary germinoma is a highly curable tumour, for which the emphasis in recent years has been to reduce morbidity while maintaining high event-free survival. Attempts to eliminate radiotherapy have been unsuccessful, but it has been possible to reduce radiation dose to the primary site (to 40 Gy) and to subclinical disease (to 24 Gy). Whilst neuropsychological issues are less of a concern in this tumour affecting predominantly older children and young adults, the issues of long-term morbidity will become increasingly important as surviving patients become older. The management of non-germinomatous germ cell tumours places greater emphasis on achievement of complete clearance of the tumour, although an initial radical approach is not recommended. The prognosis for secreting GCTs is significantly improved by platinum-based chemotherapy regimes, together with radiotherapy. Again, the survival of this group has improved sufficiently that the long-term sequelae of treatment, such as hearing impairment and infertility, have become progressively more important. Finally, the importance of close follow-up of these patients is emphasized, since recurrent disease is salvageable, and likely to be associated with less morbidity if treated early.

Many of the tumours of childhood arise with such rarity that national or international studies of treatment and outcome have not been performed. Such tumours present particular problems to the paediatric oncologist, not only because no standard or 'best' treatment is available, but also because the outcome for each child may be unpredictable. Choroid plexus tumours, reviewed by Dr Lowis, are examples of this, but thankfully the need for international cooperation has been recognized, and it is to be hoped that more effective strategies will follow.

In a brief discussion of craniopharyngioma, Dr Estlin describes the contemporary diagnosis and treatment of this interesting developmental anomaly. Surgery and radiotherapy remain the mainstay of treatment, although there are considerable differences worldwide in the philosophy of radical surgery versus limited surgery and adjuvant radiotherapy. In the long term, significant morbidity may result from hypothalamic dysfunction and obesity, and the neurocognitive sequelae following therapy need to be further characterized. Although experience with chemotherapy is limited to case reports involving few patients, its use in young children or for relapsed disease is warranted due to its efficacy as a radiation sparing agent.

Amongst the rarer paediatric CNS tumours are the mixed neuronal tumours, ganglio-gliomas and dysembryoplastic neuroepithelial tumours (DNETs). These tumours occur most commonly in the temporal lobe, and are a cause of medically intractable epilepsy in young people. Although the outcome from gross total resections is excellent, incomplete resection can still result in dramatic improvement in seizure control, and the prognosis for these tumours, especially for DNETs, is excellent in the long term.

Surgery is also the mainstay of therapy for intramedullary spinal cord tumours such as ependymoma and astrocytoma, which usually occur in later childhood. The role of adjuvant radiotherapy and chemotherapy is less certain for these tumours, although radiotherapy forms the standard of care for the postoperative management of ependymoma.

CNS tumours that result from the metastatic spread of disease from a primary outside the CNS axis are a relatively uncommon but important phenomenon in paediatric oncology. CNS disease is a well-recognized adverse factor in leukaemia treatment, but one that can usually be overcome. Even in solid tumours, the presence of CNS disease does not necessarily mean incurability, and aggressive management of metastatic Wilms' tumour in particular offers a significant chance of cure. Sadly CNS disease is often seen in the context of widely disseminated disease for which curative therapy is not possible: early recognition of this complication is important, however, to prevent morbidity in patients who are near the end of life.

In the final section of our book is a description of the late effects associated with treatment of CNS tumours in children. The principles of neurorehabilitation and neuro-psychology and palliative care are then discussed.

Drs Glaser and Butler have given an excellent account of the late effects of patients after brain tumours. Long-term effects of treatment become more important each year as the number of patients cured of their disease rises. Morbidity from brain tumours has long been recognized in the population, but until the last decade has been under-recognized in the individual, partly as a result of the absence of systematic approaches to late effects management. Physical sequelae, growth, endocrine and reproductive late effects are now managed reliably and well in most centres, but the amelioration of more complex problems relating to intellectual disability, socialization, behaviour, and their effects on employability for the individual will continue to prove difficult for many years. Dr Curran's explanation of 'how the brain works' will help many of us to approach such problems in a more systematic manner.

The care for children at the end of life remains a major part of all oncology practice, and Dr Mackie's chapter on the palliative care and symptomatic needs of children with CNS tumours highlights the importance of an holistic approach in this patient population. The cooperation of healthcare professionals with national organizations such as ACT (Association for Children with Life-threatening or Terminal Conditions and their Families) and NCH-SPCS (National Council for Hospice and Specialist Palliative Care Services) has allowed the development of optimal decision making and symptom care in relation to palliative care for children with CNS tumours. In particular, guidance for the treatment of various problems ranging from raised intracranial pressure to persistent neuropathic pain, nausea and agitation, are discussed in the context of providing support for both the child and their family or carers.

Paediatric CNS tumours pose many challenges for the future, including the need for improvements in survival rates and also the avoidance or minimization of neurocognitive late effects. The invading edge of CNS tumours may be seen as a relative sanctuary site in terms of chemotherapy penetration. New drugs and new approaches are needed, and it is important that knowledge of the clinical and cellular pharmacology of such agents is employed for their optimal use. For example, preclinical studies of the novel topoisomerase 1 inhibitor topotecan have identified the potential importance of pharmacokinetic variables and scheduling in relation to tumour response (Estlin 2002). Classes of anticancer agent such as inhibitors of angiogenesis and signal transduction inhibitors are currently under-going early clinical evaluation in adult oncology, and efforts must be made to secure the rational evaluation of these therapies for children with CNS tumours. Optimization of scheduling of radiotherapy using hyperfractionated accelerated radiotherapy (HART) may offer the possibility of improving chances of cure, and/or reducing the risk of damage to the patient.

This book, an assembly of contributions from authors with detailed knowledge of many areas relating to paediatric neuro-oncology, aims to assist in the understanding of the most important problems seen in daily practice. There is a need to understand the basis for treatment of such tumours, the principles of surgery, radiotherapy, chemotherapy and supportive care. More important is the constant recognition that our patients are children, with widely varying needs both now and in the future. The care of children will continue to require multidisciplinary input, and many skills, beyond those held by any one individual, will be needed by health care workers involved with these patients.

REFERENCE

Estlin EJ (2002) Novel targets for therapy in paediatric oncology. *Curr Drug Targets Immune Endocr Metabol Disord* **2**: 141–150.

INDEX

prognosis, 281–2
radiotherapy, 279–80
recurrent disease, 280–1
surgical management, 156, 159–60, 279
treatment, 279–82
late effects, 281–2
craniotomy, awake, 158
creatine, 19
cure rate, 3
cyclizine, 337
cyclophosphamide
ependymoma, 227, 229
high-dose, 252
high-grade astrocytoma, 212
cytosine arabinoside (cytarabine), 213
clinical studies, 183

D
daunorubicin, 213
death, place of, 339–40
dehydration, 338
denaturing high-performance liquid chromatography (dHPLC), *134*, 135
dendrites, mossy fibre stage, 319–20
dependence on others, 304
dermoids, neuroimaging, 19, 28, 92
desmoplasia, 246
desmoplastic infantile ganglioglioma, 286–7
neuroimaging, *61*, *62*, 94
development
brain
environmental factors, 319–20
stress, 321
brain injury during, 324
childhood illness, 304
memory, 319
psychosocial, 319
quality of life, 304
stress effects, 321
developmental age, 325
dexamethasone
chemosensitivity effects, 182
raised intracranial pressure, 246
spinal cord compression, 196, 198–9, 299
diabetes insipidus
craniopharyngioma, 277, 278
spinal cord compression, 198
diagnosis
endoscopy, 159
histopathological, 6
diazepam, 191, 336
disease
classification, *140*, 141
management, *140*, 141–5
staging, *140*, 141
distraction techniques, 336

DNA methylation, 135–6, *137*
inhibitors, 145
doxorubicin
craniopharyngioma, 280
high-grade astrocytoma, 213
dribbling, involuntary, 338
dural astrocytoma pathology, 118–19
dural ganglioglioma pathology, 118–19
dysembryoplastic neuroepithelial tumour (DNET),
64, *65*, 95, 284–5, 348
histology, 284
imaging, 284
pathology, 116–17
resection, 160–1
surgery, 284–5
treatment, 284–5

E
education
late sequelae, 309–10
rehabilitation, 324
special needs, 309, 310
electrolyte imbalance, 190
spinal cord compression, 198–9
embryoid bodies, 263
embryonal tumours, 120–3
emotional functioning, 320
employment, late sequelae, 310
encephalomyelitis, acute disseminated (ADEM),
193
encephalopathy, 190–3, *194–5*
endocrine dysfunction, late effects, 305–7
endocrine imbalance
craniopharyngioma, 278
low-grade astrocytoma treatment, 209
replacement therapy, 281
spinal cord compression, 198–9
end-of-life decisions, 332–3
endoscopy, 159–60
endothelial-specific integrin/survival signals, 144
enkephalins, 317, 320–1
environmental agents, 10
environmental factors in brain development, 319–20
ependymoma, 221–30, 292–3, 347
age, 224–5
anaplastic, 222
chemotherapy, 227, *228*, 229, 293
postoperative, 226–7
classification, 222
cytogenetic studies, 223
diagnostic features, 223–4
dissemination, 224
genetics, 114
grading, 225
histopathology, 221–3
imaging, 224, 292

355

vomiting, 337
intramedullary spinal cord tumours, 289–94, 348
  imaging, 290
  management, 290–4
  presenting symptoms, 289–90
  surgery, 290
  tumour types, 290–4

J

JC polyoma virus late gene VP1 DNA, 10

K

karyotyping
  choroid plexus tumours, 115
  glioblastoma, 112–13
ketamine, 336
Klinefelter syndrome, germ cell tumours, 258
knock-out mice, 136

L

lactate, 19–20
laminectomy
  decompressive, 299
  late effects, 308
Langerhans cell histiocytosis, *78–9*, 99
language, 322
large cell medulloblastoma, 121
learning patterns, 316–17
leptomeningeal disease
  PNET, 247
  spinal, *84–7*, 101–2
leukaemia
  acute lymphoblastic (ALL), 9, 10, 297
  acute non-lymphoblastic, 308
  CNS involvement, 297
  radiotherapy, 309
  secondary, 308
leukoencephalopathy, 303
  methotrexate, 309
levomepromazine, 337
lexicon, 322
Lhermitte–Duclos disease, 15
  pathology, 116
life insurance, 310
Li–Fraumeni syndrome, 15, 345
  choroid plexus tumours, 115, 274
  primitive neuroectodermal tumours, 15
  second malignancy, 307
limb paralysis, 323
limbic structures, 316
limbic system, 316, 318–19
lipid peaks, 19, 20
lipoma, 19
location of tumours, 107–8
long-term potentiation/depression, 316
lorazepam, 336, 337

M

magnetic resonance imaging (MRI), 18–19
  functional, 156–7
  intraoperative, 158, *159*
  spinal cord compression, 197
magnetic resonance proton spectroscopy (MRS), 19
malignancy
  second, 307–8
  spread, 144–5
management of children, 3, 4–5
  curative treatment, 332
  see also chemotherapy; palliative care; radiother-
    apy; surgical management
MAPK cascade, 143–4
massage, 337
medulloblastoma, 245
  craniospinal medulloblastoma, 251
  cytogenetics, 248
  ErbB dysregulation, 249
  Gorlin syndrome, 14, 245, 307–8
  high-dose chemotherapy, 252
  Li–Fraumeni syndrome, 15
  metastases, 144, 154, 247
  molecular targeted therapies, 142
  mouse models, 139
  neuroimaging, 19, 20–1, *27*, *32–5*
  oncogene amplification, 135, *136*
  PDGFR systems, 143–4
  prognosis, 170, 248–9
  prognostic factors, 121
  radiotherapy, 169–71
    hyperfractionated, 251
  signal transduction pathways, *142*
  spread, 246
  staging, 247
  surgery, 154
  treatment impact on IQ, 309
  Turcot syndrome, 13, 14
medulloepithelioma pathology, 123
memory
  developmental aspects, 319
  emotional content, 318
  hippocampus role, 318–19
  neurochemical control, 317
  non-declarative, 317
  retention, 318
  stress effect, 318
  structural aspects, 317–18
meningioma
  cytogenetics, 125
  neurofibromatosis type 2, 12
  pathology, 124–5
Mer$^{+/-}$ phenotype, 185
metastases, 297–9, 348–9
  brain, 297–8
  leukaemia, 297

357